Constable & Lim
Colour Atlas of Ophthalmology

Sixth Edition

Constable & Lim
Colour Atlas of Ophthalmology

Sixth Edition

Ian J Constable
AO, MBBS, DSc (Hon), FRCSE, FRANZCO, DIP Am. Board Ophth
Lion's Professor of Ophthalmology, University of Western Australia
Director, Lion's Eye Institute, Perth, Australia

Tien Yin Wong
MBBS, MMED (Ophth), MPH, PhD (Johns Hopkins), FRCS (Edin), FRANZCO, FAMS
Medical Director, Singapore National Eye Centre
Senior Consultant Ophthalmologist, Singapore National Eye Centre and National University Hospital
Vice-Dean of Clinical Sciences, Duke-NUS Medical School, National University of Singapore

Vignesh Raja
MBBS, MS (Ophth), FRCS (Glasg), MRCS (Edin),
FRCOphth (Lon), FRANZCO
Head of Department, Department of Ophthalmology
Sir Charles Gairdner Hospital, Australia

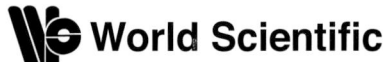

NEW JERSEY • LONDON • SINGAPORE • BEIJING • SHANGHAI • HONG KONG • TAIPEI • CHENNAI • TOKYO

Published by

World Scientific Publishing Co. Pte. Ltd.
5 Toh Tuck Link, Singapore 596224
USA office: 27 Warren Street, Suite 401-402, Hackensack, NJ 07601
UK office: 57 Shelton Street, Covent Garden, London WC2H 9HE

Library of Congress Cataloging-in-Publication Data
Names: Constable, Ian J., author. | Wong, Tien Yin, author. | Raja, Vignesh, author. |
 Preceded by (work): Lim, Arthur Siew Ming. Colour atlas of opthalmology.
Title: Constable & Lim colour atlas of ophthalmology / Ian J. Constable,
 Tien Yin Wong, Vignesh Raja.
Description: Sixth edition. | New Jersey : World Scientific, 2018. | Includes index. |
 Preceded by: Colour atlas of opthalmology / Arthur Lim Siew Ming,
 Ian J. Constable, Tien Yin Wong. 5th ed. 2008.
Identifiers: LCCN 2018015315| ISBN 9789813236615 (hardcover : alk. paper) |
 ISBN 9813236612 (hardcover : alk. paper) | ISBN 9789813237292 (pbk. : alk. paper) |
 ISBN 9813237295 (pbk. : alk. paper)
Subjects: | MESH: Eye Diseases | Atlases
Classification: LCC RE71 | NLM WW 17 | DDC 617.70022/2--dc23
LC record available at https://lccn.loc.gov/2018015315

British Library Cataloguing-in-Publication Data
A catalogue record for this book is available from the British Library.

1st English Edition	— 1979	English Edition (Second) — 1987
Malay Edition	— 1981	English Edition (Paperback) — 1987
Spanish Edition	— 1981	English Edition (Reprint) — 1991
English Edition (Reprint)	— 1982	German Edition — 1991
Italian Edition	— 1984	Portuguese Edition — 1991
Chinese Edition	— 1984	English Edition (Third) — 1995
English Edition (Reprint)	— 1984	English Edition (Reprint) — 1999
English Edition (Paperback)	— 1985	English Edition (Fourth) — 2001
French Edition	— 1985	English Edition (Reprint) — 2003
Finnish Edition	— 1987	English Edition (Reprint) — 2004

Copyright © 2019 by World Scientific Publishing Co. Pte. Ltd.

All rights reserved. This book, or parts thereof, may not be reproduced in any form or by any means, electronic or mechanical, including photocopying, recording or any information storage and retrieval system now known or to be invented, without written permission from the publisher.

For photocopying of material in this volume, please pay a copying fee through the Copyright Clearance Center, Inc., 222 Rosewood Drive, Danvers, MA 01923, USA. In this case permission to photocopy is not required from the publisher.

For any available supplementary material, please visit
https://www.worldscientific.com/worldscibooks/10.1142/10892#t=suppl

Printed in Singapore by Mainland Press Pte Ltd.

PREFACE TO THE SIXTH EDITION

This practical outline of ophthalmology has been widely distributed over 38 years to those in the front line charged with detecting and providing initial therapy for blinding eye disease. These practitioners can now, with easy internet access even in remote settings, search the web worldwide for ophthalmic information and even join in tele-ophthalmic services for advice. However, they are still dependent on detailed history and examination skills to provide crucial information and timely treatment. This atlas continues to address those skills. We have added a series of brief videos to better illustrate the most important tasks. The rapid advances in technology and therapies require frequent adjustment on the part of all of us involved in eye care. No one communicated these messages better than the late Dr. Arthur Lim and we dedicate this new edition to his memory. We hope that this updated sixth edition will continue to be of value to general practitioners, medical students, optometrists, nurses, paramedics and residents starting ophthalmology training. The authors acknowledge the clinical and technical staff of the Lions Eye Institute, Perth and the Singapore National Eye Centre for the many fine images and videos in this book.

Ian Constable
Tien Yin Wong
Vignesh Raja

PREFACE TO THE FIFTH EDITION

Once in a lifetime, authors are encouraged by the popularity of the book they have written and the enthusiasm and excellent reviews of major journals. Furthermore, we are delighted that the demand for the book has spread around the world and has resulted in translations into eight languages: Malay, Spanish, Italian, Chinese, French, Finnish, German and Portuguese.

In recent years, we have witnessed spectacular ophthalmic innovations, including the development of new ophthalmic procedures and the creation of new drugs. We are happy that we have managed to include many of these innovations in this new edition without increasing its size so that it can be carried around in the clinics. We are pleased that this book has now been produced in videos and CD-ROM format. We hope that this updated fifth edition will continue to be of value to general practitioners, medical students, optometrists, nurses and paramedics everywhere.

ASM Lim
TY Wong
IJ Constable

PREFACE TO THE FOURTH EDITION

We are delighted with the numerous enthusiastic reviews that we have received from international journals of the first three editions of this book. We are of course pleased that the book has been translated into eight languages: Malay, Spanish, Italian, Chinese, French, Finnish, German and Portuguese, and that it continues to be popular. In the last few years, new procedures and drugs have emerged. We have therefore updated every chapter to include the latest in ophthalmic management, but have taken pains not to increase the size of the book so that it can be easily carried around by medical students and residents in the clinics. We are also delighted that this book has been produced on video and CD-ROM.

CONTENTS

Preface to the Sixth Edition..v
Preface to the Fifth Edition...vii
Preface to the Fourth Edition..ix

Chapter 1	History and Examination 1
Chapter 2	Lid, Lacrimal Apparatus and Orbit 31
Chapter 3	Conjunctiva, Sclera and Cornea..................... 47
Chapter 4	Cataract 73
Chapter 5	Glaucoma 83
Chapter 6	Uveitis: Iris, Ciliary Body and Choroid............... 98
Chapter 7	Retina and Vitreous 108
Chapter 8	Diabetic Retinopathy and the Eye in Systemic Diseases 144
Chapter 9	Neuro-Ophthalmology.............................. 170
Chapter 10	Eye Diseases in Children........................... 189
Chapter 11	Ocular Injuries....................................... 208
Chapter 12	Refractive Errors.................................... 222
Chapter 13	Ophthalmic Medications 231
Chapter 14	Global Blindness and Its Prevention 239

Index..245

LIST OF VIDEOS

1. Visual field — (Chapter 1, page 23)
2. Chalazion incision and curettage — (Chapter 2, page 43)
3. Cataract removal and insertion of an intraocular lens — (Chapter 4, page 82)
4. Trabeculectomy — (Chapter 5, page 97)
5. Vitrectomy for retinal detachment — (Chapter 7, page 126)
6. OCT: Macular telangiectasia type 2 showing an intraretinal cyst and a break in the photoreceptor layer — (Chapter 7, page 130)
7. Intravitreal injection with anti-VEGF — (Chapter 7, page 137)
8. Vitrectomy for diabetic vitreous haemorrhage — (Chapter 8, page 165)
9. Removal of an embedded corneal foreign body — (Chapter 11, page 216)
10. LASIK surgery for myopia — (Chapter 12, page 230)

To access Videos 1 to 10 for this book, please follow the instructions below.

1. Go to: https://www.worldscientific.com/
2. Register an account/login.
3. Key in this link: https://www.worldscientific.com/r/10892-supp.
4. Access will be activated after step 3.

For subsequent access, please use this link:
https://www.worldscientific.com/worldscibooks/10.1142/10892#t=suppl.

For enquiries, please email: sales@wspc.com.sg.

1
HISTORY AND EXAMINATION

INTRODUCTION

In the assessment of a patient with eye disease, it is important to take a good history, examine the eyes with adequate illumination and test the visual function. Macular diseases and glaucoma have become more common as causes of severe visual loss. In these cases, a fundal examination with dilatation of the pupils in a darkened room is necessary in order to assess the macula and optic disc.

Altered vision or pain in the eye usually indicates eye disease and must be explained. A detailed history, thorough clinical examination, and in some cases, relevant imaging are required for accurate diagnosis and timely treatment.

HISTORY

Past ocular and systemic history can provide useful clues to diagnosis as can family history.

Note previous allergies and current medications.

OCULAR SYMPTOMS

These include blurred vision, distorted vision, double vision, floaters, flashes, central or peripheral field defect, ocular pain, itching, watering, photophobia and mucopurulent discharge. Altered colour vision and poor night vision may also occur.

Decreased Visual Acuity

Decreased visual acuity must always be investigated and the cause found. The cause of a sudden loss of vision could be vascular in nature, such as retinal vein occlusion, retinal artery occlusion or vitreous haemorrhage. It could also be due to acute glaucoma, retinal detachment or inflammatory conditions such as acute uveitis and optic neuritis.

Gradual loss of vision is usually caused by a refractive error, such as myopia or presbyopia, or to degenerative conditions, of which cataract is the most common. It could also be due to macular degeneration or chronic glaucoma.

Distorted Vision

This may be due to macular distortion from an epiretinal membrane, drusen or a choroidal new vessel in wet macular degeneration. Astigmatism and corneal scars can also cause it.

Double Vision (Diplopia)

It is important to note if double vision is true separation of the images or just overlapping, where it may in fact be due to distortion of the image from one eye.

Binocular diplopia is due to extraocular muscle nerve paralysis or muscle injury or dysfunction as in myasthenia gravis.

Monocular diplopia is caused by diseases of the eyeball including cataract, corneal opacity and iris defects.

Floaters

These are small semitranslucent particles of varying shapes which tend to move across the field of vision with eye movements. They are noticeable by almost every adult against a white background and are due to vitreous gel degradation. A sudden onset of floaters with flashes may mean vitreous detachment or vitreous blood from a retinal tear or diabetic retinopathy.

Flashes

Single flashes in one eye, sometimes with eye movement and usually projected to the side, are due to stimulation of the retina by vitreous traction or impending vitreous detachment. Retinal tear must be excluded.

Flickering lights or colour sensations are usually of cerebral origin and most often due to transient vascular changes such as in migraine. They may be bilateral and homonymous in the corresponding part of each visual field.

Eye Pain and Headaches

Scratchy surface pain may be due to dry eyes but occurs with a foreign body or inturned eyelashes, corneal epithelial defects and ulcers.

Deep aching pain may be due to acute glaucoma, iritis, scleritis, trauma and endophthalmitis. These are blinding conditions and severe pain must never be ignored.

Uncorrected refractive error, migraine and neuralgia referred to the eye are common causes of eye ache and may involve more diffuse headache.

Itchy Eyes

Itchy eyes and surrounding skin is often due to allergy. Itch may also occur with blepharitis.

Watering Eyes

In infants, watering is usually due to congenital blockage of the nasolacrimal duct. A rare but important cause is congenital glaucoma.

In adults, watering is caused by blockage of the drainage system or excess production from irritation of the surface, such as with a foreign body, trichiasis, entropion, conjunctivitis and keratitis.

Photophobia

Excess sensitivity to light can be due to a large pupil or damaged iris, acute corneal changes, iritis, cone dystrophy or ocular albinism.

EXAMINATION

Visual Acuity

The assessment of distant and near visual acuity is important, as it reflects the state of the macular function (central vision). The visual acuity can be tested by asking the patient to cover one eye with a cardboard or the palm of his hand. By testing the ability of the patient to see objects such as a clock or newspaper in his own environment, it is possible to get a gross assessment of the visual acuity as blind, grossly defective, subnormal or normal.

Distant visual acuity

It is usual to record a patient's distant visual acuity more accurately using the Snellen chart. This is read at 6 m, with the letters diminishing in size from above. The patient has normal vision if he is able to read the line of letters designated as 6/6 at or near the bottom of the chart. The scale for decreasing distant visual acuity is 6/9, 6/12 (industrial vision and requirement for driving), 6/18, 6/24, 6/36 and 6/60 (legal blindness in some countries). Thus, the normal subject can read the 6/18 line at 18 m. Countries which do not use the metric system, including the USA, record Snellen chart findings in feet — 20/20 down to 20/200. Other countries record decimal fractions — 0.1 to 1.0.

Clinical trials and many retinal clinics now use a logMAR (logarithm of the minimum angle of resolution) Bailey–Lovie chart. A Snellen score of 6/12 or 20/40 means that the subject can resolve details down to 2 minutes of the visual angle or a logMAR score of 0.3. This is recorded as the number of actual letters read on the logMAR chart.

If the patient is unable to read the letters, he is asked to count the examiner's fingers, which are held a metre away. If his answers are correct, he has a distant visual acuity of "counting fingers" at a metre. If he is unable to count the fingers, the examiner should move his hand in front of the patient's eyes. The visual acuity is then said to be "hand movement". If he can see only light, the visual acuity is recorded as "perception of light". If he cannot see any light, the visual acuity is recorded as "no perception of light", which is total blindness.

Four Ways to Record Visual Acuity Used in Different Countries

Feet	Metric	Decimal	LogMAR
20/200	6/60	0.10	1.00
20/160	6/48	0.125	0.90
20/125	6/38	0.16	0.80
20/100	6/30	0.20	0.70
20/80	6/24	0.25	0.60
20/63	6/19	0.32	0.50
20/50	6/15	0.40	0.40
20/40	6/12	0.50	0.30
20/32	6/9.5	0.63	0.20
20/25	6/7.5	0.80	0.10
20/20	6/6	1.00	0.00
20/16	6/4.8	1.25	−0.10
20/12.5	6/3.8	1.60	−0.20

Each line on the logMAR chart represents a change of 0.1 log unit in the acuity level, with each of the five letters having a value of 0.02 log unit. Therefore, a patient reading correctly all the letters on a specific line will score the full 0.1 log unit. For every extra letter on subsequent lines read correctly, the patient will score an extra −0.02.

Patients with less than 6/60 vision are classified as legally blind. Patients who can see 6/12 have sufficient vision to work in most industries and are said to have "industrial vision", which is also the legal visual requirement for driving.

Pinhole

Distance vision is tested without and then with distance glasses. By looking through a pinhole an eye with blurred vision is improved if the defective vision is due to a refractive error. Visual acuity usually does not improve with the pinhole if it is due to organic eye disease.

Near visual acuity

The common near visual acuity tests are the Jaegar test and the N chart, usually read at a distance of 30 cm. The Jaegar test is recorded as J1, J2, J4, J6, etc., and the N chart as N5, N6, N8, N10, etc. Standard small newsprint is approximately J4 or N6. Each eye is tested in turn with the other covered. Middle-aged patients (presbyopic age) must be tested with their reading glasses.

Difficulties in examination

It is often difficult to test visual acuity in young children, as well as patients who are illiterate, uncooperative or malingering. Frequently only an estimate can be made. The E chart, picture cards or small coloured objects may be used. It can be difficult to determine whether a patient is malingering without the use of special tests.

VISUAL FIELDS

Confrontation Testing

The visual fields can be recorded approximately by using the confrontation test. The patient covers the eye which is not being tested with his palm and fixes the other on the examiner's nose or eye. A target is then brought into his field of vision from the side, and the point at which the patient sees the object is noted. The eye is tested in the different meridians, usually in each quadrant.

Alternatively, the examiner's fingers are held at a distance of 1 m and the patient is asked to count them in the different quadrants, i.e. the superior temporal, the inferior temporal, the superior nasal and the inferior nasal quadrants.

EXTERNAL EYE EXAMINATION

This is done with good illumination from either a window or a bright torch. A magnifying glass facilitates examination and should be used whenever available.

The position and appearance of the eyelids should be noted, especially with regard to their position in relation to the limbus. Also note whether there is eyelash crusting, watering, oedema, discharge or inflammation. Common problems include drooping of the upper eyelid (ptosis), lid retraction, inability to close the lids (lagophthalmos), eversion of the lid margins (ectropion) and inversion of lid margins (entropion).

The conjunctiva and sclera should be almost white, with only a few small vessels. The transparent disc-like cornea is best seen with a good oblique light from a torch. Staining with fluorescein dye will help to show ulcers or abrasions of the cornea. The fluorescence is highlighted by blue light. The colour and pattern of the iris should be observed. A dense cataract can be seen through the pupil as a white reflex.

Eversion of the Upper Eyelid

It is sometimes necessary to evert the upper lid to examine the tarsal conjunctiva if the patient is suspected of having a foreign body under the lid. This is also done for diagnosis of the conjunctival follicles of the upper lid, as in trachoma. To evert the lid, ask the patient to look downwards and apply slight pressure on the lid with a cotton bud or blunt rod. The lid margin is then gently pulled upwards to evert it.

PUPIL RESPONSES

The response to light directed at one pupil in a darkened room is known as the direct pupillary response. The reaction to light by the fellow pupil is called the consensual pupillary response.

If a darkened room is not available, the pupillary response can be tested by having the patient cover both his eyes with his palms. The contraction of the pupil is observed when the palm is removed from one eye. This indicates the response of the pupil to direct light.

The reaction to accommodation is tested by asking the patient to fix his eyes on an object at a distance and then to focus on another object about 10 cm away from him. The pupil constricts on convergence and near point focus.

EXTRAOCULAR MUSCLES

The extraocular muscles are examined by observing the position of the eyeballs with the patient looking straight ahead. Any gross malposition of the eyes can easily be seen. One eye may be observed to be turned inwards (convergent squint) or outwards (divergent squint). Occasionally, one of the eyes may be seen to be higher than the other (vertical squint).

Corneal Light Reflex

The corneal light reflex is a useful method of determining whether one of the eyes is turned inwards or outwards, or vertically displaced. Normally, when the patient is asked to look at a torch, a light reflex is seen at the centre of the pupil. If one of the eyes is misaligned, the reflex will not be at the centre of the pupil. In a convergent squint, the light reflex will be at the outer side of the cornea, and in a divergent squint, at the inner side of the cornea. A general guide is that if the reflex is at the limbus, the degree of convergence or divergence is approximately 40°. If it is halfway between the centre of the cornea and the limbus, it is approximately 20°. The corneal light reflex is also a useful means to exclude pseudosquint, where there is an appearance of a convergent squint because of broad medial epicanthal lid folds. In pseudosquint the corneal light reflex is central in both eyes.

Ocular Movements

When the extraocular muscles are severely paralysed, the restriction in movement is tested by asking the patient to look in different directions (positions of gaze). If the extraocular muscles are less severely affected, special techniques have to be used involving measurement with prisms.

The Six Cardinal Positions of Gaze and Their Corresponding Primary Extraocular Muscle Actions

Movement	Right Eye	Left Eye
Right	Right lateral rectus	Left medial rectus
Up and right	Right superior rectus	Left inferior oblique
Down and right	Right inferior rectus	Left superior oblique
Left	Right medial rectus	Left lateral rectus
Up and left	Right inferior oblique	Left superior rectus
Down and left	Right superior oblique	Left inferior rectus

OPHTHALMOSCOPY

The ophthalmoscope is used to observe abnormalities in the ocular media, optic disc, retinal vessels, fundal background and macula.

Red Reflex

With the lens power of the ophthalmoscope turned to 0 and the ophthalmoscope held 1 m away from the patient's eye, a red reflex is seen through the pupil. Alternatively, the lens power disc can be turned to about +5 dioptres and the eye examined approximately 10 cm away. The reflection of the light of the ophthalmoscope from the fundus creates a bright-red pupil. Any opacity in the cornea, lens (cataract) or vitreous will be seen as a dark area. In retinal detachment, the reflex appears grey instead of red.

Fundus

Examination of the fundus may be done with the direct ophthalmoscope and is best done in a darkened room. The refractive error in both the patient and the examiner has to be compensated for by adjusting the lens power of the ophthalmoscope. Alternatively, the examiner and the patient may use their glasses or contact lenses, in which case no adjustment will be required. The patient is then instructed to look at a distant object.

When the right fundus is examined, the ophthalmoscope is held in the right hand. The examiner uses his right eye to examine the patient's right eye approaching from the right side. The patient's left fundus is examined with the examiner's left eye and the patient is approached from the left. It is important to get near enough so that the examiner's forehead touches his own thumb which is used to lift the upper lid of the eye being examined.

It is best to approach the eye from the temporal side so that a good view of the disc can be seen before the pupil contracts when light is shone on the macula. The nasal retinal vessels and the temporal retinal vessels are examined before the macula. Because of the extra sensitivity of the macula to light, which results in rapid constriction of the pupil, examination of the macula is difficult and requires a dilated pupil.

Difficulties in Examination of the Fundus

Examination of the fundus can be difficult because of:

- Uncooperative patient
- High myopia
- Opacity in the cornea, lens or vitreous
- Poor ophthalmoscope or old batteries
- Bright room

- Small pupils
- Nystagmus

In high myopia, examination is simplified by looking through the patient's glasses or contact lenses. As the lenses of an ophthalmoscope can sometimes be fogged with dust or mould, especially in the tropics, they may have to be cleaned to enable adequate examination of the fundus.

The Small Pupil

In order to see the fundus clearly, the pupils should be dilated. Examination in a darkened room may be adequate for patients who have naturally large pupils. For patients with small pupils, examination can be difficult and a short-acting mydriatic such as tropicamide, which acts in less than 30 min and has an effect of about 4 hr, should be used. Long-acting mydriatics are no longer used because of their length of action: homatropine (one day) and atropine (one week).

SPECIAL TECHNIQUES

Modern technology has enabled examination of the eye and ocular conditions with greater precision. The techniques and equipment described here are commonly used by ophthalmologists, optometrists and allied health workers.

Tests for Extraocular Muscles

The cover–uncover test is done by covering one of the patient's eyes while the other eye looks at an object. When the cover is removed, the uncovered eye may move to look at the object. By observing the movement of the eye, the presence of a squint may be confirmed. It can be measured with a rack of prisms held in front of the corneal reflex.

A number of tests can be carried out to analyse diplopia with the use of red–green goggles to dissociate the eyes. The synoptophore is a machine with specially designed pictures to measure the angle of a squint accurately and to test the ability of the patient to see with both eyes together (binocular single vision).

Binocular Slit-Lamp Microscopy

The binocular slit-lamp microscope enables accurate observation of the eye up to a magnification of 40 times. It consists of two parts: an oblique light which can be adjusted to a slit, and a binocular microscope. The anterior segment is seen in minute detail. If the pupil is dilated the lens and anterior vitreous are visible. Examination of the retina with the slit lamp requires a +78D to +90D hand-held lens to create an indirect image, or else a flat corneal contact lens. A range of different contact lenses are available for viewing the optic disc and macular, the peripheral fundus and the iridocorneal filtration angle of glaucoma patients (gonioscopy).

Tonometry

A tonometer is used to measure intraocular pressure. The most widely used tonometer is the Goldmann applanation tonometer fitted to the slit lamp. The Schiotz corneal indentation tonometer is portable but less accurate and is now rarely used. Portable digital tonometers are convenient as they do not require a slit-lamp mounting. Non-contact tonometers use a puff of air and do not require local anaesthesia.

Visual Field Assessment

Perimetry

Perimetry gives a more accurate record of the visual fields than the confrontation test. The ability of the patient to see a small 5 mm target on an arc moving into view from the periphery at different meridians is recorded on a chart. One problem in comparative field studies is the lack of standardisation. The Goldmann bowl perimeter overcomes this with controlled lighting and standard target sizes.

The central 30° part of the field of vision can be plotted using a small 1–5 mm target on a screen (Bjerrum or tangent screen) placed 1 m or 2 m away and noting when the test target appears. The normal blind spot is found 15° lateral to the fixation point. This manual method has been replaced by automated computerised perimetry (Humphrey field analyser). It is now the gold standard and is used widely for routine screening and for serial visual field testing for glaucoma and pituitary tumours.

Tests for colour vision

The Ishihara test plates are most commonly used for colour vision. This test is very sensitive. Patients who are able to see colours for general purposes may in fact be found to have a colour defect. Patients who fail the Ishihara test but who respond accurately to the Lantern colour matches or Farnsworth–Munsell 100-hue test should not be prevented from pursuing their occupation of choice. This includes pilots, who generally need to have perfect or near-perfect vision. The Farnsworth–Munsell D-15 hue test is quick and useful for screening.

Indirect ophthalmoscopy

The head-mounted binocular indirect ophthalmoscope is widely used by ophthalmologists. Its advantages include a binocular, stereoscopic view, a wide field and the ability with scleral depression to examine the retinal periphery. It is particularly valuable in assessing patients with opacity in the ocular media, high myopia, retinal tears and detachment or tumours.

Colour Fundus Photography and Fluorescein Angiography

Fundus colour imaging and fluorescein angiography are methods which supplement the examination of the fundus and provide digital records. Wide-angle fundus imaging is very popular as a general screening tool.

In fluorescein angiography, fluorescein dye is injected intravenously and serial fundus images are taken with blue light to reveal the retinal circulation and the retinal pigment epithelium. The deeper choroidal layers can be imaged by red light after intravenous indocyanine green (ICG angiography).

Optical Coherence Tomography

This non-invasive imaging technique images the reflected light off each retinal interface and provides very fine details of the retinal layers and optic disc or the anterior segment and iridocorneal angle.

Optical coherence tomography (OCT) is now the first-line method for assessment of macular and optic nerve diseases. Diabetic maculopathy, macular oedema and age-related macular degeneration therapy are followed with serial OCT to assess the therapeutic response to therapy. Macular holes and epiretinal membranes are readily diagnosed by OCT.

Refraction

The refractive power of the eye can be measured objectively with a retinoscope. Subjective refraction is done with a trial frame and a set of lenses. Alternatively, the lenses may be mounted on a series of rotating discs (phoropter). Computerised scanning machines now measure the refraction with remarkable accuracy (autorefraction).

Ultrasonography

A-scan ultrasonography is used for measuring the thickness of the cornea (pachymetry) and for the axial length of the eye. This is essential data for calculating the required lens power prior to intraocular lens implantation in cataract surgery.

B-scan ultrasonography is used to evaluate the state of the posterior segment of the eyeball when the ocular media are opaque from corneal opacities, dense cataract or vitreous haemorrhage. It is particularly useful in severe ocular injuries and vitreous haemorrhage prior to vitrectomy. Ocular tumours are also followed by B scans after radiation treatment.

Corneal Diagnostic Equipment

A range of modern instruments are available for precise evaluation of the cornea. Corneal topography and power is mapped in minute detail prior to surgical correction of refractive error with the excimer laser. Corneal thickness maps and corneal endothelial cell population are also important data evaluated prior to corneal transplantation.

CT Scan and Magnetic Resonance Imaging

The CT scan is used for many ophthalmic conditions, but especially for detecting orbital tumours and localisation of intraocular foreign bodies. It is also widely used for investigation of neuro-ophthalmic disorders.

Magnetic resonance imaging (MRI) is a non-invasive imaging procedure that does not involve the use of ionising radiation. It utilises the interactions of three physical properties, namely a powerful magnetic field, radiowaves and the electric charge of atomic nuclei in tissue.

The CT scan is better for bone and fractures. MRI possesses greater sensitivity to soft tissue contrast. MRI is used to diagnose and monitor demyelinating lesions in multiple sclerosis and cerebral tumours. MRI with contrast also allows analysis of the vasculature and stroke lesions. The MRI scan does not detect calcification well and is therefore less valuable in the diagnosis of retinoblastoma.

Macular Potential Acuity

It is frequently important to predict the visual outcome prior to surgery, especially for cataract. This can be done by testing visual acuity with the pinhole and by careful examination of the macula. OCT will rule out macular disease. Special tests have been used in the past including the potential visual acuity meter (PAM), the laser interferometer and the blue field entoptoscope.

Electrophysiology

Clinical electrophysiological studies include electroretinography (ERG), electrooculography (EOG) and visual evoked response (VER). These are used to evaluate decreased visual function from diseases of the retina and the visual pathway. ERG provides a mass response to light stimulation of the retina and is useful in the diagnosis of retinal dystrophies such as retinitis pigmentosa. Macular pathology is evaluated with multifocal ERG. EOG measures retinal pigment epithelial function under conditions of light and dark adaptation. VER records occipital lobe responses to pattern stimuli and is a measure of the entire visual pathway. It is diminished in optic nerve disease.

Visual Acuity

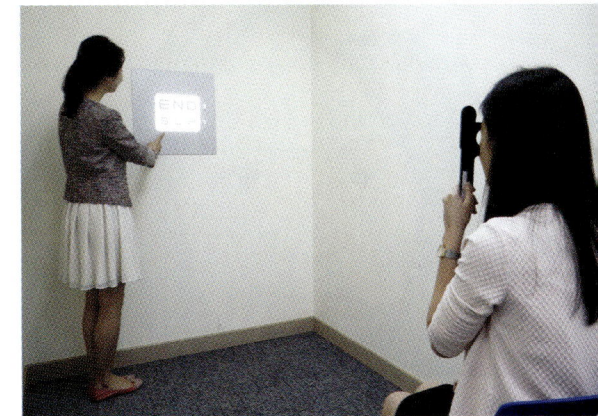

Fig. 1.1. Distant visual acuity examined at 6 m.

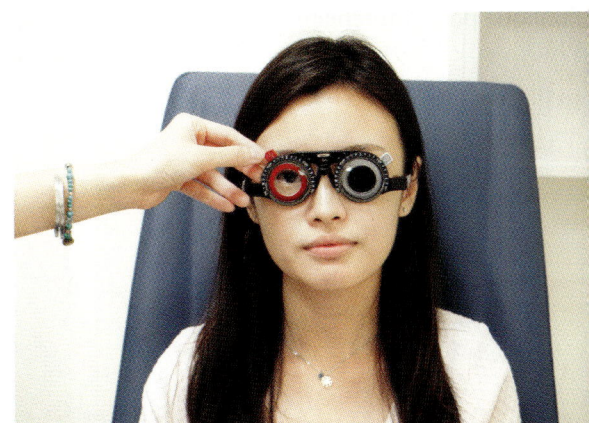

Fig. 1.2. Refraction.

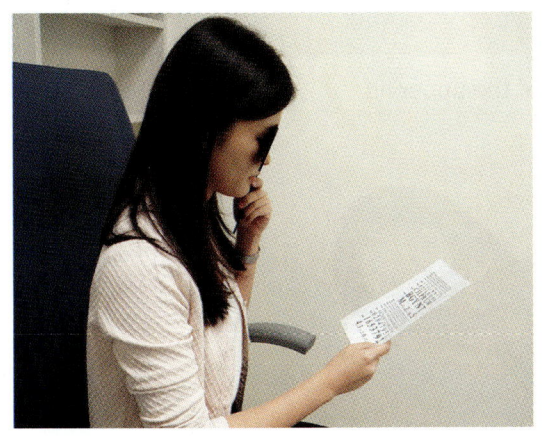

Fig. 1.3. Near visual acuity examined at about 30 cm.

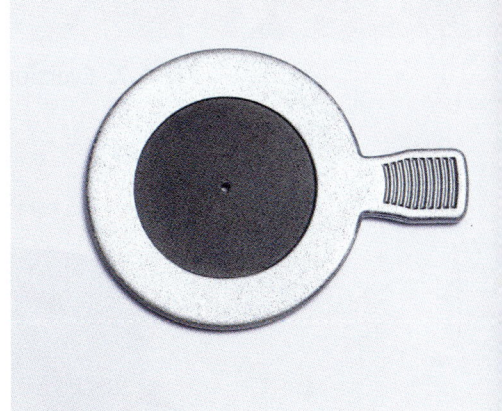

Fig. 1.4. Pinhole.

Examination of the Anterior Segment

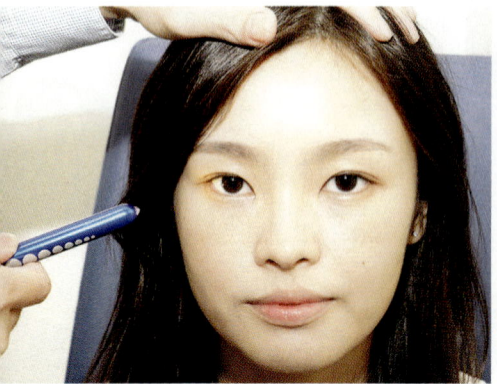

Fig. 1.5. Good focal illumination with an oblique pocket torchlight.

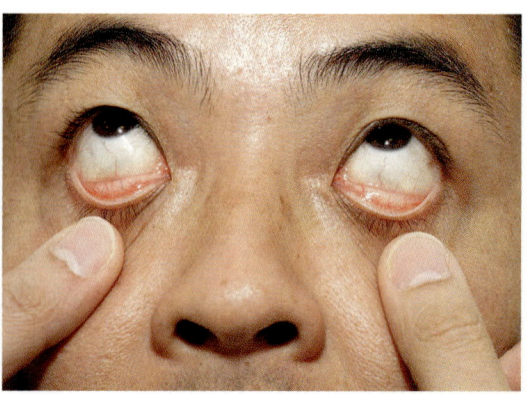

Fig. 1.6. The lower lids are pulled down with the patient looking up for examination of the lower conjunctival fornix.

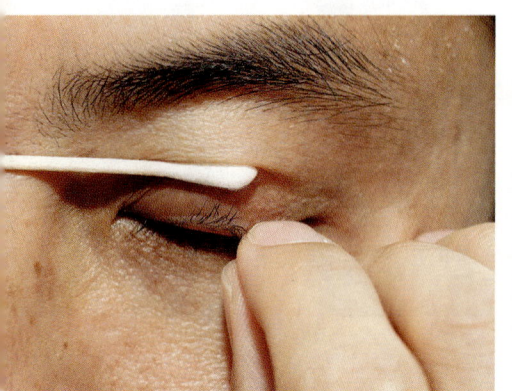
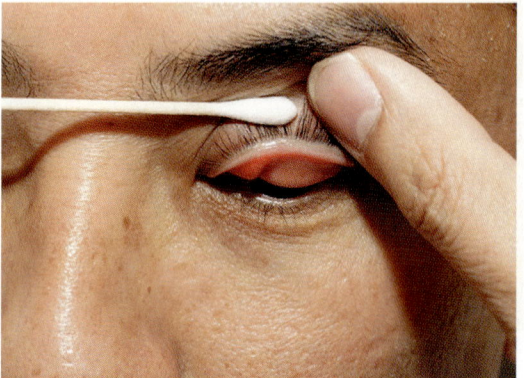

Fig. 1.7. Eversion of the upper lid.

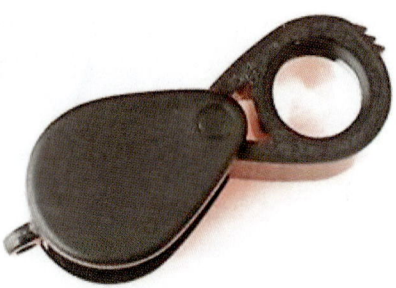

Fig. 1.8. An ordinary magnifier helps identify abnormalities.

Extraocular Muscles

Corneal reflexes at the centre of the pupils signify normal ocular alignment and muscle balance.

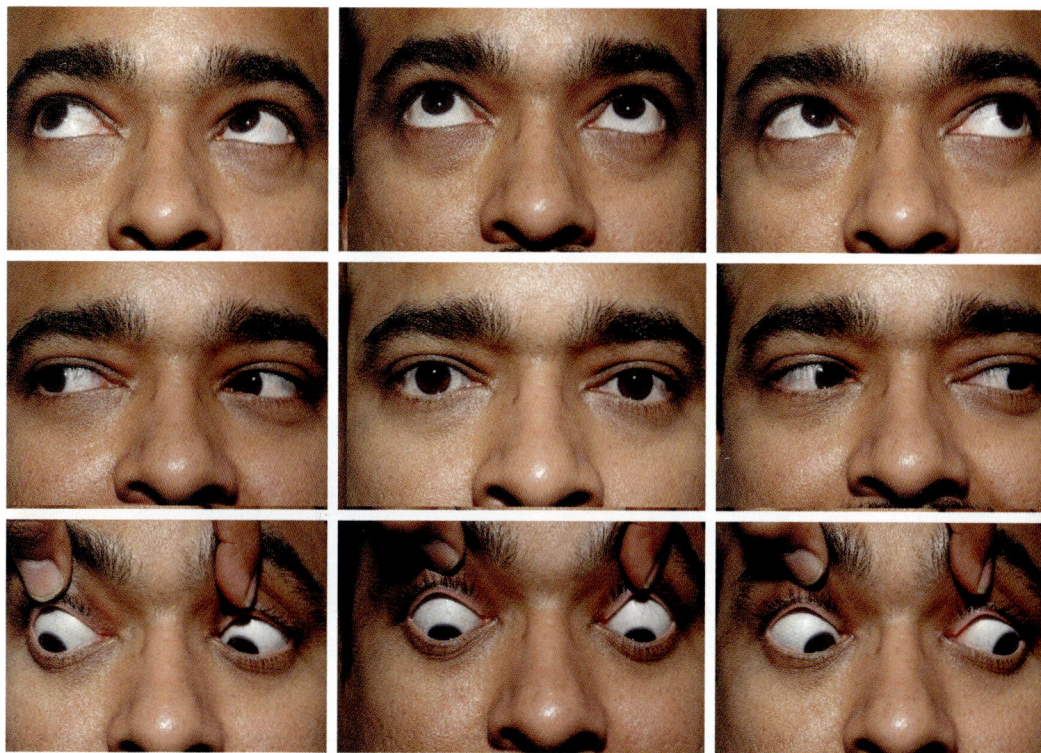

Fig. 1.9. The nine fields of gaze examined to assess extraocular muscle function. Each of the six extraocular muscles move the eye into one of the six cardinal positions on either side. *Up and right*: Right superior rectus and left inferior oblique. *Right*: Right lateral rectus and left medial rectus. *Down and right*: Right inferior rectus and left superior oblique. *Up and left*: Right inferior oblique and left superior rectus. *Left*: Right medial rectus and left lateral rectus. *Down and left*: Right superior oblique and left inferior rectus.

Fundus Reflex

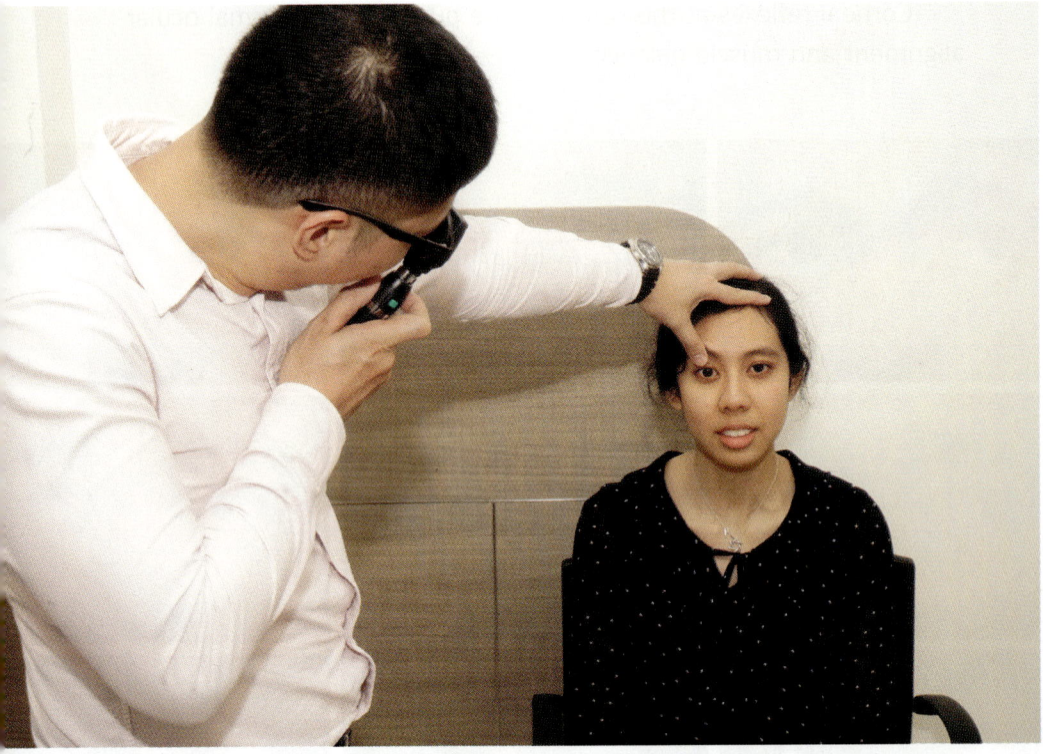

Fig. 1.10. Examination of the red reflex at 1 m using the (direct) ophthalmoscope.

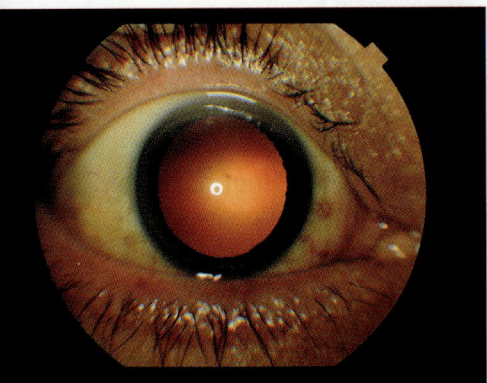

Fig. 1.11. Normal red reflex.

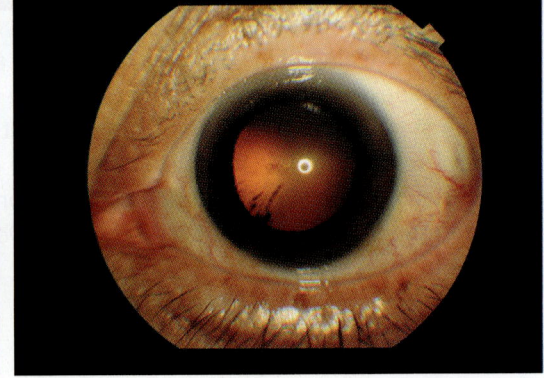

Fig. 1.12. Red reflex with peripheral lens opacity.

Ophthalmoscopy

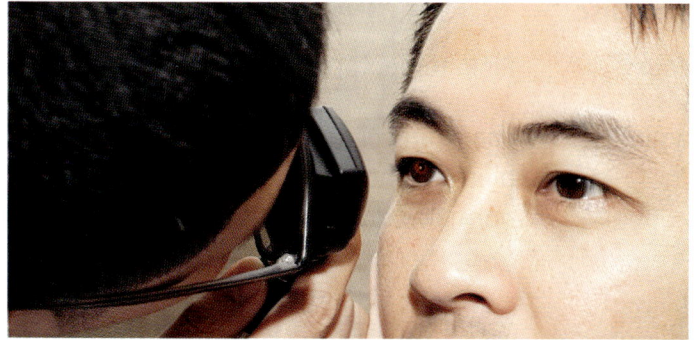

Fig. 1.13. The right fundus examined with the right eye of the examiner from the right side of the patient.

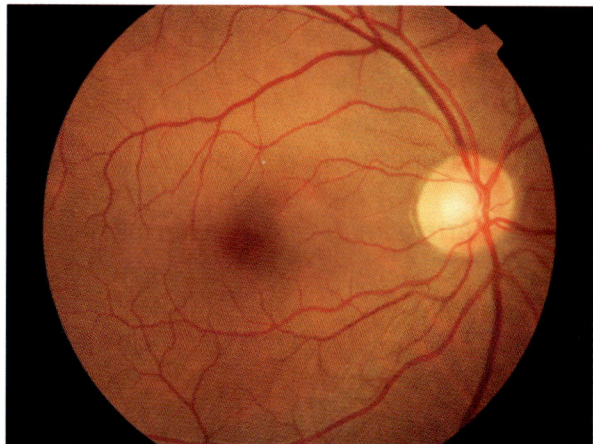

Fig. 1.14. Normal fundus.

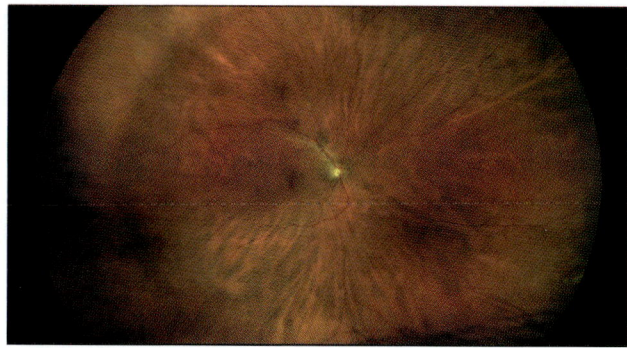

Fig. 1.15. Normal fundus — wide-angle image.

DESCRIPTION OF THE FUNDUS

Optic Disc

Colour: Pink, temporal side usually paler.

Margin: Sharp and flat. Nasal margin may be relatively blurred and raised (in hypermetropia). Many normal variations, including pigmentation and myopic crescent.

Cup: Varies in size and depth. Situated at centre of disc and slopes temporally.

Cup–disc ratio: Vertical ratio of diameter of cup to that of optic disc.

Retinal Vessels

Colour: Arteries more red than veins.

Diameter: Arteries narrower than veins. Ratio approximately 2:3.

Crossing: Arteries cross anterior to veins at arteriovenous crossings.

Fundus Background

Colour: Red fundal background because of choroidal vessels and retinal pigment layer. Darker in pigmented races. In lightly pigmented persons, large choroidal vessels seen against white sclera.

Macular Area

Normally darker than rest of fundus. At centre, normal foveal light reflex.

Visual Fields

Fig. 1.16. Visual fields by confrontation. The patient looks at the examiner's right ear while the test object is being moved in from the periphery.

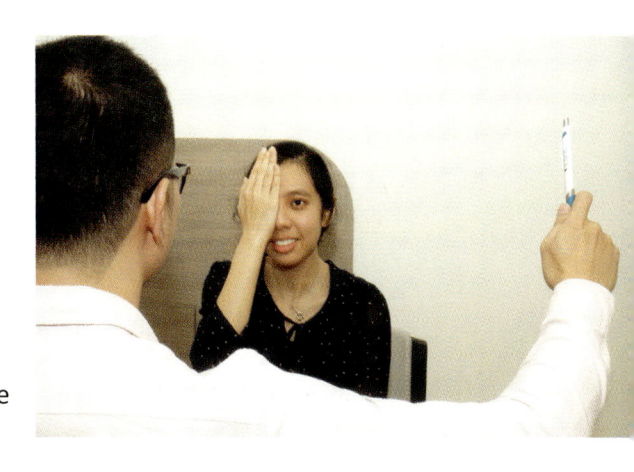

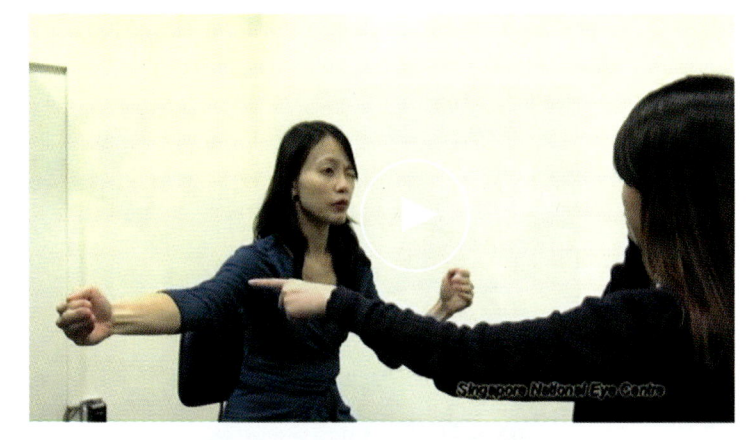

Video of visual field.

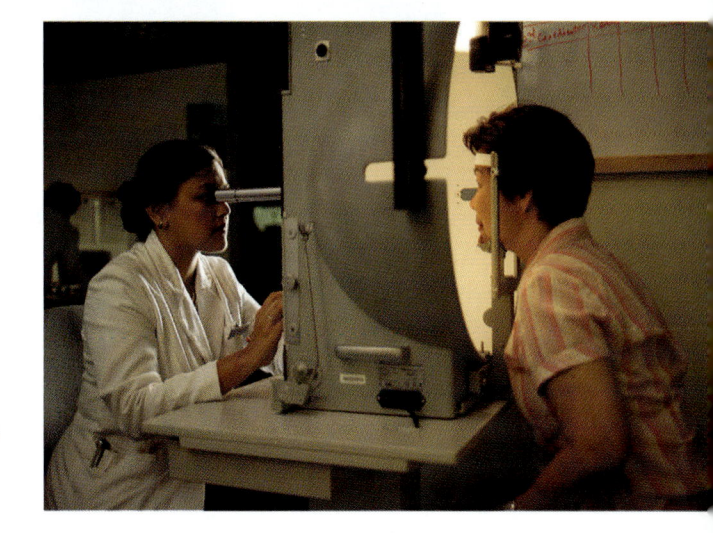

Fig. 1.17. Perimetry permits accurate recording of peripheral visual fields.

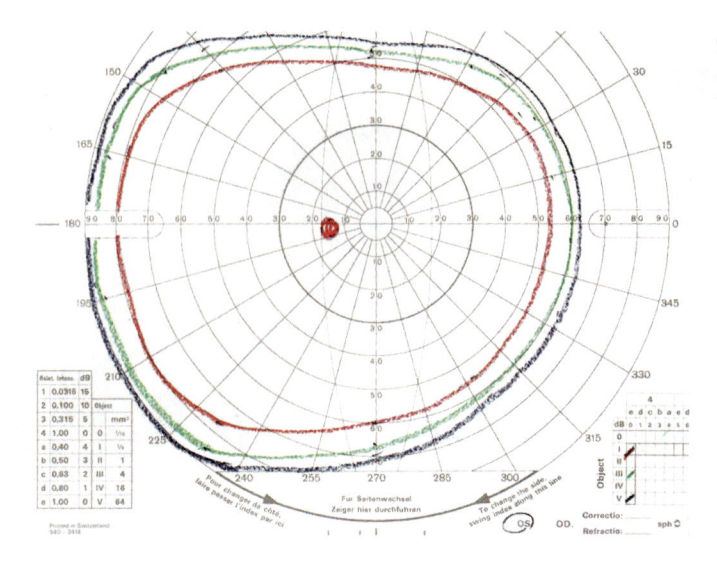

Fig. 1.18. Perimetry chart plotting the peripheral field.

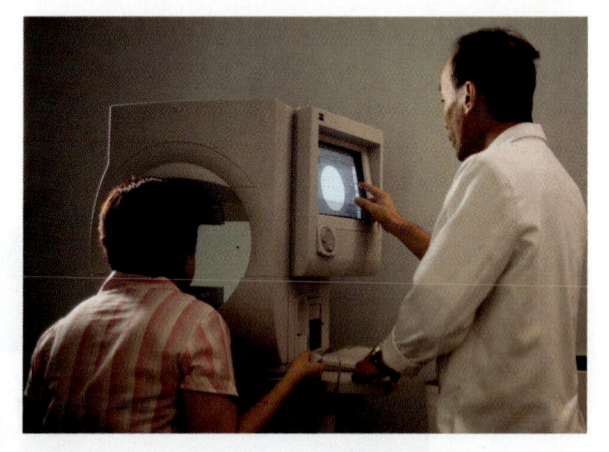

Fig. 1.19. Humphrey automated visual field testing.

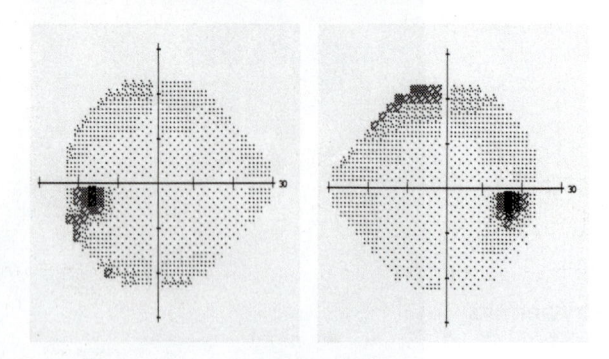

Fig. 1.20. Computerised field central 30° (used for glaucoma).

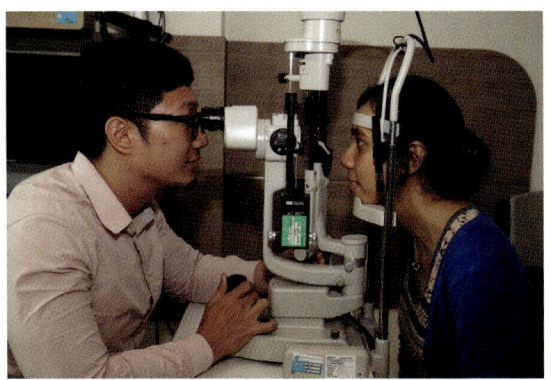

Fig. 1.21. Slit-lamp microscopy permits not only magnified examination of the anterior segment but also the filtration angles, the intraocular pressure with an applanation tonometer, and the vitreous and retina with a special contact lens.

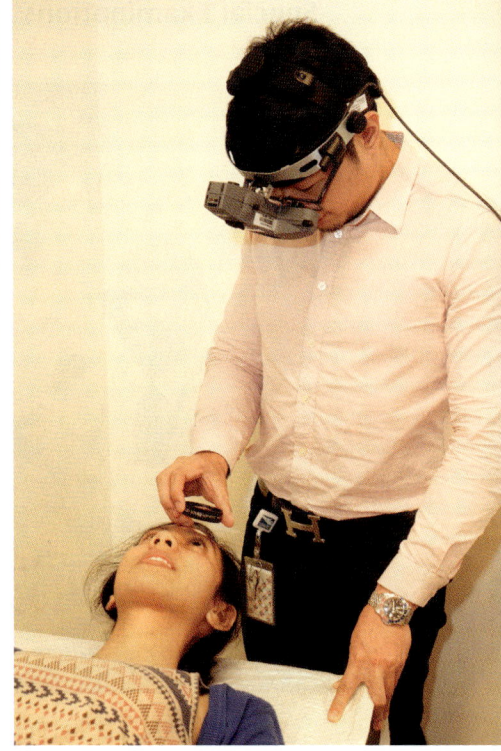

Fig. 1.22. Indirect ophthalmoscopy permits good binocular examination of the retinal periphery, and is especially useful in retinal detachment or cloudy media.

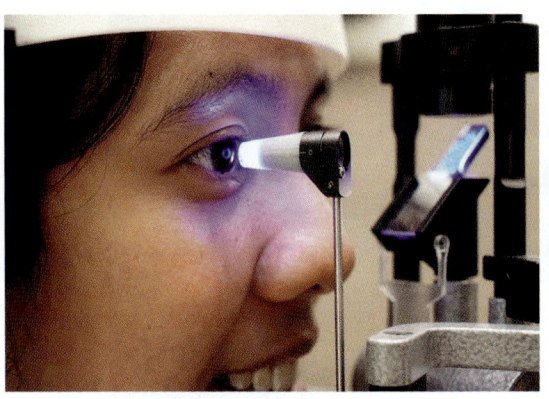

Fig. 1.23. Applanation tonometry using fluorescein and blue cobalt light is the most accurate method of measuring intraocular pressure.

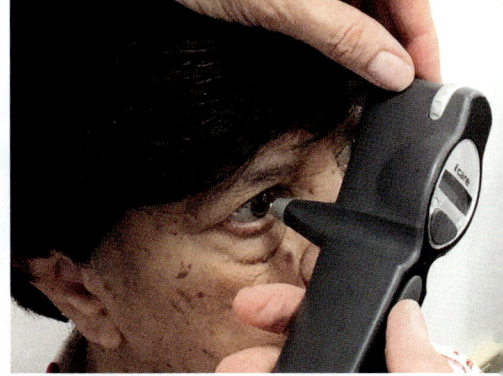

Fig. 1.24. Electronic portable tonometry (I-care).

25

Special Examinations

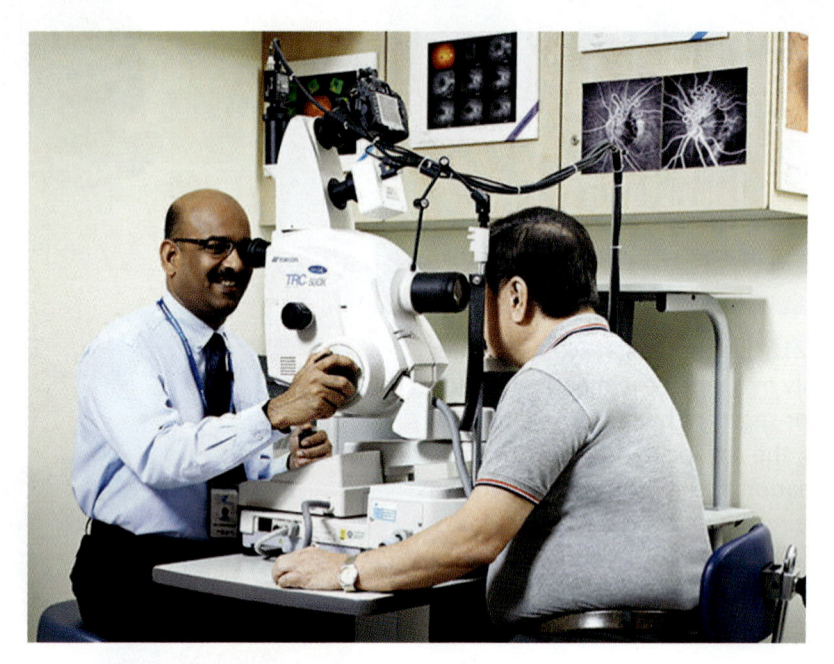

Fig. 1.25. Digital colour fundus camera.

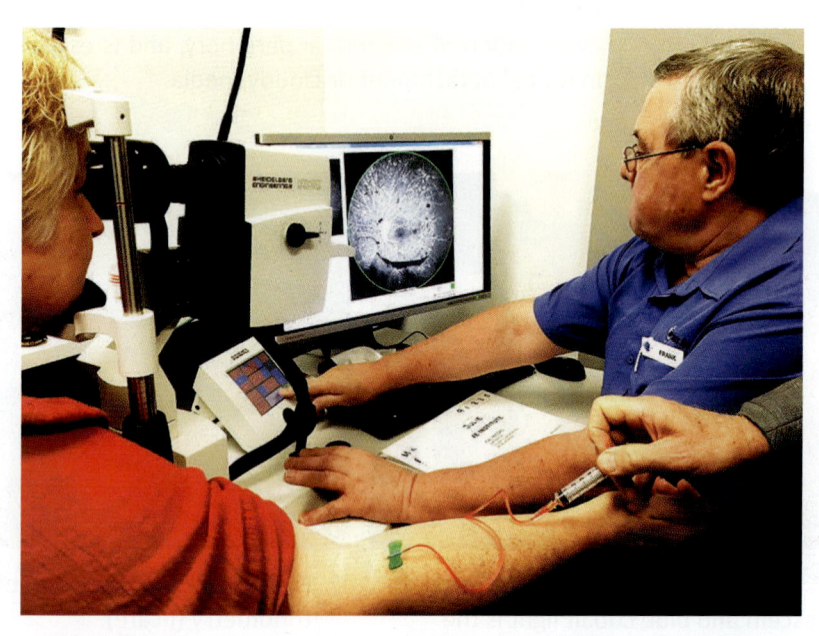

Fig. 1.26. Fluorescein angiography showing proliferative diabetic retinopathy.

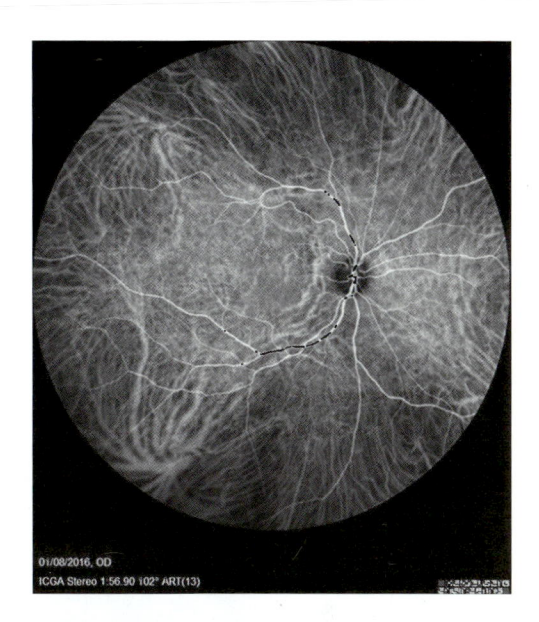

Fig. 1.27. Indocyanine green angiography (ICGA) showing deep choroidal as well as retinal circulation.

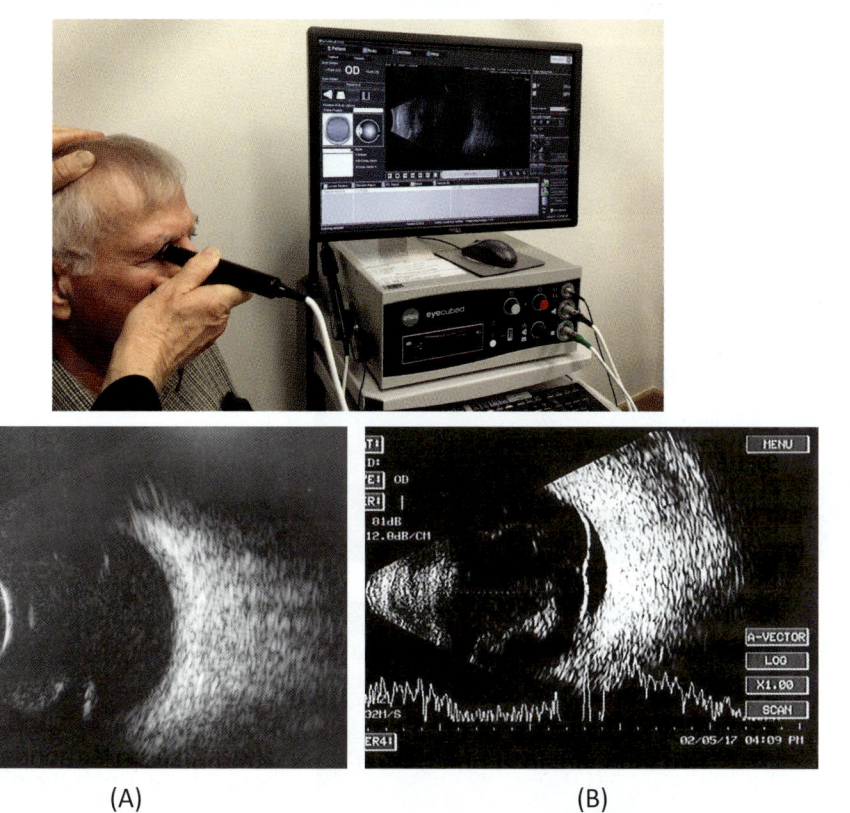

(A)   (B)

Fig. 1.28. B-scan ultrasonography is used in ophthalmology, especially when the ocular media are opaque. (Note vitreous haemorrhage A and retinal detachment B.)

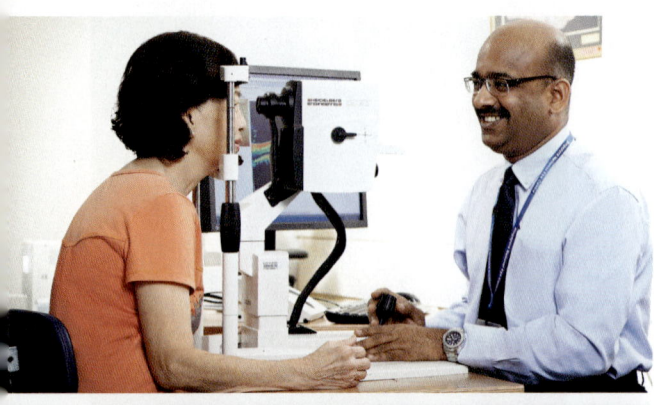

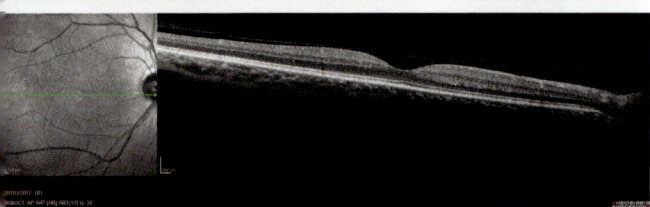

Fig. 1.29. Spectral domain optical coherence tomography (OCT) has become a key diagnostic test for retinal disease and glaucoma.

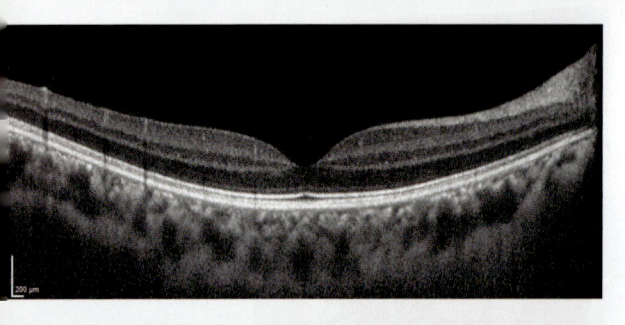

Fig. 1.30. Optical coherence tomography (OCT) of the posterior pole, showing normal macula.

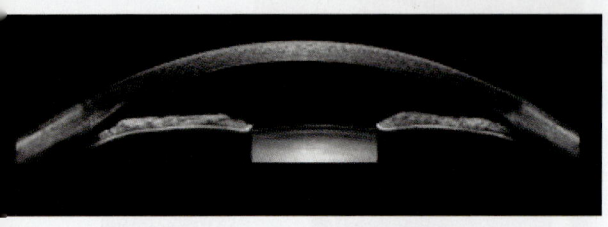

Fig. 1.31. OCT of a normal anterior segment and iris/corneal angle.

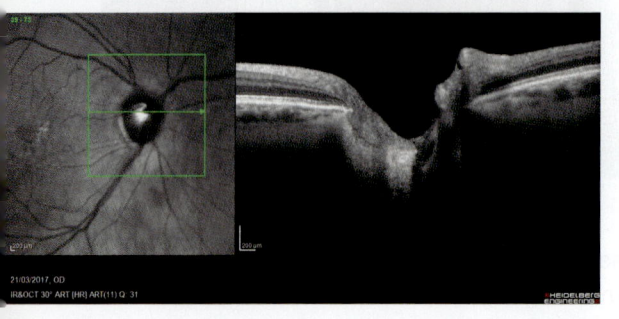

Fig. 1.32. OCT of optic disc and nerve fibre layer thickness used for glaucoma diagnosis and management.

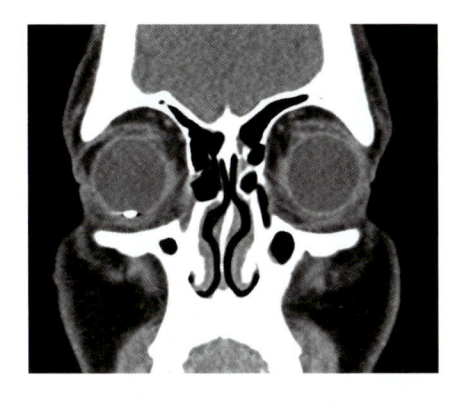

Fig. 1.33. CT scan is used to confirm the diagnosis of an intraocular foreign body (seen here) and orbital fractures.

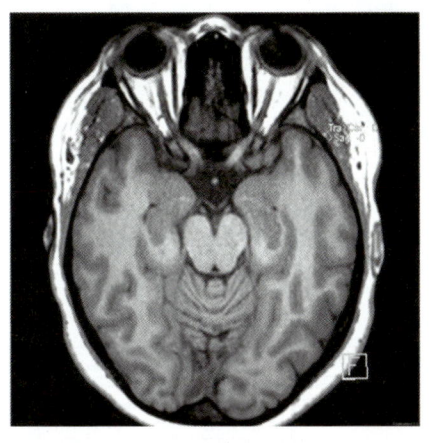

Fig. 1.34. Nuclear magnetic resonance (MRI) scan showing normal soft tissues of the eye, orbit and brain.

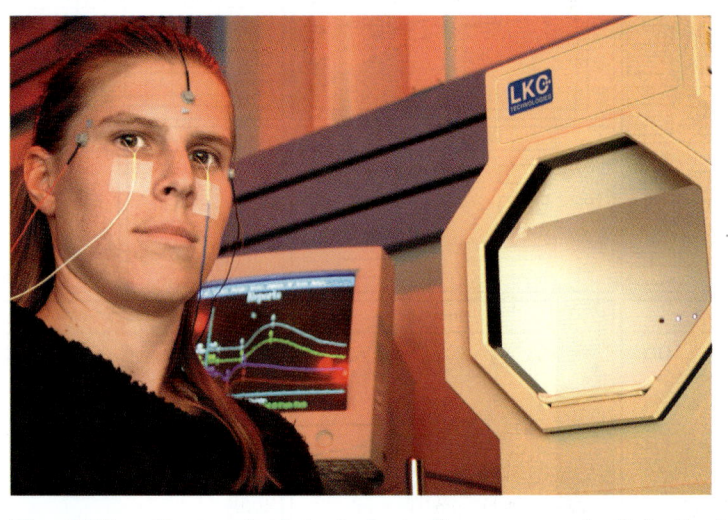

Fig. 1.35. Electrophysiological studies are used clinically in many retinal conditions. The figure shows electrode placements and a widefield light stimulator to record an electroretinogram (ERG), with the normal pattern shown on the screen.

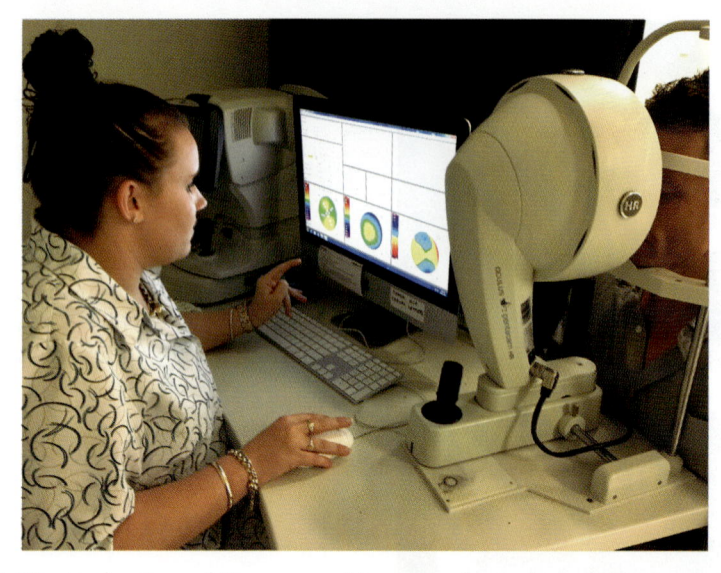

Fig. 1.36. Evaluation of the corneal topography is done with the Orbscan or Pentacam.

OCULUS - PENTACAM

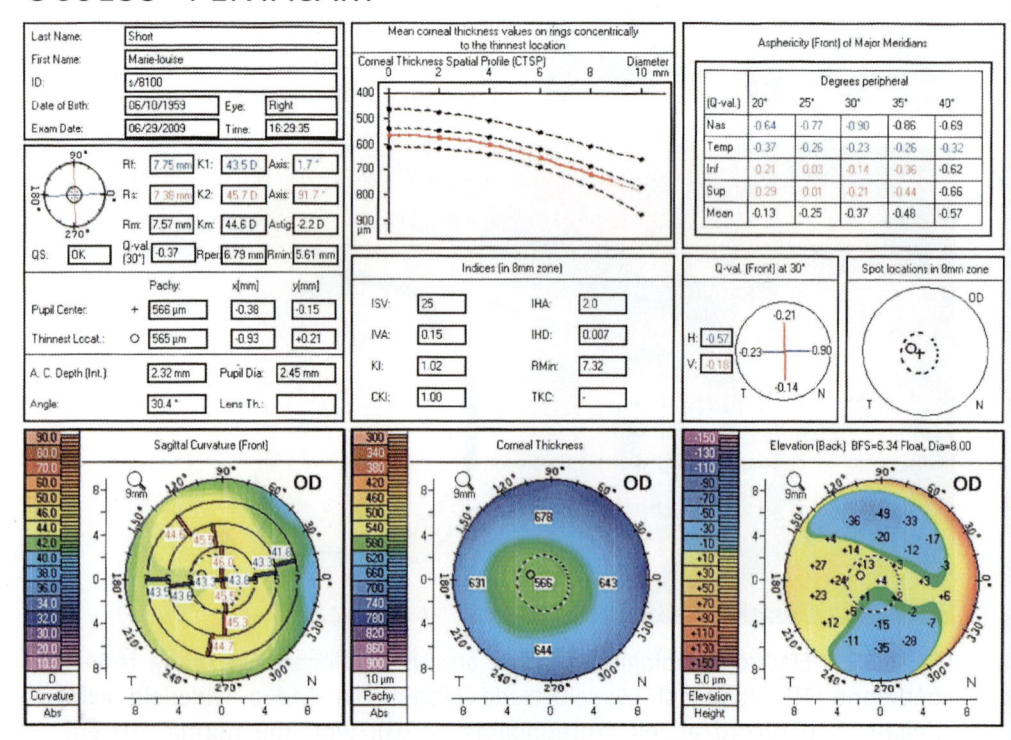

Fig. 1.37. Computer-generated map of the corneal surface.

2
LID, LACRIMAL APPARATUS AND ORBIT

INTRODUCTION

Most eyelid conditions are related to inflammation, infection, allergic disorders, malposition, eyelid deposits or tumours.

A common lacrimal disease is obstruction of the lacrimal drainage system — either congenital or acquired — which results in persistent watering or epiphora.

Orbital diseases can result from inflammation, infection, neoplasm, trauma or congenital malformation. The most common condition of the orbit is inflammatory orbital disease: thyroid-related orbitopathy or idiopathic orbital inflammatory pseudotumour.

EYELID INFLAMMATION

Blepharitis (Inflammation of the Lid Margin)

Blepharitis is inflammation of the eyelid, resulting in ocular irritation and discomfort. The two main types of blepharitis are anterior and posterior blepharitis.

Anterior blepharitis affects the anterior lid margin, near the base of the eyelashes. It may be staphylococcal or seborrhoeic, meaning that there are dandruff scales. Staphylococcal blepharitis shows hard scales and crusting at the base of the eyelashes. Long-standing staphylococcal blepharitis may result in scarring and notching of the lid margin, loss of eyelashes (madarosis) or misdirected lashes which may turn inwards, rubbing against the eye (trichiasis). Seborrhoeic blepharitis is more common and is frequently associated with dandruff or seborrhoeic dermatitis. It presents with a greasy lid margin and sticky lashes. There are small, white, soft scales at the roots of the eyelashes.

Posterior blepharitis affects the posterior eyelid margin, and is otherwise known as meibomian gland disease. The lid margin is often hyperaemic with telangiectatic vessels and capping of meibomian gland openings with oil globules. Pressure on the eyelid may express toothpaste-like secretions from the meibomian gland. Patients often have sore and gritty eyes from an unstable tear film.

Treatment is frequently difficult and tedious, as the condition is chronic. Treatment of anterior and of posterior blepharitis both involve a warm compress and good lid hygiene. The crusts may be initially softened by a warm wet towel or a soap-impregnated sponge and then removed by scrubbing the lid margins with a cotton bud soaked in baby shampoo or sodium bicarbonate. Topical antibiotic ointments are suitable for anterior blepharitis, whilst oral antibiotics like doxycycline are indicated for chronic posterior blepharitis. Topical steroids may be useful in controlling meibomian gland inflammation in posterior blepharitis but should be used with caution.

Chalazion (Meibomian Cyst)

A chalazion results from a chronic granulomatous inflammation of the meibomian or Zeis gland, caused by retained secretion because of a blockage of the duct. Initially, a chalazion presents as a small, painless nodule within the tarsal plate, which can gradually enlarge, sometimes being associated with inflammation or bacterial infection. A small chalazion can be treated conservatively, with a hot compress. It may require oral antibiotics if associated with bacterial infection. Surgery is necessary for a large or non-resolving chalazion, and involves incision and currettage of the cyst from the posterior side. (See video.)

EYELID INFECTION

Bacterial

Stye (hordeolum externum)

A stye is an acute staphylococcal abscess of an eyelash follicle which presents as a small, inflamed, tender nodule, with a lash at its apex. Treatment is with a hot compress, oral and topical antibiotics, and epilation of the involved lash.

Viral

Herpes simplex

Herpes simplex infection of the eyelid presents with eyelid and facial tingling lasting for up to 24 hr followed by the development of crops of vesicles. These vesicles break down over the next 48 hr to form erythema with lid ulcers and eyelid swelling. The ulcers may involve the lid margin and result in herpetic blepharoconjunctivitis. Treatment is with topical aciclovir ointment five times daily for five days.

Herpes zoster ophthalmicus

Herpes zoster ophthalmicus affects the skin supplied by the ophthalmic division of the fifth cranial nerve. Initially, erythematous areas with a maculopapular rash appear, followed by skin vesicles. Patients present with pain and a burning sensation. If the nasociliary nerve is affected, the vesicles appear on the side of the nose — Hutchinson's sign — which implies a strong risk of ocular involvement. In this case, the eye is at risk from complications which include corneal dendritic ulcer, iritis and secondary glaucoma.

Treatment is urgent. Systemic antiviral drugs (acyclovir, famcyclovir or valacyclovir) are indicated in all cases during the acute stage. General hygiene for the skin blisters and the application of local antibiotics to prevent secondary infection are also important. A topical antiviral to the eye is needed if keratitis develops. Ocular complications may require regular ophthalmic care. Prolonged pain over the scalp and eye (post-herpetic neuralgia) may be a serious problem in those diagnosed late and who miss out on early systemic antiviral therapy.

Molluscum contagiosum

This is a skin infection affecting the eyelid caused by the DNA poxvirus, and is mainly seen in young children. It presents with pale, waxy umbilicated nodules, which can sometimes cause follicular conjunctivitis if they are on the eyelid margin. Spontaneous resolution occurs within a few months. Excision is necessary only if there is chronic follicular conjunctivitis.

ALLERGIC DISORDERS OF THE EYELID

Allergic or Contact Dermatitis

In allergic contact dermatitis of the eyelids, the skin around the eyelids becomes oedematous, inflamed and scaly. There is intense itching. It may be due to allergy to cosmetics or a variety of ophthalmic medications, especially sulphonamides, but also a wide range of antibiotics, glaucoma drops and even preservative in artificial tears.

Treatment consists of identifying and stopping the offending cosmetics or medication and a cold compress for symptomatic relief. The application of local steroid cream to the skin of the eyelids and oral antihistamines may hasten resolution.

Atopic Dermatitis (Eczema)

In atopic eczema, the skin of the eyelids shows thickening, crusting and vertical fissures. The patients usually suffer from asthma, hay fever and generalised dermatitis. Other ocular associations are blepharitis (most common), keratoconus, cataract and retinal detachment. Treatment involves use of emollients to moisturise the skin and topical steroid ointment.

EYELID MALPOSITION

Ptosis (Drooping Upper Lid)

Ptosis is a condition where the upper lid droops from its normal position. It can be unilateral or bilateral, complete or partial, and congenital or acquired. In bilateral ptosis, the patient's head is characteristically tilted backwards in order to see under the drooped upper eyelids.

Congenital ptosis is usually due to dystrophy of the levator palpebrae superioris muscle, and may lead to amblyopia if severe and untreated.

The causes of acquired ptosis are:

1. Neurogenic: Defective nerve supply to the upper eyelid — Horner's syndrome, third nerve palsy.
2. Myogenic: Myopathy of the levator palpebrae superioris — myasthenia gravis, myotonic dystrophy, other myopathies.
3. Aponeurotic: Otherwise known as senile ptosis, where there is degeneration of the levator palpebrae superioris muscle.
4. Mechanical: Trauma to the lids, inflammation and the mass effect of a tumour.

Treatment of congenital ptosis is an operation to shorten the levator palpebrae superioris, usually with good cosmetic results. Treatment of other types of ptosis depends on the cause.

Testing for muscle fatigue and its reversal with a Tensilon injection to exclude myasthenia gravis must always be considered.

Lid Retraction

Lid retraction can involve the upper lid, the lower lid or both. Instead of covering the upper edge of the cornea, the upper lid is retracted upwards several millimetres. The most common cause of upper lid retraction is thyroid eye disease.

Control of thyroid function is necessary before any surgical management is considered. In severe, chronic cases, bridging of the lids (tarsorrhaphy) or recession of the levator muscle may be done.

Entropion (Inversion of Lid Margin)

This condition mainly affects the lower lid, causing the eyelashes to constantly rub against the cornea. This may lead to chronic conjunctivitis, corneal punctate erosion, corneal abrasion or even ulceration.

The cause may be age-related, owing to horizontal lid laxity; or cicatricial, owing to scar tissue on the conjunctival surface. Cicatricial entropion is a common complication of the end stage of trachoma, severe chemical injury and lid trauma. Lubricants and lid taping might provide temporary relief but surgical eversion of the lid is usually required.

Trichiasis (Inturned Eyelashes)

Misdirected eyelashes rubbing against the globe is called trichiasis. Trichiasis can cause a unilateral red eye from chronic irritation of the cornea or conjunctiva. It is frequently associated with entropion. For a permanent cure, the hair follicles of the inturned lashes can be destroyed by focal electrodiathermy or cryotherapy. Alternatively, the eyelid may be everted surgically.

Ectropion (Eversion of the Lid Margin)

Ectropion affects the lower eyelid in older patients. The eyelid is lax and sometimes everted. The patient usually complains of tearing (epiphora) due to failure of the tears to gain access to the lacrimal drainage apparatus. This is sometimes accompanied by exposure conjunctivitis or inferior keratitis.

The causes of ectropion are age-related with lax tissues; cicatricial, owing to contraction of eyelid scarring; and paralytic, secondary to a facial nerve palsy.

Surgical management of ectropion becomes necessary when the patient has ocular discomfort, persistent epiphora or signs of exposure keratopathy. The choice of operation depends on the cause of the ectropion.

EYELID DEPOSITS AND TUMOURS

Eyelid tumours may be benign or malignant. Benign tumours include xanthelasma, papillomas and sebaceous cysts. Malignant tumours may be primary (e.g. basal cell carcinoma, squamous cell carcinoma) or part of a systemic neoplasm (e.g. lymphoma).

Xanthelasma

Xanthelasma is a fatty deposit under the skin, usually bilateral and occurring at the medial part of the upper lid. Less commonly, it develops on the lower lid. Hyperlipidaemia is a known association. It is a local condition which has no symptoms. Surgical removal is for cosmetic reasons only.

Basal Cell Carcinoma (Rodent Ulcer)

Basal cell carcinoma (BCC) constitutes 90% of the malignant eyelid tumours, and usually appears on the lower lid margin as a raised nodule with a characteristic pearly, rolled edge. This is common in Caucasians living in hot climates. There is often a family history. If left untreated, the lesion may ulcerate and infiltrate into the adjacent tissues. It may, although rarely, invade the orbital tissues or bone and lead to loss of the eye or even reach the surface of the brain. Although BCC is locally invasive, it does not metastasize.

The choice of treatment is between surgery and radiotherapy. Surgery is more commonly performed and involves wide excision with a 2–4 mm margin, followed by eyelid reconstruction. Moh's micrographic surgery may be used for diffuse tumours with indefinite margins or those involving the medial canthus. This shaving technique minimises the sacrifice of normal tissue with complete excision of tumour margins. Careful follow-up is essential in order to prevent recurrence.

Squamous Cell Carcinoma

Squamous cell carcinoma (SCC) is less common than BCC, but more aggressive, with spread to regional lymph nodes. SCC may infiltrate deeper into the orbit and intracranial cavity via perineural pathways. Management involves extensive surgery, radiotherapy or even orbital exenteration in aggressive cases.

LACRIMAL SYSTEM

Blockage of the lacrimal drainage system can be congenital or acquired.

In congenital blockage, spontaneous resolution occurs in over 95% within the first year. If it persists, probing of the lacrimal system under anaesthesia is required.

Acquired blockage may occur in the punctum, canaliculus or nasolacrimal duct, resulting in chronic tearing. Very often, the blockage occurs in the nasolacrimal duct, which may cause the lacrimal sac to become chronically infected (chronic dacryocystitis). The patient complains of persistent watering in the eye with reflux of mucopurulent material when pressure is applied on the lacrimal sac.

If the condition persists, an operation (dacryocystorhinostomy) to create a new drainage channel may have to be performed. In acute dacryocystitis, systemic antibiotics and surgical drainage of the pus are required.

ORBIT

Infection

Orbital cellulitis

This condition is usually unilateral. It presents with intense pain, lid oedema, conjunctival injection and chemosis, proptosis and restriction of eye movements. It often occurs as a result of the spread of infection to the orbit from one of the surrounding paranasal sinuses. Sometimes there is optic disc oedema. The patient usually has systemic manifestations of fever and malaise.

Rarely, the infection may spread backwards and cause cavernous sinus thrombosis, a condition which can be fatal.

Treatment is urgent. Intensive medication with intravenous antibiotics usually clears the infection. An X-ray of the sinuses should be taken, and an ear, nose and throat specialist consulted for consideration of drainage of the sinuses.

Preseptal cellulitis

Preseptal cellulitis can simulate orbital cellulitis. It presents with swollen and inflamed eyelids, but there is no proptosis, ocular movements are not affected, and the patient is generally well. The condition is mild and treatment with systemic antibiotics is effective.

Inflammation

Thyroid eye disease

This is the most common cause of proptosis (forward protrusion of the eyeball). It can result from an overactive euthyroid or an underactive thyroid. This condition is more common in females. The pathogenesis involves an autoimmune reaction wherein an antibody against the thyroid gland cross-reacts with orbital fibroblasts, causing inflammation of extraocular muscles and orbital tissue.

The features of thyroid eye disease include puffy eyelids, red and gritty eyes, eyelid retraction, proptosis, and restriction of extraocular muscles causing diplopia. In extreme cases, compressive optic neuropathy and sight-threatening exposure keratopathy may occur. On an MRI scan, there is a characteristic enlargement of the belly of the extraocular muscles, sparing the tendon.

Treatment involves management of thyroid dysfunction, systemic steroids and low dose radiotherapy. Orbital decompression surgery is rarely needed but fibrotic extraocular muscle contracture and chronic diplopia may require strabismus surgery after the acute stage has passed.

Idiopathic orbital inflammatory disease

Orbital pseudotumour is a non-specific orbital inflammatory disease which may be acute, recurrent or chronic. It is mostly unilateral in adults and occurs less commonly in children, sometimes bilaterally. An acute painful onset of double vision and proptosis in one eye should strongly raise suspicion of this condition. A CT or MRI scan shows orbital infiltration with thickening of extraocular muscles including the tendon (which is in contrast to thyroid eye disease). Treatment involves systemic steroids.

Tumours Involving the Orbit

Space-occupying lesions in the orbit, which usually present with axial or eccentric proptosis, may arise from any of the orbital structures — vascular tissue, lacrimal gland, neural tissue, lymphatic tissue, smooth muscle. Metastatic tumour of the orbit or spread from adjacent structures including nasopharyngeal cancer can also occur.

Vascular lesions in the orbit include orbital varices, lymphangioma and capillary or cavernous haemangioma.

The common lacrimal gland tumours are pleomorphic lacrimal gland adenoma and lacrimal gland carcinoma.

Tumours from the optic nerve — optic nerve glioma and optic nerve sheath meningioma — commonly result in visual loss and proptosis. Plexiform neurofibroma, seen in neurofibromatosis type 1, is a peripheral nerve tumour of the orbit which usually presents in early childhood with periorbital swelling and a characteristic S-shaped lid.

Lymphomas of the orbit are mainly of non-Hodgkin's type B-cell origin and can involve any part of the orbit. Diagnosis involves MRI scan and biopsy as well as the appropriate systemic and haematological investigations.

Rhabdomyosarcoma is the most common soft tissue sarcoma and primary orbital malignancy in children, with an average age of onset of around seven years. It presents with rapidly progressive unilateral proptosis.

Owing to the variety of causes of orbital lesions, investigations and treatment often involve other specialist teams, including neurologists, endocrinologists, radiologists and ENT surgeons. Local space-occupying lesions can be treated by surgical removal via an orbitotomy, whilst other diffuse lesions may need radiotherapy, chemotherapy or a combination of the two.

Inflammation of the Eyelid

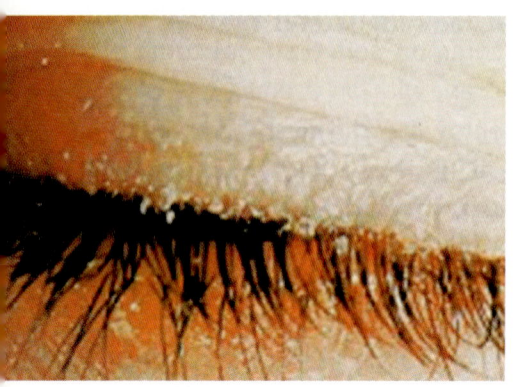

Fig. 2.1. Squamous blepharitis (crusting at the base of the lashes).

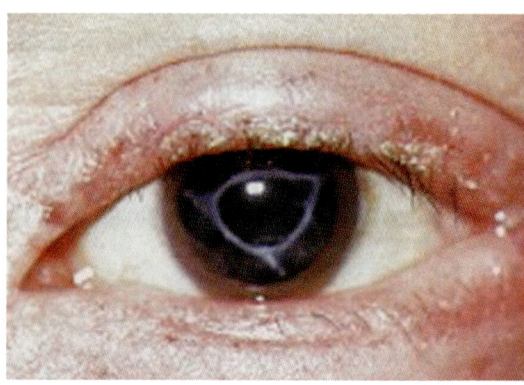

Fig. 2.2. Ulcerative blepharitis.

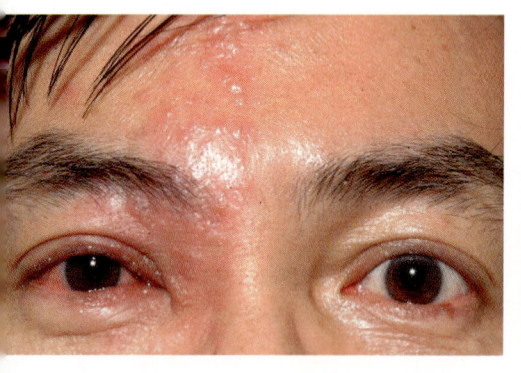

Fig. 2.3. Herpes zoster ophthalmicus with vesicles affecting the right upper eyelid and forehead.

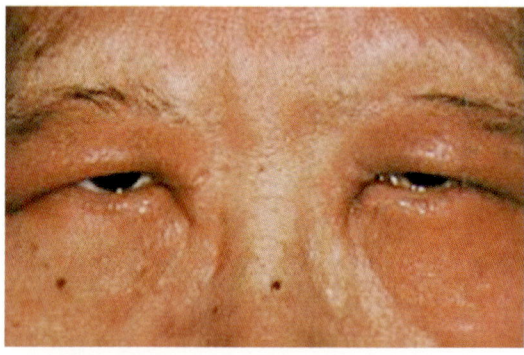

Fig. 2.4. Bilateral allergic blepharitis resulting from sulphacetamide eye drops.

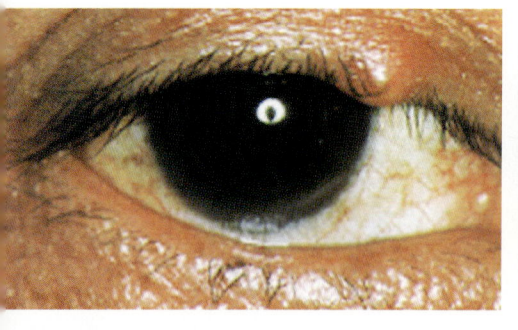

Fig. 2.5. Stye (an abscess of the eyelash follicle).

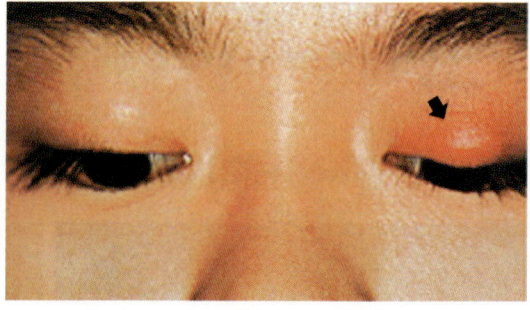

Fig. 2.6. Inflamed chalazion (meibomian gland swelling) of the left upper lid.

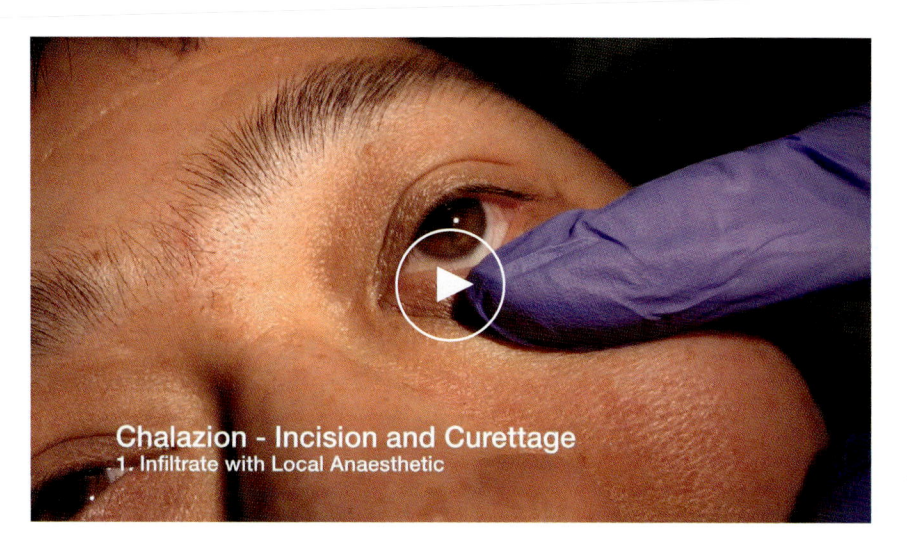

Video of chalazion incision and curettage.

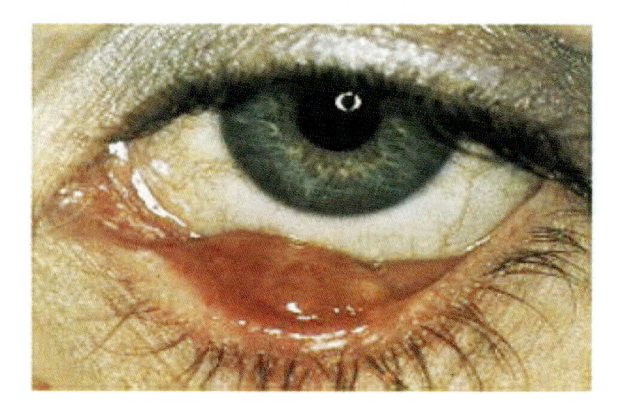

Fig. 2.7. Chronic chalazion which has ruptured through the conjunctiva and appears as a granulomatous lesion.

Malposition of the Eyelid

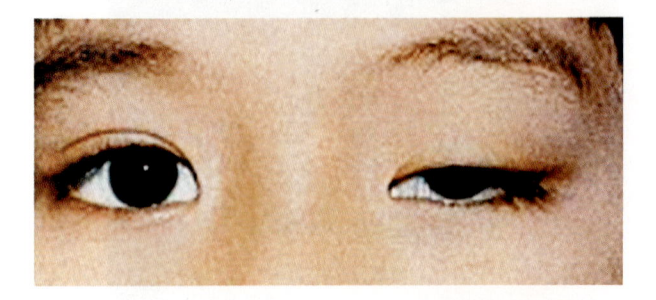

Fig. 2.8. Left congenital ptosis (drooping of the eyelid).

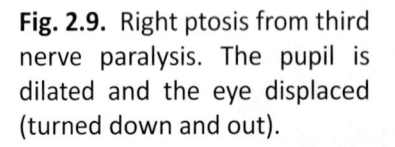

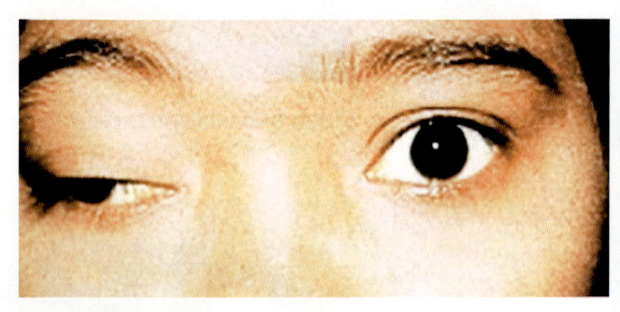

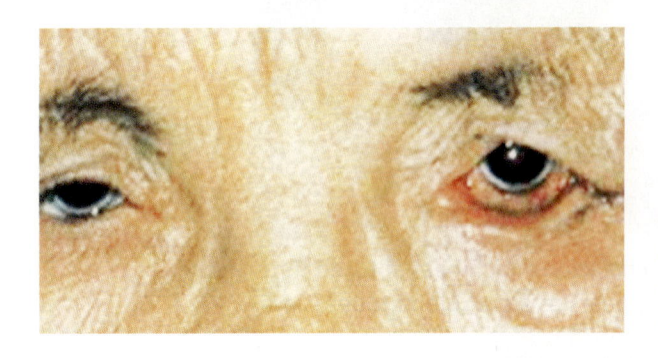

Fig. 2.9. Right ptosis from third nerve paralysis. The pupil is dilated and the eye displaced (turned down and out).

Fig. 2.10. Ectropion of the left lower lid (eversion of the eyelid) with a red eye due to exposure keratitis.

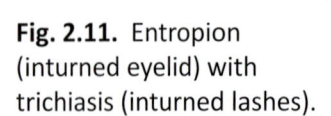

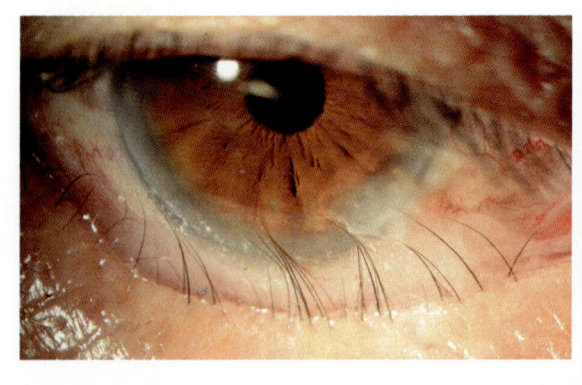

Fig. 2.11. Entropion (inturned eyelid) with trichiasis (inturned lashes).

Deposits and Tumours of the Eyelid

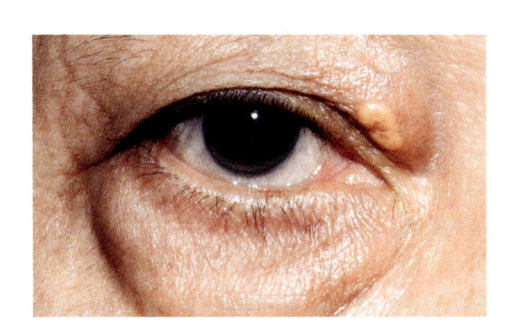

Fig. 2.12. Xanthelasma (fatty deposits on the eyelid).

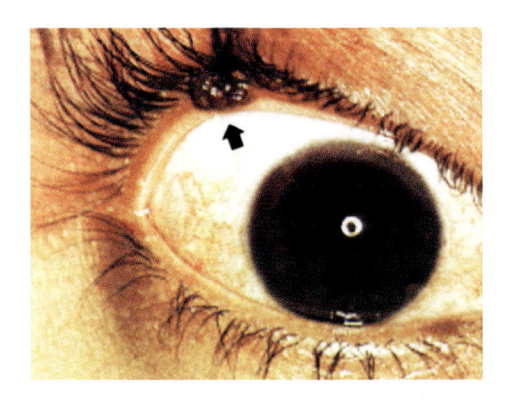

Fig. 2.13. Benign compound naevus at the upper eyelid margin.

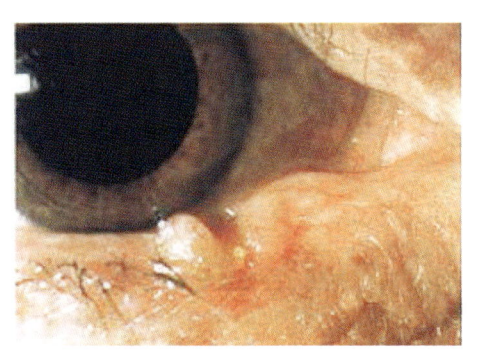

Fig. 2.14. Basal cell carcinoma at the lid margin, with a central ulcer and raised edges.

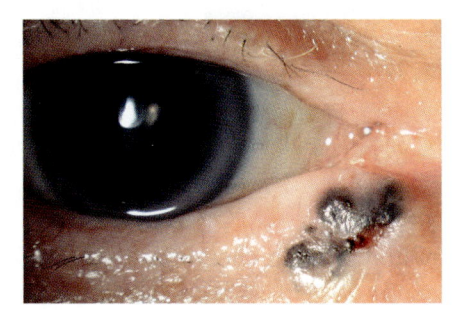

Fig. 2.15. Ulcerated, pigmented tumour of the right lower lid. Biopsy will differentiate malignant melanoma from basal or squamous cell carcinoma.

Orbital Lesions

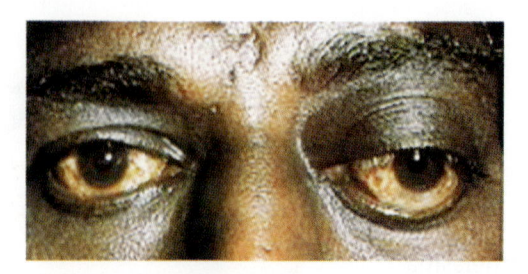

Fig. 2.16. Left exophthalmos caused by a retrobulbar tumour. (Note the left lower lid, 4 mm away from the limbus.)

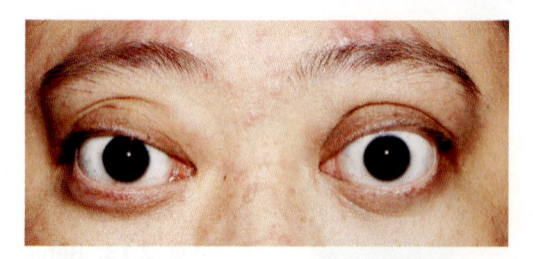

Fig. 2.17. Exophthalmos with lid retraction in thyroid exophthalmos.

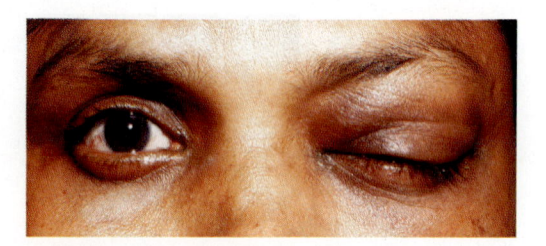

Fig. 2.18. Left orbital cellulitis with lid oedema, exophthalmos and chemosis (oedema of conjunctiva).

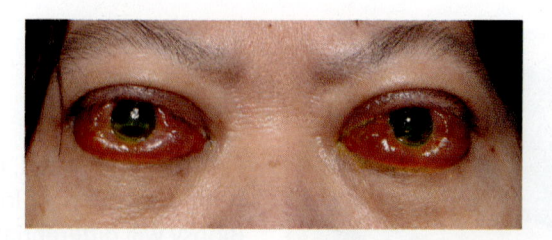

Fig. 2.19. Bilateral orbital infiltration with chemosis of protruding conjunctiva.

3
CONJUNCTIVA, SCLERA AND CORNEA

INTRODUCTION

Red eyes from infection or allergy are common and relatively harmless. However, a unilateral red eye requires careful ocular examination, as the common causes are acute glaucoma, acute iritis, keratitis, corneal ulcer or a foreign body. These conditions can lead to blindness if untreated.

Corneal diseases may lead to visual loss because of scarring. Of particular importance are contact-lens-associated microbial keratitis, herpes simplex infection and trachoma. Corneal transplantation may restore vision to patients with central corneal opacities and corneal endothelial decompensation.

CONJUNCTIVITIS

Bacterial Conjunctivitis

Acute bacterial conjunctivitis is a common cause of bilateral red eyes. The symptoms include acute onset of redness and grittiness with yellowish mucopurulent discharge and sticky eyelids, especially in the morning. The sensation of grittiness or of having a foreign body in the eyes is due to the rubbing of the inflamed palpebral conjunctiva against the cornea. The signs depend on the severity of the infection. Patients present with eyelid oedema, and red and congested conjunctiva with purulent discharge, usually bilateral. The diagnosis is usually straightforward, especially when the condition occurs during an epidemic. Application of local antibiotic eye drops

4–6 times a day (chloramphenicol, tobramycin, ciprofloxacin or ofloxacin) and frequent washing with warm water should cure the condition in 5–7 days. Antibiotic ointment may be used at night for prolonged effect and to prevent the lids sticking together in the morning. Patching of the eyes is not recommended. If there is no improvement within two days of commencing treatment, or for severe or resistant cases, conjunctival swabs, Gram stain and culture should be done. It is recommended to continue with the eye drops for two days after the infection has cleared clinically. The risk of transmission should be reduced by frequent handwashing.

Viral Conjunctivitis

Viral conjunctivitis may be unilateral or bilateral. It presents with redness, watering, irritation and mild photophobia. The discharge is less than that seen in bacterial conjunctivitis. Follicles are seen in the palpebral conjunctiva of the eyelids. Corneal involvement in the form of punctate epithelial keratitis and focal sub-epithelial infiltrates are common and can result in blurring of vision. The pre-auricular lymph node can be tender and swollen on the side of involvement. The onset of viral conjunctivitis is preceded by flu-like symptoms, sore throat and malaise. Most cases are due to the adenovirus and can appear in epidemics, but can also result from the herpes simplex virus. There is no specific treatment. Artificial tears can be used for comfort. When there is corneal involvement, steroid drops can be used carefully if the patient is managed by an ophthalmologist. Antibiotic drops may be prescribed to prevent secondary bacterial infection.

Preventive measures to limit the spread of infection, such as washing the hands between patients and not sharing towels, must be taken during epidemics. Patients should also wash their hands to prevent direct spread, and isolation from the family is required.

Allergic Conjunctivitis

Allergic conjunctivitis also presents with bilateral red eyes. It is associated with intense itchiness and watering. Sometimes it is associated with vasomotor rhinitis, hay fever, a history of allergic rashes and a reaction to drugs or cosmetics. In addition, it is sometimes due to topical medications or even the preservative in them.

Treatment includes stopping the possible causative medications, then artificial tears, mast cell stabilisers (sodium cromoglycate) and decongestive or antihistamine eye drops. Mild topical steroids (fluoromethalone) are effective but should not be used routinely or long-term except in the occasional severe cases.

Vernal Conjunctivitis (Spring Catarrh)

A less common specific allergic conjunctivitis is spring catarrh. It occurs seasonally, usually in spring, and is more common in boys. Large flat papillary conjunctival thickenings form on the upper tarsal conjunctiva. A thick ropy mucous discharge is seen. Corneal complications include punctate epithelial erosions, plaques and even ulcers. Treatment involves use of topical mast cell stabilisers (sodium cromoglycate), antihistamines, steroids and acetyl cysteine to dissolve mucous filaments.

Dry Eye

Dry eye (keratoconjunctivitis sicca) is due to defective or deficient tear formation. It can be classified as having aqueous-deficient and evaporative causes. Aqueous-deficient dry eye results from decreased production of tears. Evaporative dry eye results from alteration of the lipid layer which may destabilise the tear film by increasing evaporation, causing it to break up quickly after each blink and creating small dry spots on the corneal epithelium.

Patients present with a sensation of dryness, discomfort, irritation, burning, redness, reflex watering and pain, as with chronic non-specific conjunctivitis. Signs include reduced tear meniscus, blepharitis, redness, decreased tear film break-up time and punctate epithelial erosions or filaments on the cornea. Severe dry eye can result in keratinisation of the conjunctiva and cornea.

The most common form is idiopathic and is seen mainly in older patients. It may also follow viral conjunctivitis, contact lens wear, LASIK and cataract surgery, and a range of systemic and local medications. A more severe but less common form is often associated with systemic conditions such as Sjoegren's syndrome (triad of dry eyes, dry mouth and parotid enlargement), connective tissue diseases (rheumatoid arthritis, systemic lupus erythematosus, scleroderma), sarcoidosis and Stevens–Johnson syndrome. Occasionally, serious corneal complications, including bacterial infection, corneal stromal melting and even corneal perforation, may develop in severe dry eye.

Treatment

If the condition is mild, tear substitutes will help. There are a wide range of ocular lubricants (see chapter on "Ophthalmic Therapeutics") available, of varying viscosity. Application may need to be very frequent. Spray-on formulations and gel at night also help. Some patients improve with oral fish oil capsules, others with vitamin A ointment. An associated inflammatory element may require preservative free drops, lid massage for blepharitis or cyclosporine drops. There are newer drops like diquafosol and lifitegrast which help increase tear production. Avoiding low humidity such as air-conditioning and the use of wrap-around glasses or swimming goggles at night may also help. Occlusion of the punctum with plugs may also be tried. For severe dry eye with no relief from artificial tears, autologous serum eye drops can be tried.

Evaporative dry eye is often associated with chronic blepharitis, in which case, daily hot towel compresses and massage of the lid margins with lid care soap or baby shampoo is also necessary.

UNILATERAL RED EYE

A unilateral red eye is a potentially dangerous condition. It may be due to serious ocular conditions such as acute closed-angle glaucoma, acute iritis, keratitis, corneal ulcer or a foreign body. Less commonly, it is due to scleritis. Of particular importance is acute closed-angle glaucoma, which presents with a unilateral red eye with a mid-dilated pupil, associated with headache, severe pain in the eye and blurred vision. Prompt consultation with an ophthalmologist or at the hospital emergency department is required.

Unilateral conjunctivitis is usually associated with an underlying cause, such as a blocked nasolacrimal duct or trichiasis (inturned eyelashes). A unilateral red eye with follicles in the tarsal conjunctiva should raise the suspicion of a viral or chlamydial infection. It is important to carry out a thorough investigation of a unilateral red eye to establish the cause.

Subconjunctival Haemorrhage

This condition also presents as a unilateral red eye. Rubbing of the eyes and severe coughing may cause capillary rupture, resulting in haemorrhage into the subconjunctival space, but it is more often spontaneous.

Treatment is normally not required except to reassure the patient that the haemorrhage will take one to two weeks to absorb. Occasionally, the condition recurs. If it does, investigations to exclude a blood dyscrasia may be carried out.

TRACHOMA

This is a major worldwide blinding condition caused by infection brought about by an organism known as *Chlamydia trachomatis*. It has a varying pattern in different countries. In poor overcrowded communities, it can be endemic, with up to 90% of some populations showing signs of trachoma. In some areas, 10% of those with chronic recurrent infection become blind.

Chlamydia presents a different clinical picture in developed societies, where it causes less serious conjunctivitis but affects the genitals as well as the eye and is called trachoma inclusion conjunctivitis (TRIC).

The clinical features of trachoma vary considerably. At the initial stage, it may be asymptomatic, or may present with acute conjunctivitis. The signs of active infection are white round follicles on the conjunctival surface of the upper lids associated with a velvety papillary hypertrophy. Follicles at the limbus leave small depressions known as Herbert's pits, which are permanent diagnostic signs of previous trachoma. A layer of new blood vessels and connective tissue (pannus) usually invades the upper cornea. Intense inflammation of the tarsal conjunctiva occurs, progressing to conjunctival scarring, seen as fibrous white bands known as Arlt's lines. If that is compounded by cyclical reinfection and superimposed bacterial infection, entropion (inturned eyelid), trichiasis (inturned eyelashes) and blindness due to an opaque cornea, corneal bacterial ulceration or even endophthalmitis may result.

In active trachoma, antibiotics should be given to the patient and all family members. A single dose of Azithromycin 1 g is recommended. If mass surveys reveal that over 20% of the population are actively infected, treatment is given to the whole population to eliminate the infectious pool of chlamydia. Surgical correction of entropion and trichiasis relieves discomfort and decreases the risk of visual loss from corneal scarring and infection. If there is corneal scarring, it is not usually possible to improve vision with corneal graft surgery owing to subsequent graft rejection in a very dry eye with corneal vascularisation.

In spite of advances in modern medicine, trachoma remains one of the most difficult eye diseases to eradicate in the developing countries, mainly because of crowded and unhygienic living conditions, including a lack of water supply, dust and flies. The WHO advocates the SAFE strategy for management of trachoma: Surgery to relieve entropion and trichiasis, Antibiotics (Azithromycin), Facial cleanliness and Environmental improvement with good sanitation and clean water. Trachoma invariably becomes less of a threat with improved living conditions that follow economic development but remote populations in arid environments still suffer the effects.

RAISED CONJUNCTIVAL LESIONS

Pinguecula

This is a tiny, cream-coloured, slightly raised, opaque lesion on the conjunctiva, usually on the nasal side of the cornea but sometimes on the temporal side. A pinguecula usually causes no symptoms. It is common in the tropics, and is related to exposure to the sun. No treatment is required except for reassurance that it is not a growth. Surgical removal for cosmetic reasons is seldom required.

Pterygium

A pterygium is a triangular fleshy wing of the conjunctiva which grows onto the cornea, usually on the nasal side. Some pterygia are vascular, thick and fleshy, while others are avascular and flat. A pterygium is usually bilateral and harmless but may cause mild astigmatism. Patients often complain of dryness, soreness and redness over the raised exposed area. Visual disturbance may result from induced astigmatism. It is very rare for a pterygium to grow across to the pupillary area. Pterygia are common in the tropics, amongst outdoor workers, sport and surfing enthusiasts, and are associated with exposure to the UV in sunlight. Excision may be considered if the pterygium is symptomatic or cosmetically worrying. To prevent recurrence, the pterygium excision is combined with a free conjunctival graft from under the upper lid of the same eye to cover the bare sclera.

Conjunctival Pigmentary Deposits (Naevus)

Benign conjunctival melanin deposits are common but usually harmless. The lesions occasionally grow in size during puberty. Although they may be removed for cosmetic reasons, they are usually just monitored by serial observation. Malignant conjunctival melanoma is very uncommon.

Ocular Surface Squamous Neoplasia (OSSN)

This includes benign and malignant lesions of the corneal and conjunctival epithelium. Usually a mass is visible on the conjunctiva or limbus of the cornea, which appears fleshy and pink with feeder vessels. Impression cytology and excision biopsy are performed to confirm the diagnosis. Topical chemotherapy (5-fluorouracil or mitomycin C) and cryotherapy may also be used to prevent recurrence after excision.

CORNEAL ULCERS

Corneal ulcers are usually due to the herpes simplex virus or bacterial infection and may be associated with dry eye, trauma or contact lens wear.

Herpes Simplex Dendritic Ulcers

Herpes simplex infection can be primary or recurrent. Primary infection usually occurs in childhood and is self-limited. Recurrent infection occurs owing to reactivation of the herpes simplex virus that is dormant in the sensory ganglia of the brain stem and spinal cord (the trigeminal ganglion in the case of ocular involvement).

Herpes simplex causes epithelial keratitis, usually in the form of a dendritic ulcer. The eye is usually irritable, red, watering and photophobic. A typical branched dendritic ulcer stains with topical fluorescein. Corneal sensation is usually reduced. Iritis and elevated intraocular pressure can also occur. Treatment involves topical antiviral agents like aciclovir 3% ointment or ganciclovir 0.15% gel. In some cases, the infected loose epithelium may be removed with a cotton bud after application of topical anaesthetic eye drops. Oral antivirals are usually not necessary unless the patient is immunocompromised. Steroids are contraindicated for viral dendritic ulcers.

A serious complication known as disciform keratitis is a deep stromal, disc-like area of oedema and inflammation of the cornea. Keratic precipitates are seen underneath the corneal oedema. Iritis with increased intraocular pressure may also result. Reduced corneal sensation is present. Disciform keratitis is thought to arise from an immune reaction to viral antigens. The condition tends to recur especially during periods of stress or fever. Repeated episodes can result in corneal stromal scarring. Treatment involves topical steroids and topical antiviral ointment with a slow taper. A small minority of those who lose vision from stromal scarring may be considered for corneal transplantation but herpetic recurrence in the graft affects the prognosis.

Small Marginal Corneal Ulcers

These are frequently associated with ulcerative blepharitis and are believed to be due to hypersensitivity to staphylococcal antigens. Treatment with antibiotic eye drops in combination with steroids is effective.

Bacterial Corneal Ulcers

A bacterial corneal ulcer may occur when there is a breakdown of the corneal epithelium. The risk factors include trauma, contact lens wear (especially prolonged wear and unhygienic maintenance of the contact lenses) and ocular surface disease. The signs and symptoms are those of a unilateral red eye which is painful, watering and photophobic with mucopurulent discharge. The eye shows a corneal ulcer with a white infiltrate. The vision is blurred. The ulcer is caused by bacterial infection from a variety of organisms. The commonest are Staphylococcus, Streptococcus and *Pseudomonas aeruginosa*. Gonococcus and Haemophilus are important causes in children. Bacterial keratitis leads to permanent scarring or even perforation. Pseudomonas is the most dangerous, as it can lead to a large destructive corneal ulcer rapidly. When a bacterial corneal ulcer is suspected, corneal scraping and conjunctival swabs are done for microscopy, Gram stain and culture. In contact-lens-related keratitis, the contact lenses and cleaning solution should also be sent for culture and sensitivity. Treatment involves monotherapy with fluoroquinolone drops (ciprofloxacin, ofloxacin, levofloxacin) or intensive fortified topical antibiotics such as cephazolin, gentamicin, and vancomycin subsequently modified according to micobiological findings. Dilation of the pupil with atropine prevents posterior synechiae (adhesion of the iris to the lens) and provides pain relief from ciliary spasm. In severe cases, subconjunctival injections and systemic antibiotics are sometimes also required.

Severe Corneal Ulcers

Severe corneal ulcers can often be prevented by adequate initial treatment of minor injuries. Early application of drops or ointment (broad-spectrum antibiotics) is particularly important in rural areas where ophthalmic care is not immediately available. Severe and neglected corneal ulcers lead to blindness from corneal scarring, corneal perforation, secondary glaucoma or endophthalmitis. In severe cases, therapeutic corneal grafting may occasionally be required after the infection is eradicated to manage corneal melting and the risk of perforation.

Fungal Corneal Ulcers

Corneal ulcers caused by a wide variety of fungi have a more insidious and protracted course. They are particularly likely to occur in susceptible eyes with depressed immunity after prolonged treatment with steroid or antibiotic drops and in eyes after injury involving organic material. Scrapings may reveal the fungus. Local and sometimes systemic antifungal agents, including natamycin, voriconazole and amphotericin-B, are used for treatment. Eradication is often difficult and corneal grafting may be required. The prognosis for vision is often poor.

Acanthamoeba (Protozoan) Keratitis

Indolent corneal infection caused by protozoa typically occurs in people washing contact lenses in tap water, swimming in contaminated fresh water or wearing contact lenses in saunas. Patients present with disproportionate symptoms and less florid signs. Signs include circumcorneal congestion with corneal stromal infiltrates and characteristic perineural infiltrates along the corneal nerves. Sometimes, these infiltrates may join together to form a ring abscess in the cornea. It is made worse with steroid drops. Investigations include corneal scraping and staining with the periodic acid–Schiff (PAS) stain as well as culture with non-nutrient agar. *In vivo* confocal microscopy can also be useful. Treatment can be prolonged with a guarded prognosis and involves the use of topical amoebicides like PHMB 0.02% (polyhexamethylene biguanide, which is usually employed as a swimming pool disinfectant), Brolene (propamidine) and antifungals like ketoconazole and voriconazole.

Non-Ulcerative (Interstitial) Keratitis

In the active stage, interstitial keratitis is bilateral and presents with clouded vascularised corneas. In the later stages, the eyes are quiet with residual opacity of varying intensity in the deep corneal layers and "ghost" or empty blood vessels, which are best seen under the slit-lamp microscope. Congenital syphilis is the usual cause, but other infective conditions, such as tuberculosis, leprosy and the herpes virus, may also cause interstitial keratitis.

The acute stage responds rapidly to local steroids. Antibiotics may be used in addition. Defective vision due to long-term corneal opacity can be improved with corneal graft surgery.

CORNEAL OPACITY

If the corneal scarring is in the periphery, the vision remains good, but when it is central, it can interfere severely. Common causes are healed herpes keratitis, chronic trachoma, trauma and keratomalacia from vitamin A deficiency. In many cases, a corneal graft can restore vision.

Arcus Senilis

This is a white ring at the periphery of the cornea, caused by lipid deposits in the stroma. The central cornea is never affected. This condition is sometimes found in young adults (arcus juvenilis). It is harmless.

Band Keratopathy

This results from calcium deposition, mainly in the anterior cornea. Conditions that lead to a dystrophic cornea, such as chronic uveitis, chronic keratitis, intraocular silicone oil and a blind prethisical eye, are the usual causes. Metabolic causes of increased serum calcium and phosphate also may predispose to band keratopathy. Treatment involves scraping and chelation of the corneal calcium with ethylenediaminetetraacetic acid (EDTA).

Spheroidal Degeneration

This condition is otherwise called Labrador keratopathy and shows golden-yellow granules on the superficial cornea with opacification. It is usually seen in people who work outdoors. The granules do not cause visual impairment unless the visual axis is involved. Treatment involves use of sunglasses to limit UV exposure and occasionally debridement.

Corneal Dystrophies

Corneal dystrophies affect both eyes symmetrically and are usually detected early in young patients. A family history of corneal dystrophy may be present.

Hereditary corneal dystrophies of various types cause minute opacities in the central cornea. Dystrophies can involve corneal epithelium, stroma or endothelium. Common epithelial dystrophies are Reis–Bucklers corneal dystrophy (which affects the Bowman layer), Map-dot-fingerprint dystrophy and Meesmann epithelial dystrophy, which can cause ocular discomfort and recurrent corneal erosions. Common stromal dystrophies include granular dystrophy, macular dystrophy and lattice dystrophy, which can all cause varying degrees of visual loss. Severe visual loss from corneal dystrophy may need corneal grafting. Endothelial dystrophies include Fuchs' endothelial dystrophy and congenital hereditary endothelial dystrophy (CHED).

Fuchs' endothelial dystrophy presents on routine examination with diffuse irregularity of the corneal endothelium visible on retroillumination on the slit lamp. Progressive endothelial compromise may slowly lead to diffuse corneal oedema, thickening and stromal opacity and severe visual loss. The condition usually occurs in the middle-aged or the elderly and is more common in Caucasians than in Asians. It is caused by dystrophic changes in the corneal endothelium. Sometimes, it worsens after a cataract extraction. Traditionally, corneal decompensation has been treated with full-thickness corneal transplantation, but nowadays patients undergo Descemet's membrane endothelial keratoplasty (DMEK) or deep stromal automated endothelial keratoplasty (DSAEK) with excellent outcomes.

Congenital hereditary endothelial dystrophy (CHED) can be confused with congenital glaucoma and is an uncommon entity. Severe corneal clouding is noted at birth or within the first two years of life, with the symptoms of photophobia and watering. Treatment usually involves full-thickness corneal grafting but the risk of graft rejection is high in children.

Keratoconus

Keratoconus is a dystrophic condition in young adults where the cornea becomes conical in shape and thin owing to weakening of the tissue collagen. Presentation is usually in the second decade of life. About 15% of patients have a family history. The patient becomes highly short-sighted, with severe irregular astigmatism. Vision is initially improved with glasses but later contact lenses are needed to overcome irregularity and astigmatism. Collagen cross-linking with riboflavin activated by UV light is used to stabilise or slow progression. Plastic corneal inlays (INTACS — intracorneal ring segments) inserted in a tunnel formed by laser can overcome some of the refractive error and improve vision for a few years. If the condition is advanced, corneal transplantation may be required and is highly effective.

Corneal Transplantation

Corneal grafting is a surgical procedure in which a donor cornea is used to replace a diseased recipient cornea. Progress in transplantation research and microsurgical techniques has improved graft survival and visual prognosis in recent years. The graft may be full- or partial-thickness, or an endothelial monolayer.

The primary reason for corneal transplantation is usually visual improvement (optical indication). Common indications include post-cataract-surgery bullous keratopathy (corneal decompensation), keratoconus, corneal dystrophies and corneal opacities. Corneal grafts can also be used for severe corneal ulcers (therapeutic indication) or for impending corneal perforation (tectonic indication). The prognosis is less favourable for corneal scarring that is vascularised or due to herpes keratitis. Severe dry eye and poorly controlled glaucoma are contraindications.

Full-thickness corneal grafting

This has been the conventional corneal grafting surgery. Corneal tissue is harvested from a donor within 12–24 hr of death. The donor corneas are evaluated and stored in eye banks. Contraindications for corneal donation include death from an unknown cause, HIV, syphilis, TB, hepatitis, CJD (Creutzfeldt–Jakob disease) and various malignancies.

Full-thickness corneal grafting for conditions like keratoconus, corneal dystrophies and traumatic corneal scarring usually has a good prognosis. Prognosis is guarded in severe herpetic eye disease, corneal vascularisation, ocular surface disease causing severe dry eye, lid malpositions, severe glaucoma and chronic uveitis.

The donor tissue is first prepared under sterile conditions and is usually about 0.25–0.50 mm larger than the excised host corneal tissue. The donor corneal button is anchored to the host cornea using interrupted or continuous 10-0 sutures. Patients are treated with topical steroids and antibiotics in the initial post-op period, with the topical steroids to continue for at least a year in order to minimise graft rejection. Graft failure and graft rejection can occur at any time, and this needs intensive treatment with topical steroids and immunosuppression with systemic steroids and immune modulators like cyclosporine or tacrolimus.

Partial-thickness corneal grafting (lamellar graft)

To decrease complications like graft rejection and to allow faster visual rehabilitation, partial-thickness excision of only the corneal epithelium and corneal stroma is sometimes able to be done, leaving behind intact deep stroma and endothelium. This is suitable for eyes with anterior corneal opacities.

Endothelial keratoplasty

This is a relatively new variation of the conventional full-thickness corneal graft, wherein only the diseased endothelium with Descemet's membrane is removed and replaced by donor Descemet's membrane with healthy endothelium. DSAEK involves removal of deep stromal tissue with Descemet's membrane and endothelium. DMEK involves removal of Descemet's membrane with endothelium without the stroma, and this technique has shown better visual recovery, with lower rejection rates than DSAEK.

Bilateral Red Eyes

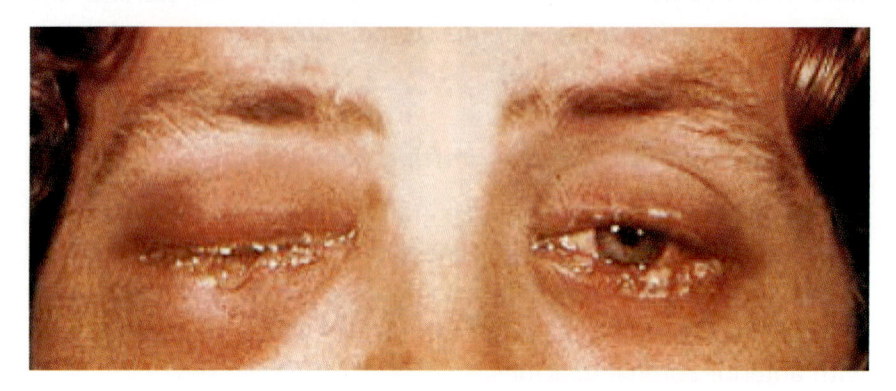

Fig. 3.1. Bilateral bacterial conjunctivitis with lid oedema and sticky mucopurulent discharge.

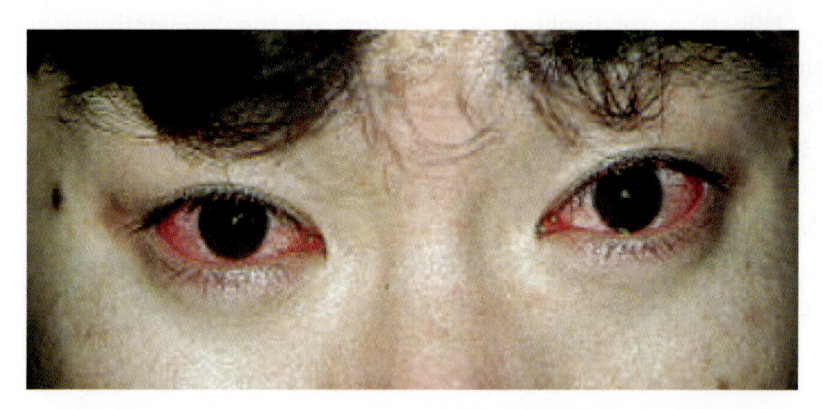

Fig. 3.2. Bilateral viral conjunctivitis presenting with watering red eyes.

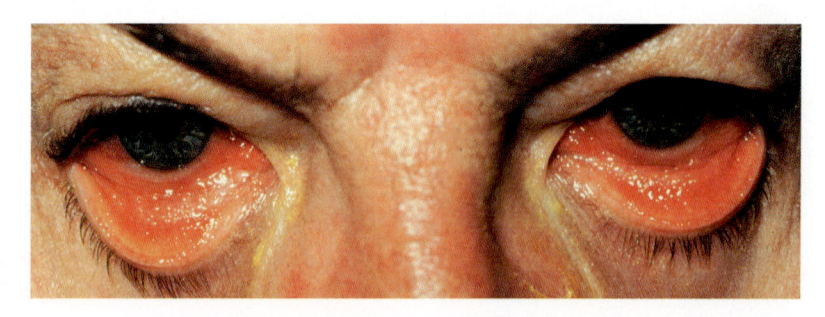

Fig. 3.3. Allergic conjunctivitis.

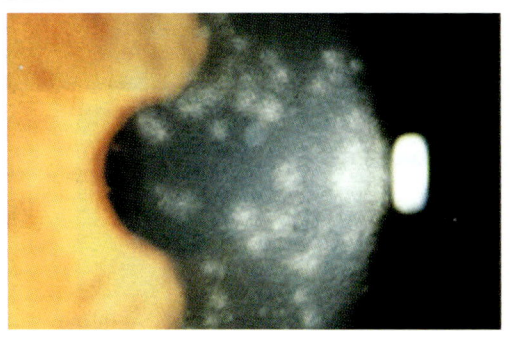

Fig. 3.4. Sub-epithelial punctate corneal infiltrates in viral keratoconjunctivitis.

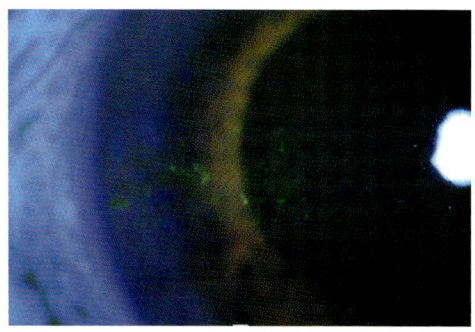

Fig. 3.5. Fluorescent staining of an exposed cornea in dry eye.

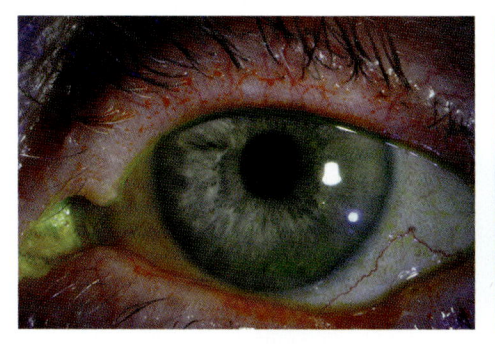

Fig. 3.6. Dry eye due to Sjogren's syndrome with deficient tear meniscus.

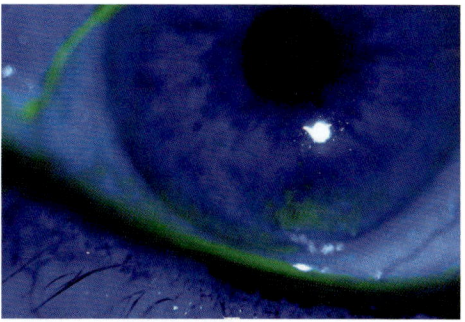

Fluorescein stain on the inferior cornea.

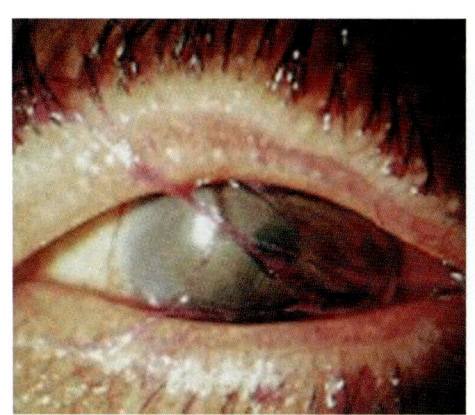

Fig. 3.7. Severe dry eye. Vital staining with rose bengal.

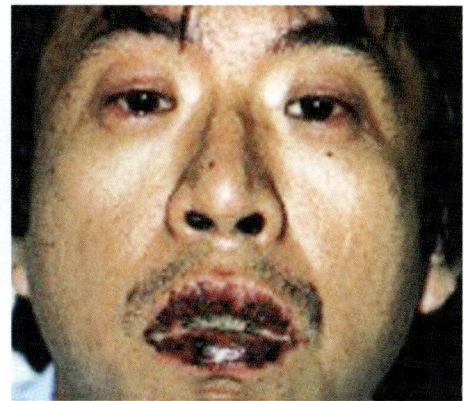

Fig. 3.8. Stevens–Johnson syndrome with severe conjunctival and buccal inflammation.

Unilateral Red Eye

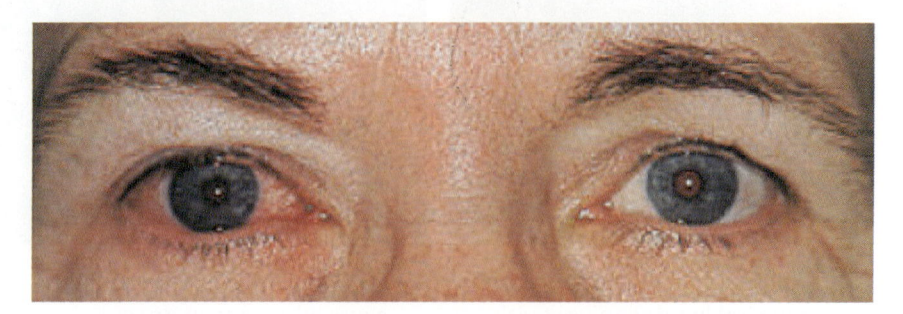

Fig. 3.9. Iritis presenting as a unilateral red right eye. The pupil is small.

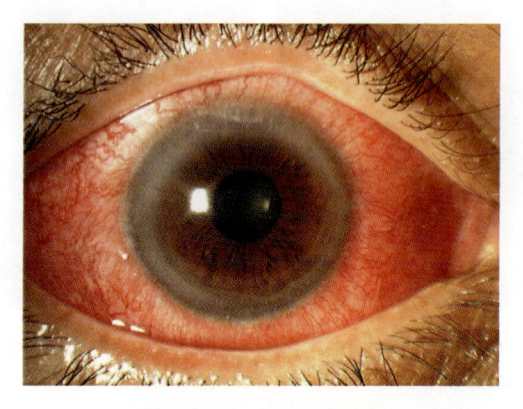

Fig. 3.10. Acute iritis.

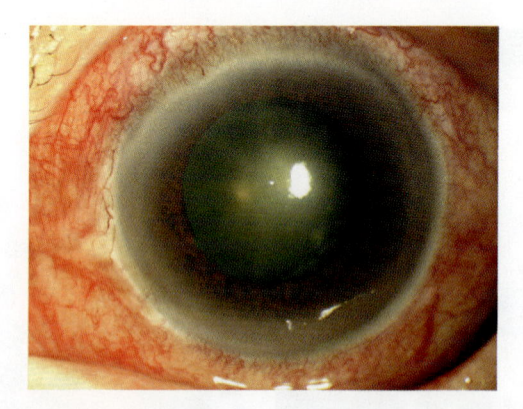

Fig. 3.11. Acute, congestive, closed-angle glaucoma, with a hazy cornea and a fixed, dilated pupil. Acute glaucoma is an important cause of sudden blindness in middle-aged patients. With early diagnosis and emergency treatment, blindness can be prevented.

Dendritic Corneal Ulcer

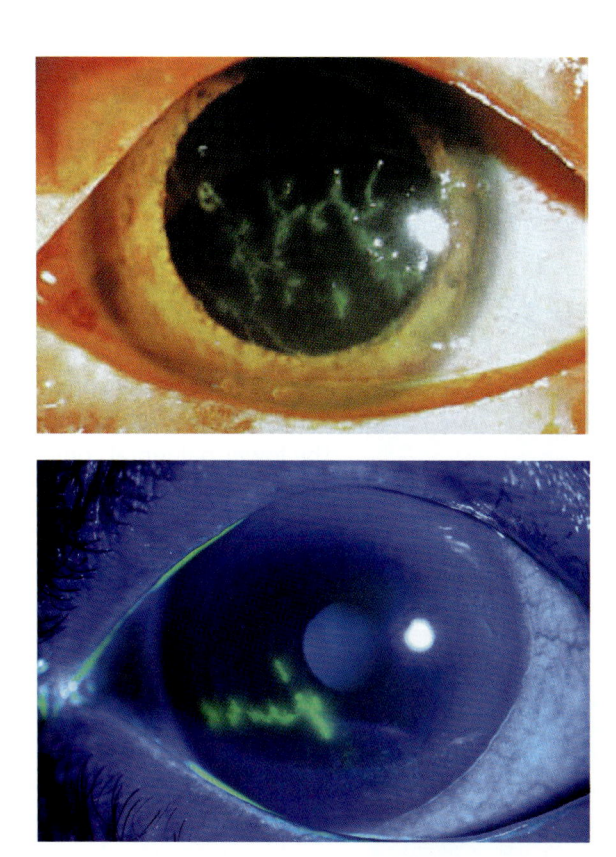

Fig. 3.12. Unilateral red eye with dendritic ulcer caused by the herpes simplex virus. The branching ulcer is best seen under magnification with a fluorescein stain.

Conjunctival Follicles and Papillae

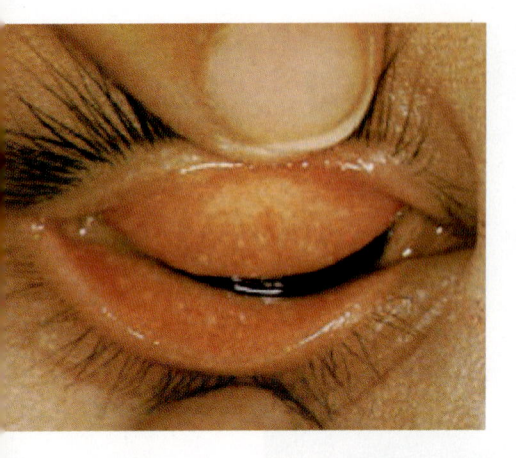

Fig. 3.13. Follicular conjunctivitis resulting from allergy. The follicles are mainly on the lower palpebral conjunctiva.

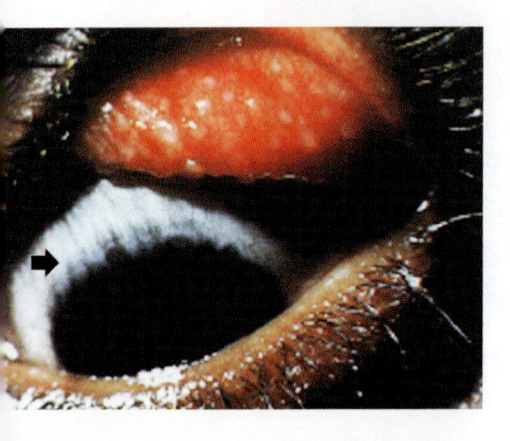

Fig. 3.14. Follicular conjunctivitis in trachoma. The follicles are on the upper palpebral conjunctiva. (Note the diagnostic Herbert's pits at the limbus.)

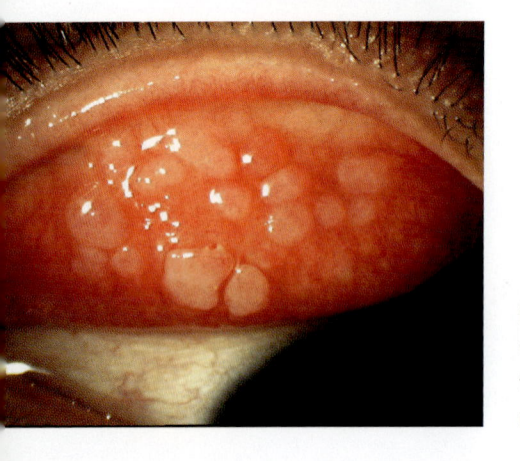

Fig. 3.15. Spring catarrh (vernal conjunctivitis) with large flattened papillary hypertrophy of the upper palpebral conjunctiva, sometimes mistaken for trachomatous follicles.

Raised Conjunctival Lesions

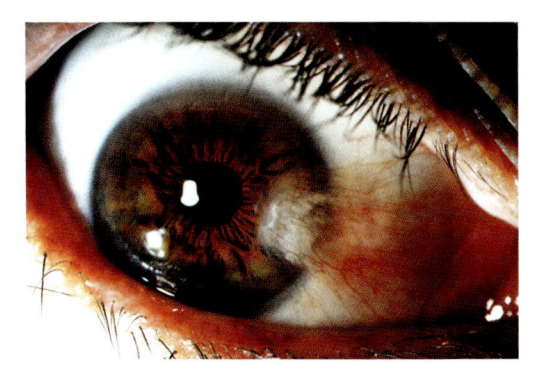

Fig. 3.16. Nasal pterygium encroaching on the cornea.

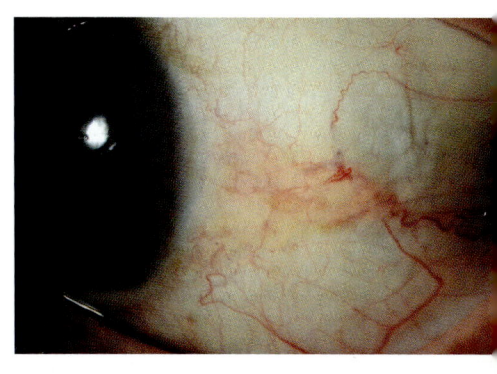

Fig. 3.17. Nasal pinguecula. (Note the cornea is not affected.)

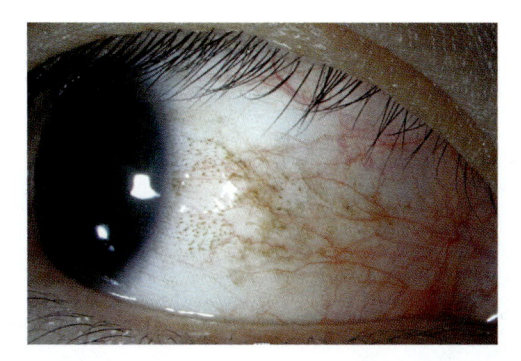

Fig. 3.18. Benign melanosis of the conjunctiva.

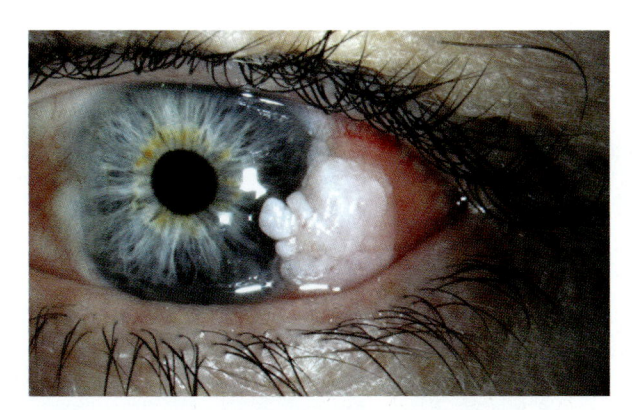

Fig. 3.19. Squamous cell carcinoma of the corneoscleral junction (limbus).

Corneal Ulcers

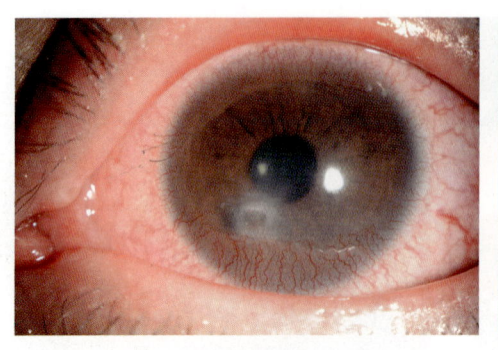

Fig. 3.20. Small corneal ulcer caused by staphylococcal infection with the use of soft contact lenses. (Note the corneal vascularisation.)

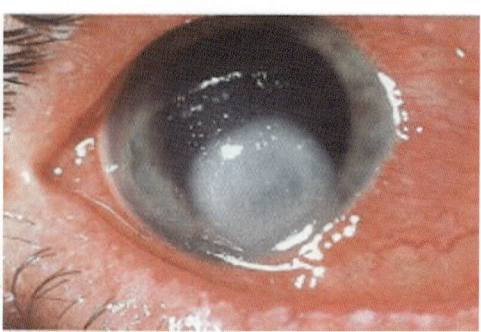

Fig. 3.21. Severe *Pseudomonas pyocyaneus* corneal ulcer.

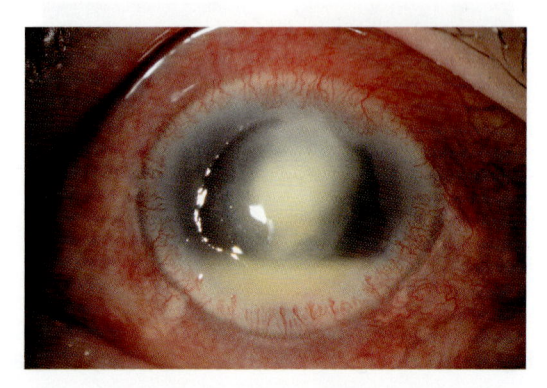

Fig. 3.22. Central pneumococcal corneal ulcer with hypopyon (the fluid level of pus in the anterior chamber).

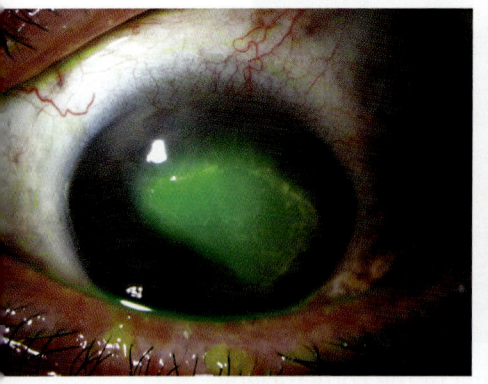

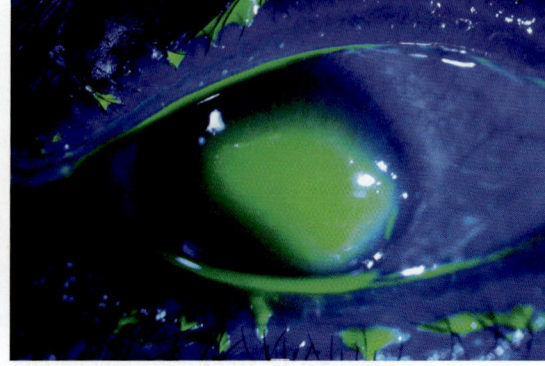

Fig. 3.23. Large bacterial corneal ulcer stained with fluorescein.

Corneal Dystrophies

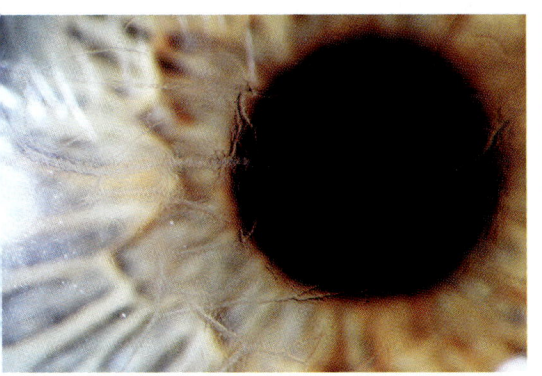

Fig. 3.24. Lattice dystrophy of the cornea.

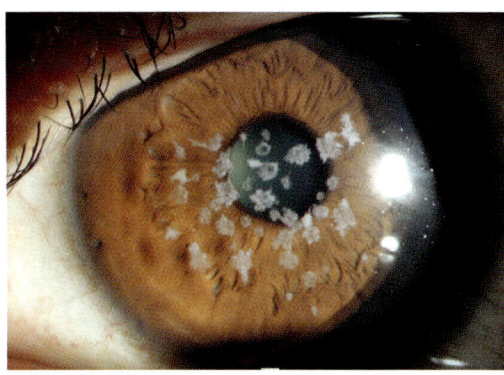

Fig. 3.25. Granular dystrophy of the cornea.

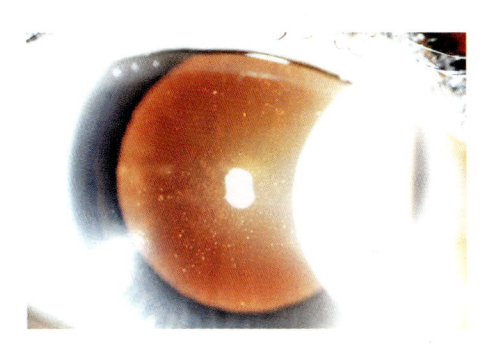

Fig. 3.26. Early Fuchs' corneal dystrophy showing endothelial abnormalities.

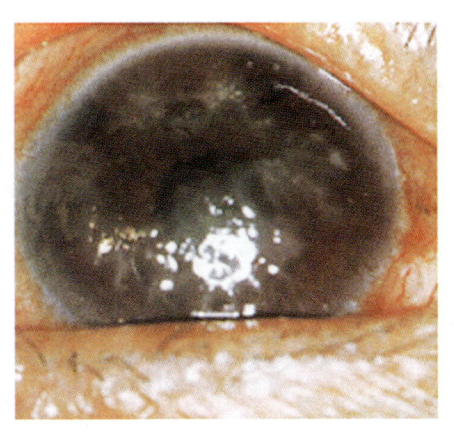

Fig. 3.27. Advanced Fuchs' corneal dystrophy with diffuse corneal oedema.

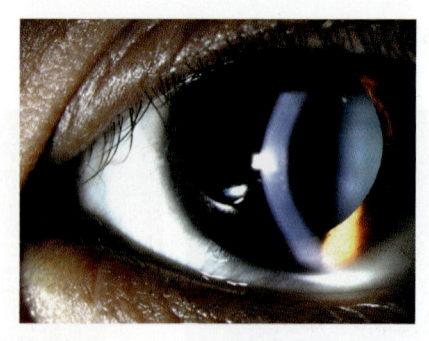

Fig. 3.28. Keratoconus with a conical slit beam shape on the cornea.

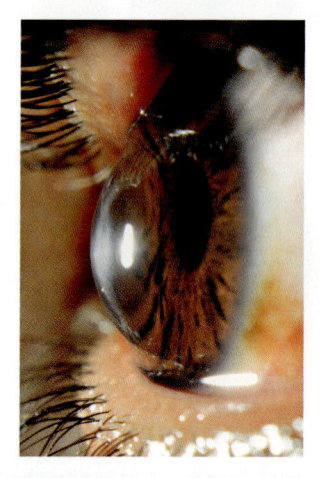

Fig. 3.29. Keratoconus with a conical cornea and opacity at the apex.

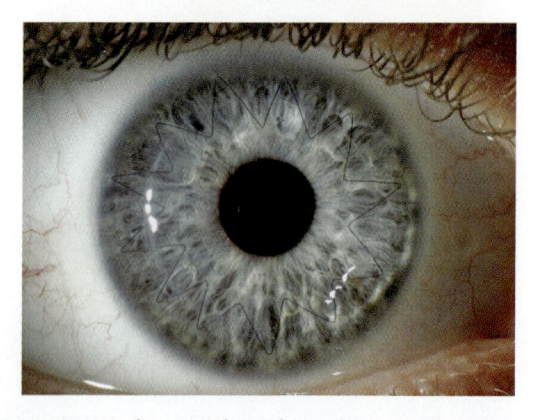

Fig. 3.30. Corneal transplant for advanced keratoconus — post-operative appearance with a running 10-0 nylon suture.

Corneal Opacities

Fig. 3.31. Interstitial keratitis showing stromal thickening, opacity and corneal ghost vessels.

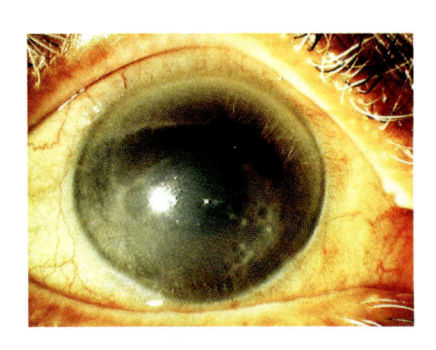

Fig. 3.32. Corneal opacity caused by herpes simplex infection (disciform keratitis).

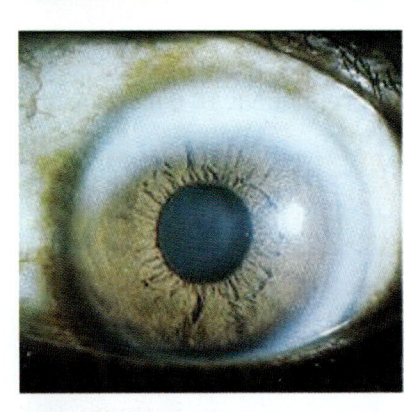

Fig. 3.33. Arcus senilis at the corneal periphery (this never affects vision).

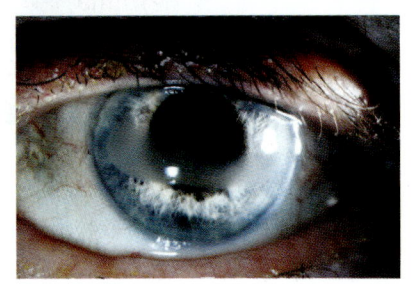

Fig. 3.34. Band keratopathy due to dystrophic calcification.

Corneal Opacity and Corneal Grafting

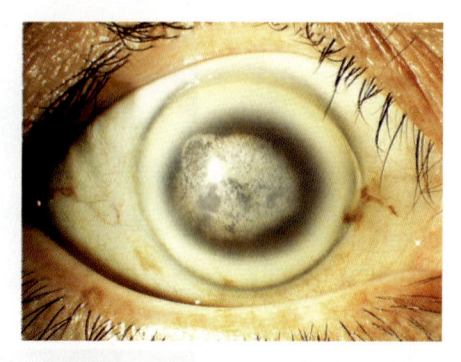

Fig. 3.35. Before surgery, dense corneal opacity causing blindness.

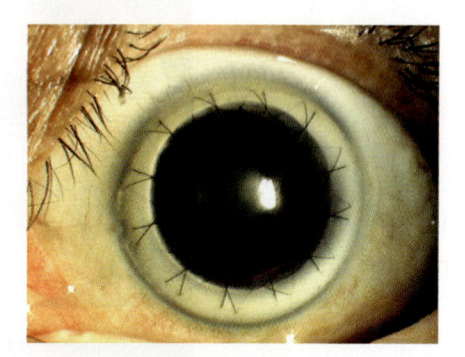

Fig. 3.36. After surgery, clear penetrating corneal graft with two continuous 10-0 monofilament nylon sutures.

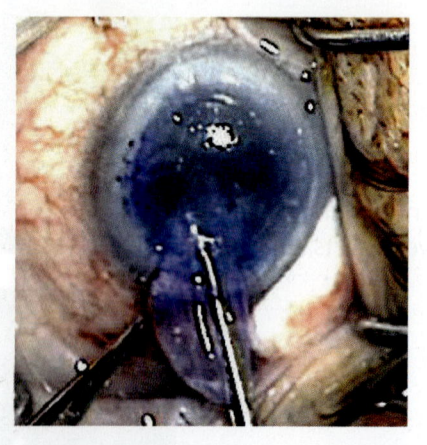

Fig. 3.37. Corneal endothelial layer transplant (DSEK) being inserted after stripping Descemet's membrane in Fuchs' corneal endothelial dystrophy.

4
CATARACT

INTRODUCTION

Clouding of the crystalline natural lens in the eye is called a cataract. Normally, the human lens converges light rays. An opacity in the lens will scatter or block these rays. If the opacity is small and at the lens periphery, there will be little or no interference with vision, but if the opacity is central and dense, visual impairment will occur.

A cataract may be congenital or acquired.

Congenital cataract arises because of infection during pregnancy TORCH (toxoplasmosis, rubella, cytomegalovirus and herpes), genetic transmission (familial, sporadic or Down's syndrome) or metabolic disorders (galactosaemia).

The most common cause of acquired cataract is ageing (senile cataract). However, presenile cataract can occur because of systemic ocular disease or trauma. The systemic diseases which are associated with acquired cataract include atopic dermatitis (eczema), diabetes, myotonic dystrophy and neurofibromatosis type 2. The most common ocular conditions that can lead to early cataract formation are trauma, acute angle closure glaucoma, chronic uveitis, high myopia, corticosteroid therapy and after vitreoretinal surgery.

Cataract can be cortical, nuclear and/or subcapsular. Based on the stage of development, it can be immature, mature (dense or white) or hypermature (liquefied, swollen or partly absorbed).

Cataract is the most common cause of gradual painless visual loss in the elderly. The usual indication for surgery is when the patient's vision has deteriorated to such an extent that it interferes with normal activities such as driving or reading. Mature cataracts can lead to complications such as uveitis and secondary glaucoma. Cataract extraction with an intraocular lens implant is the most commonly performed surgical operation in man, at more than 1 per 100 people per year in developed countries with an ageing population.

SURGERY

The timing of cataract extraction depends on the patient's visual requirements. This is highly subjective. For example, a young person may want earlier cataract removal if it interferes with his or her occupation. On the other hand, an elderly sedentary person may defer cataract surgery because of lower visual requirements. Cataract extraction is also required if the cataract is mature, as it can lead to complications. Age and poor general health are usually not contraindications for surgery, owing to of the use of local anaesthesia and early mobilisation.

Cataract surgery involves extraction of the contents of the cloudy lens and implantation of an artificial intraocular lens (IOL). The surgical removal of cataract can be carried out using three different techniques: large incision extracapsular cataract extraction (ECCE) with IOL implantation, manual small incision cataract surgery (SICS) or phacoemulsification.

In ECCE, a large corneoscleral incision of 8–10 mm is made through which the nucleus and the cortex are removed after creating an opening in the anterior capsule (can-opener capsulorhexis), with the posterior capsule left intact. Cortical remnants are aspirated and an IOL inserted in the capsular bag. The corneoscleral wound is closed using 10-0 nylon sutures.

Manual SICS is a variant of ECCE, wherein a self-sealing scleral tunnel incision is created through which the lens is expressed and an IOL implanted in the bag. The scleral incision does not need any sutures, thus significantly reducing operating time and enabling faster visual rehabilitation.

Phacoemulsification is the modern variation on the extracapsular cataract technique and is now the gold standard. In this operation, after ultrasonic disintegration of the nucleus, the surgeon aspirates the disrupted nuclear fragments and cortex through a small corneal incision (less than 3 mm). A foldable IOL implant is then inserted through this incision. The advantages of phacoemulsification include faster rehabilitation and less postoperative astigmatism. This operation is machine-dependent and is more expensive.

See video at end of chapter.

OPTICAL CORRECTION USING IOL IMPLANTS

There are many different types of IOL implants based on their physical composition, optical/refractive properties and location of implantation. IOLs have dramatically improved the visual rehabilitation in patients undergoing cataract surgery.

Based on their composition, they can be either hydrophobic or hydrophilic and are made of polymethylmethacrylate (PMMA), other soft foldable copolymers or silicone.

Based on the location of implantation, different IOLs are designed for placement in the anterior chamber, fixation on the iris, or placement in the sulcus or the capsular bag (posterior chamber IOL).

Based on their refractive properties, IOLs can be monofocal to correct for distance, toric or cylindric to correct astigmatism or multifocal to allow for both distance and near-vision correction.

The choice of IOL to be implanted in the eye is based on the patient's visual requirements and on the ocular pathology present.

The power of the IOL to be inserted is calculated from measurement of the axial length and corneal curvature of the individual eye.

POSTOPERATIVE RECOVERY

Patients are not required to be confined to bed and most can walk with help, as soon as they recover from the effects of anaesthesia or sedation. Cataract surgery is now usually performed as a day case procedure. Vision improvement occurs within one day. Patients can usually return to all but extreme work environments in three to four days.

Cataract extraction is one of the safest, most cost-effective and satisfying operations for both the patient and the surgeon. Most patients regain their eyesight or experience a considerable improvement in vision and quality of life following successful surgery. Failure to restore normal vision is usually due to a pre-existing disease of the retina or optic nerve.

POSTOPERATIVE COMPLICATIONS

Although cataract surgery is generally simple and effective, a number of intraoperative and postoperative complications can occasionally occur.

The intraoperative complications that can have an adverse effect on the outcome include rupture of the posterior capsule, vitreous loss, escape of lens fragments or the IOL into the vitreous cavity and suprachoroidal haemorrhage, which can cause expulsion of intraocular contents.

The postoperative complications include a refractive surprise, periocular bruising, ptosis, wound leak, corneal oedema, raised intra-ocular pressure, malposition of the IOL implant, cystoid macular oedema, retinal detachment and the most serious and devastating — postoperative endophthalmitis.

DISLOCATED LENS AND TRAUMATIC CATARACT

The natural lens may subluxate or completely dislocate in a number of clinical settings, including Marfan syndrome, or as a complication of ocular trauma. Lens removal is then a more complex procedure, often requiring removal of the lens capsule and vitrectomy. The intraocular lens is then sutured into the sclera behind the iris, captured at the pupil by the iris, or else an anterior chamber IOL may be inserted.

IMPACT OF CATARACT ON SOCIETY WORLDWIDE

Cataract is still the most common cause of avoidable blindness in the developing world. There is an ongoing need for eye surgeons to continue to put together international collaborative plans like Vision 2020 to deal with the problem. Unnecessary global blindness can be prevented with low-cost extracapsular cataract extraction and posterior chamber lens implantation.

Quality cataract surgery is the rule in the hands of experienced surgeons who have been well-trained in the technique of both extra-capsular cataract extraction and phacoemulsification with posterior chamber implantation. With a good operating microscope and modern phacoemulsification machines, excellent visual recovery is achieved in over 95% of patients.

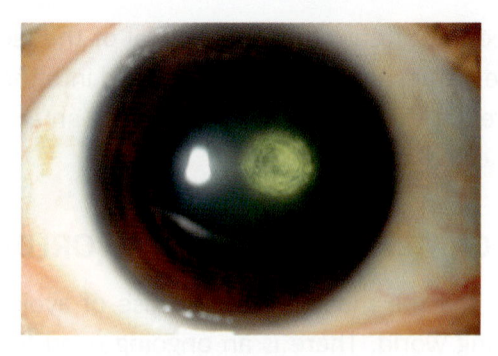

Fig. 4.1. Cataract centred on the visual axis. Vision is worse in bright sunlight or while reading when the pupil constricts.

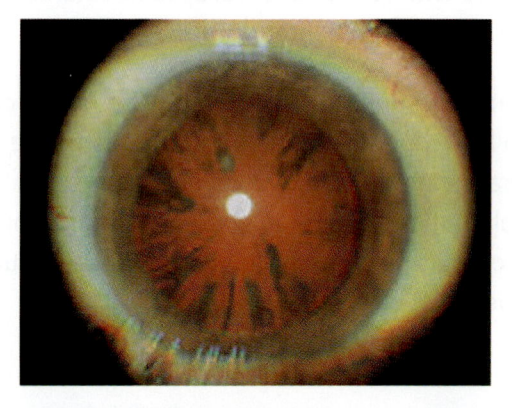

Fig. 4.2. Peripheral cortical cataract. Vision is usually affected later.

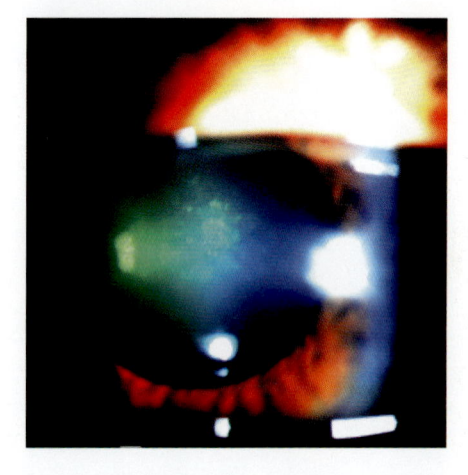

Fig. 4.3. Early posterior subcapsular cataract associated with systemic steroid therapy.

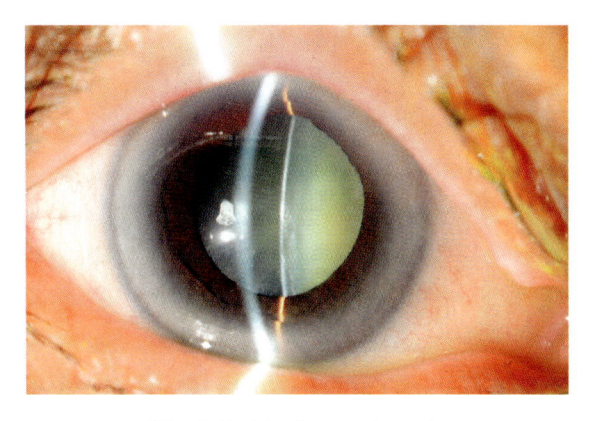

Fig. 4.4. Nuclear cataract.

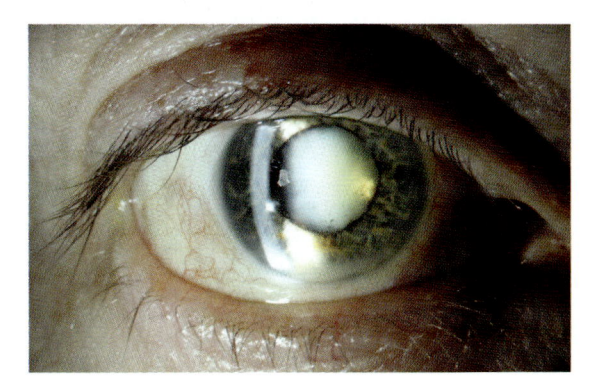

Fig. 4.5. Mature cataract where the entire lens becomes white. Maturity can lead to uveitis or secondary glaucoma.

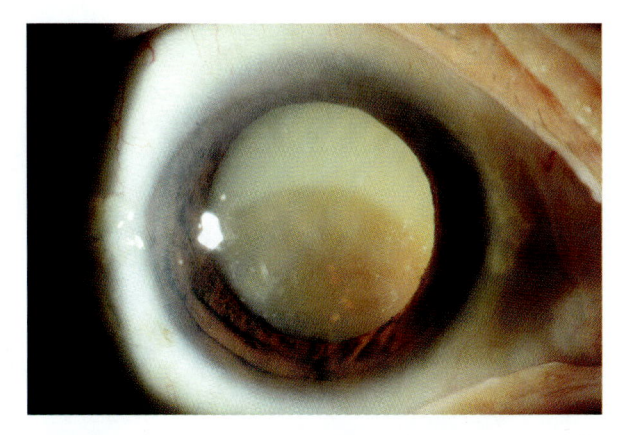

Fig. 4.6. Hypermature cataract with liquefaction of the cortex. (Note the brown nucleus which has sunk downwards.)

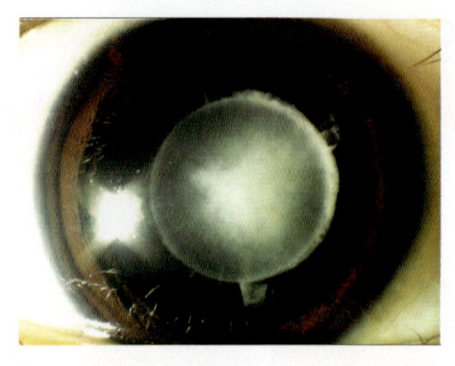

Fig. 4.7. Congenital cataract affecting the nucleus during development.

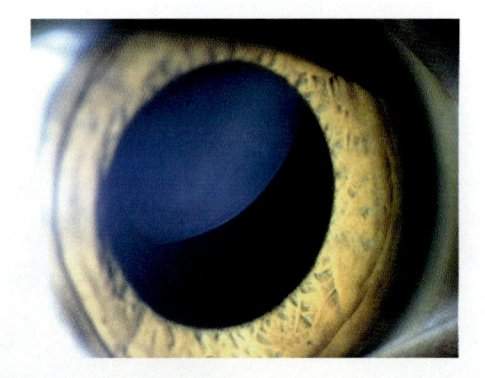

Fig. 4.8. Subluxation superiorly of the lens in Marfan syndrome.

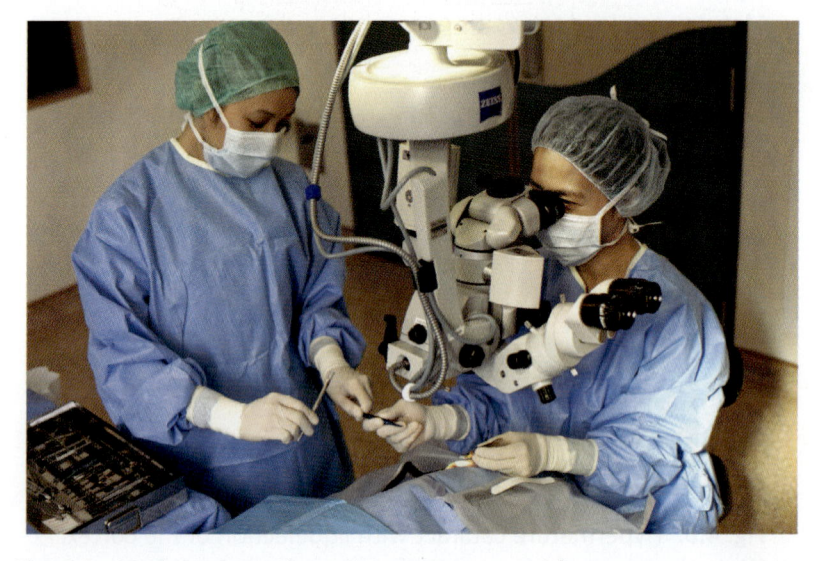

Fig. 4.9. Modern operating microscope — used for most eye surgeries.

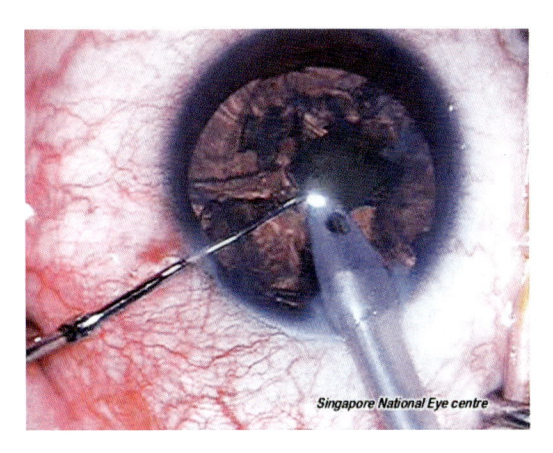

Fig. 4.10. Phacoemulsification of the nuclear fragments of cataract.

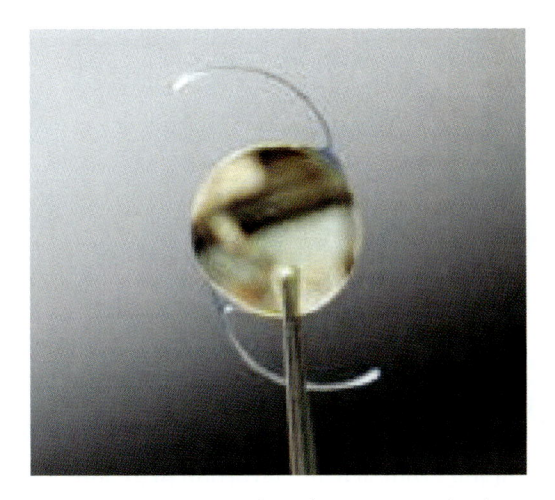

Fig. 4.11. Posterior chamber intraocular lens.

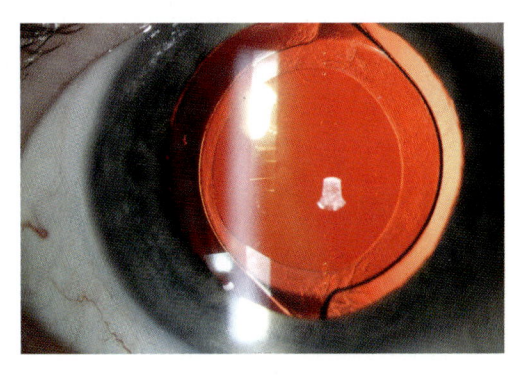

Fig. 4.12. Posterior chamber intraocular lens within the capsular bag.

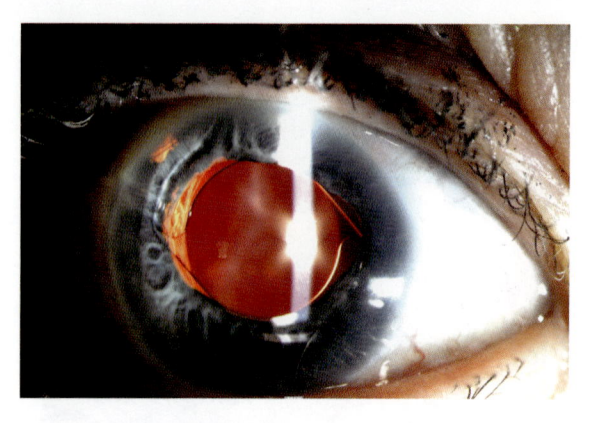

Fig. 4.13. Anterior chamber intraocular lens (used rarely for eyes with no capsular support).

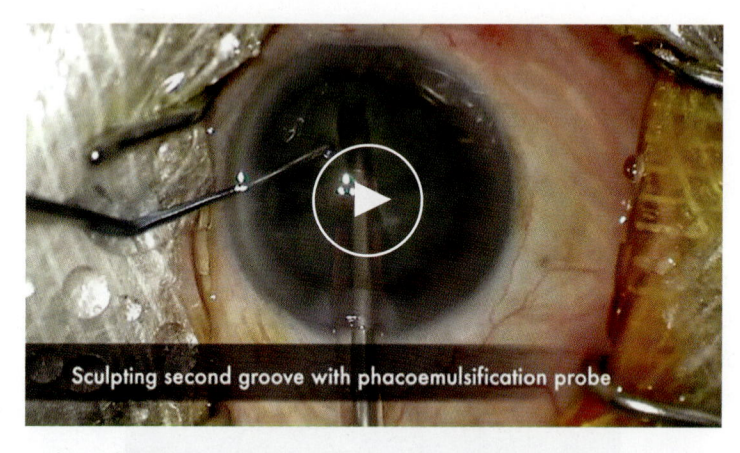

Video of cataract removal and insertion of an intraocular lens.

5
GLAUCOMA

INTRODUCTION

Glaucoma is a common cause of global blindness, affecting an estimated 60 million people worldwide in 2010, with the number rising to 80 million in 2020. It affects 2–4% of the adult population over 40 years of age. Because of this, screening and early diagnosis of glaucoma has become an important responsibility for all medical and allied health practitioners.

In the normal eye, there is a delicate balance between the rate of aqueous production and of aqueous outflow, such that a normal intraocular pressure (IOP) is maintained. IOP is the only known treatable risk factor in glaucoma, which is associated with visual field loss and progressive optic neuropathy.

Glaucoma can be classified as congenital or acquired. Based on the anterior chamber angle, it is further classified into open-angle and closed-angle glaucoma.

Open-angle glaucoma develops insidiously. It leads to slow and progressive damage to the optic nerve because of raised IOP and progresses to visual field loss with few or no symptoms. Open-angle glaucoma has been referred to as the "thief of sight". It is more common among Caucasians and Afro-Caribbeans.

In contrast, acute closed-angle glaucoma, which develops suddenly, is associated with pain, sudden visual loss and congestion of the eye. It frequently presents as a painful unilateral red eye, but can also occur as a chronic disease. It is more common in the Asian population.

Both types of glaucoma can be further subdivided into primary and secondary causes.

PRIMARY OPEN-ANGLE GLAUCOMA

Primary open-angle glaucoma (POAG) is a bilateral condition of adult onset characterised by elevated IOP, open anterior chamber angle, optic nerve damage and visual field loss. Risk factors for POAG include age, race, myopia, family history, diabetes, oestrogen lack and use of contraceptive pills.

Early symptoms are usually not present and this condition is of insidious onset. Once it is established, associated symptoms may include frequent change of glasses, tearing, discomfort and difficulty with light–dark adaptation and reading.

The diagnosis is confirmed by measurement of the IOP, pachymetry to measure the central corneal thickness, gonioscopy, optic disc assessment and visual field analysis. In POAG, the IOP is usually raised above 21 mmHg in one or both eyes. If the IOP is within the normal range despite signs of optic disc damage and presence of visual field defects in the absence of any other pathology, it is referred to as normal tension glaucoma (NTG).

Intraocular Pressure

An IOP of more than 21 mmHg suggests the possibility of glaucoma. It is important to note that many patients with a raised IOP of more than 20 mmHg do not suffer any visual field loss or optic disc cupping. This condition is called ocular hypertension (OHT) and usually requires no treatment but just careful and regular reviews. Occasionally, in high-risk patients (for example with a family history), lowering of the IOP may be indicated to prevent progression to overt glaucoma. Risk factors for developing glaucoma in OHT include high IOP, age, low central corneal thickness and increased optic disc cup–disc ratio.

Central Corneal Thickness

Central corneal thickness (CCT) is an important variable in the accurate measurement of IOP and as a risk factor for glaucoma. A thinner cornea is associated with an artificially low IOP measurement and is a risk factor for glaucoma progression.

Visual Field Loss

Typical visual field changes develop in glaucoma. Early changes include increased variability of responses followed by small paracentral defects, nasal step, arcuate defects, ring scotoma and, in the end stage, loss of all but a central and temporal island of vision.

Optic Disc Changes

In glaucoma, there is usually an increase in size of the optic disc cup (increased cup–disc ratio) in association with the visual field loss. If the cup–disc ratio is greater than 0.7 or if there is asymmetry between the two eyes (such as a cup–disc ratio difference of more than 0.2), the possibility of glaucoma should be excluded. Other signs suggestive of glaucomatous damage to the optic nerve head include notching of the neuroretinal rim, bayoneting or double angulation of blood vessels on the optic nerve head, nasal displacement of blood vessels on the optic nerve head, laminar dot sign and disc haemorrhage. In advanced glaucoma, the cup enlargement reaches the edge of the disc, causing the cup–disc ratio to become almost 1.0, which is then called glaucomatous optic atrophy.

Prevention and Early Diagnosis

Diagnosis is frequently made too late, because of the lack of symptoms in primary open-angle glaucoma. To prevent this, periodic ophthalmic examination and measurement of IOP in all patients over the age of 40 is advisable. Optometrists who see most people for glasses in this age group have a particular role in detection. There is also a familial tendency in this condition. All relatives of patients with primary open-angle glaucoma should be regularly reviewed.

Treatment of POAG

The main goal of treatment is reduction of IOP to slow down the rate of progression of glaucoma. The treatment options for glaucoma can be medical, laser or surgical.

Medical

Medical treatment involves the use of different eye drops to lower the IOP. The drugs act either by inhibiting aqueous production or by promoting greater aqueous outflow.

The first-line medical therapy of choice is the prostaglandin analogues: latanoprost, travoprost, bimatoprost and tafluprost. These promote greater aqueous outflow by increasing uveoscleral outflow. The advantages of these drugs are that they have limited side effects and only need to be used once a day. The drugs promise greater pressure-lowering effects as well as better patient tolerability and compliance. There are preservative-free versions of latanoprost, bimatoprost and tafluprost that can be used for patients with preservative allergies. Common side effects of this group of drugs are hyperaemia, longer eyelashes, darkening of the iris, periorbital pigmentation and fat atrophy.

The second line of treatment involves addition of a beta blocker. Before the advent of prostaglandin analogues, beta blockers were considered the first-line of treatment. The commonly used beta blockers are timolol and betaxolol. These work by reducing production of aqueous humour and are used twice daily. Gel forms allow once-daily treatment. Common side effects include bradycardia, worsening of asthma, lethargy and depression.

Additional topical medications include carbonic anhydrase inhibitors (brinzolamide, dorzolamide) and alpha-2 agonists (brimonidine, apraclonidine). These need to be used twice daily. Carbonic anhydrase inhibitors work by reducing production of aqueous humour, whilst alpha-adrenergic agonists lower IOP by a combination of reduction in production of aqueous humour and increased aqueous outflow.

Common side effects include hyperaemia, burning sensation and allergic blepharoconjunctivitis.

Carbonic anhydrase inhibitors are also available in tablet form — acetazolamide (Diamox®), which is usually used in a dosage of 250 mg QID. Common side effects include hypokalaemia, pins and needles in fingers and toes, nausea, muscle pain, lethargy, renal stones and metabolic acidosis. There is a small, rare risk of Stevens–Johnson syndrome in patients with a sulphur allergy.

Current research also aims to develop drugs which can protect the optic nerve against the effects of high IOP (neuroprotective agents), but none is yet proven.

Laser

If medical therapy proves unsatisfactory, laser trabeculoplasty is often used. This involves laser treatment of the trabecular meshwork in an attempt to increase the aqueous outflow. Laser trabeculoplasty includes selective laser trabeculoplasty (SLT), argon laser trabeculoplasty (ALT) and micropulse laser trabeculoplasty (MLT). SLT is most widely employed nowadays. It involves the use of a double-frequency Q-switched Nd:YAG laser (532 nm) with a pulse duration of 3 nanoseconds to treat the trabecular meshwork, at either 180° or 360°, in a single session. These treatments are usually effective for 3–5 years and may need to be repeated.

Surgical

A. *Trabeculectomy*

When both medical treatment and laser are not effective, a filtering surgery, such as trabeculectomy, is performed. This creates a drainage channel which shunts the aqueous from the anterior chamber of the eye to the sub-Tenon's space, where it is absorbed by the episcleral vessels. The success of the surgery depends on the ability to limit scarring of this drainage channel and keep it patent. This is aided by the application of the antimetabolites 5-fluorouracil or mitomycin C directly to the subconjunctival tissue.

Trabeculectomy has a significant complication and failure rate. The complications include failure of filtration because of episcleral scarring, overfiltration causing hypotony, filtering bleb-related infection (blebitis), suprachoroidal haemorrhage and malignant glaucoma. The success rate is around 80% and it is still considered the gold standard.

B. *Microincisional glaucoma surgery*

Owing to the complications and unpredictable failure rate of trabeculectomy, various minimally invasive surgical interventions have been developed. They are collectively known as microincisional glaucoma surgery (MIGS). These procedures are ideally suited for patients with mild-to-moderate glaucoma as they have a better safety profile, with fewer complications. There are many trials under way to determine their long-term efficacy.

The MIGS techniques are as follows.

1. Increasing trabecular meshwork outflow.
    a. *I-stent*. This involves placement of a titanium stent in the trabecular meshwork. It can be combined with cataract surgery.
    b. *Trabectome*. This technique is an *ab interno* approach of trabeculotomy wherein a small strip of trabecular meshwork and the inner wall of Schlemm's canal are stripped by an electrocautery probe to increase the drainage of aqueous humour.
    c. *Hydrus microstent*. This titanium microstent acts like a scaffold and is inserted into the Schlemm's canal to maintain patency and improve the outflow of aqueous. It can be combined with cataract surgery. It has recently been withdrawn due to late corneal endothelial cell loss.
2. Suprachoroidal shunts.
    a. *CyPass microstent*. This is a polyamide device implanted in the suprachoroidal space, which creates a controlled cyclodialysis with flow of aqueous to the suprachoroidal space.

3. Subconjunctival stents.
   a. *XEN gel stent*. This gel implant creates an outflow channel from the anterior chamber to the subconjunctival space. It may need to be combined with antimetabolities to prevent scarring in the subconjunctival space.
   b. *ExPRESS minishunt*. A 3 mm stainless steel implant shunts fluid from the anterior chamber to the subconjunctival space under a scleral flap which is fashioned, very similar to a trabeculectomy.

C. *Glaucoma drainage devices*

When conventional filtering surgery fails or the angle and subconjunctival tissues are heavily scarred, tube or shunt surgery is carried out. The drainage tube links the anterior chamber to the sub-Tenon's space and connects to a footplate which forms a reservoir further back in the orbit.

The commonly used shunts are Molteno, Baerveldt and Ahmed. Complications include hypotony secondary to excessive drainage, malposition causing cataract because of lens touch or corneal decompensation because of corneal touch, tube erosion through the sclera and conjunctiva, and late failure to control IOP.

PRIMARY CLOSED-ANGLE GLAUCOMA

Primary closed-angle glaucoma (PCAG) is usually acute. It is common among middle-aged patients, particularly women in Oriental populations. Any middle-aged patient with a unilateral red eye and mid-dilated pupil associated with blurred vision, pain or headache should be suspected of having acute closed-angle glaucoma. This occurs because of relative pupil block, wherein there is failure of the flow of aqueous from the posterior chamber to the anterior chamber, causing the iris to bow forward, occluding the anterior chamber angle. In the Oriental population, the angle closure is thought to result from a thicker peripheral iris or plateau iris configuration, which more readily occludes the anterior chamber angle. These anatomical variations prevent aqueous from flowing into the outflow channel, leading to a sudden rise in IOP.

The patient is frequently in pain, the eye is congested and the cornea is hazy due to epithelial oedema. This is the initial cause of the blurred vision. The pupil is semi-dilated and not reactive to light. The anterior chamber is shallow, although the view is hazy. The fellow eye also shows a shallow anterior chamber with occludable angles. IOP is usually in the range of 40–60 mmHg. This can be appreciated by comparing the two eyes by finger palpation. The optic disc does not show significant cupping but is usually hyperaemic. Sustained increased pressure will cause permanent damage to the eye, resulting in severe visual loss or blindness.

Treatment is urgent. The patient should be referred to an ophthalmologist immediately.

Medical Therapy

Immediate intensive medical therapy to lower the IOP is important. Acetazolamide 500 mg should be administered intravenously along with oral acetazolamide 500 mg. Topical treatment includes topical apraclonidine and timolol, topical steroids (prednisolone or dexamethasone) and pilocarpine. Pilocarpine (1–4%) should be instilled every 10 min for the first hour, then less frequently. However, pilocarpine may not be effective alone in lowering the IOP above 40 mmHg because of pupillary sphincter ischaemia. Osmotic agents such as glycerol or intravenous mannitol may be used if the IOP fails to settle on initial treatment. An analgesic or tranquilliser should be given where appropriate. Treatment must be continued until the pressure is reduced.

Laser

Peripheral laser iridotomy done with either the argon or neodymium YAG laser is the treatment of choice for acute PCAG. It is simple and safe. Laser iridotomy should be performed in the affected eye as soon as the cornea is clear enough to permit a clear view.

Surgery

Surgical peripheral iridectomy is done when laser is not possible or available. Alternatively, early lens extraction may be considered, which would allow the iris to fall backwards after lens removal, thus widening the anterior chamber angle. A filtrating operation (trabeculectomy) may occasionally be necessary, especially for patients who have failed to respond to medical and laser therapy.

The Fellow Eye

PCAG is a bilateral disease. The fellow eye is at risk of developing an acute attack in 50% of cases over five years. A prophylactic peripheral laser iridotomy should be performed on it.

Chronic Primary Closed-Angle Glaucoma

When the filtration angle is less rapidly closed, the rise in pressure will be insidious (chronic PCAG). Accordingly, the symptoms will be milder. The patient may complain of transient blurred vision, mild headache and seeing "halos" (rainbow colours around lights). The optic disc shows increased cupping. Chronic PCAG may even simulate chronic POAG and have no symptoms until there is severe visual field loss at an advanced stage of the condition. Diagnosis of chronic PCAG is made by gonioscopy, which shows creeping angle closure and/or peripheral anterior synechiae.

SECONDARY GLAUCOMA

Secondary glaucoma may present with either an open or a closed angle.

Open Angle

Secondary open-angle glaucoma results from obstruction of the trabecular meshwork by an ocular disease process:

a. Membrane (neovascular glaucoma, iridocorneal endothelial syndrome)
b. Iris pigment (pigmentary glaucoma)
c. Pseudoexfoliative material from the lens capsule (pseudo-exfoliative glaucoma)
d. Inflammatory cells and proteins (uveitic glaucoma)
e. Red cell glaucoma from a hyphaema
f. Degenerated RBCs (ghost cell glaucoma from old vitreous haemorrhage)
g. Lens proteins (phacolytic glaucoma)
h. Raised episceral venous pressure (carotid cavernous fistula, Sturge–Weber Syndrome)

The most common secondary glaucomas are pigmentary glaucoma, pseudoexfoliative glaucoma and neovascular glaucoma.

Closed Angle

Secondary pupil block may result from:

a. Phacomorphic glaucoma (mature cataract)
b. 360° posterior synechiae secondary to uveitis
c. Subluxed lens
d. Aphakic pupillary block by the vitreous

Secondary angle closure without pupil block may occur in:

a. Ciliochoroidal effusion
b. Extensive peripheral anterior synechiae
c. Malignant glaucoma (aqueous misdirection)
d. Ciliary body tumours

Treatment of secondary glaucoma is first aimed at controlling the IOP with drops and acetazolamide. Further treatment varies widely and aims to deal with the cause.

Visual Field Loss in Open-Angle Glaucoma

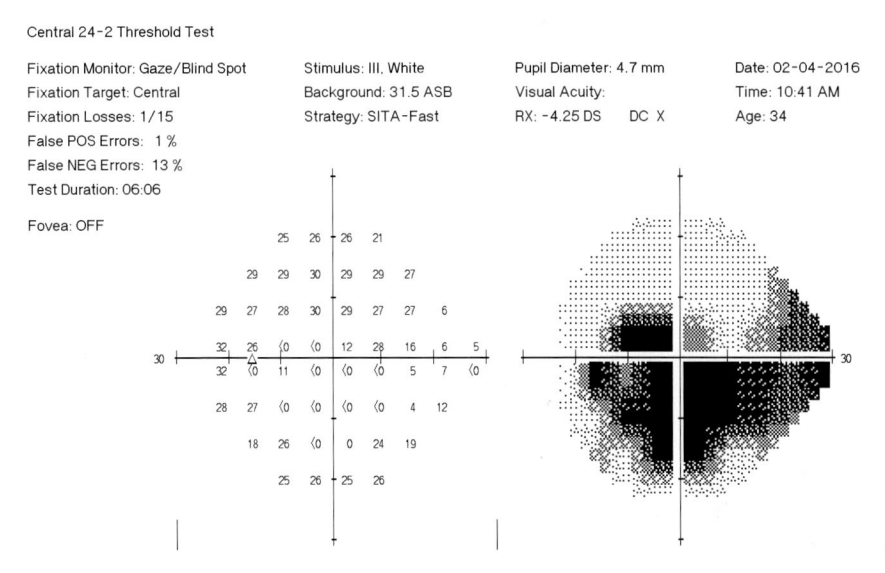

Central 24-2 Threshold Test

Fixation Monitor: Gaze/Blind Spot
Fixation Target: Central
Fixation Losses: 1/15
False POS Errors: 1 %
False NEG Errors: 13 %
Test Duration: 06:06

Fovea: OFF

Stimulus: III, White
Background: 31.5 ASB
Strategy: SITA-Fast

Pupil Diameter: 4.7 mm
Visual Acuity:
RX: -4.25 DS   DC X

Date: 02-04-2016
Time: 10:41 AM
Age: 34

Fig. 5.1. Arcuate scotoma in glaucoma.

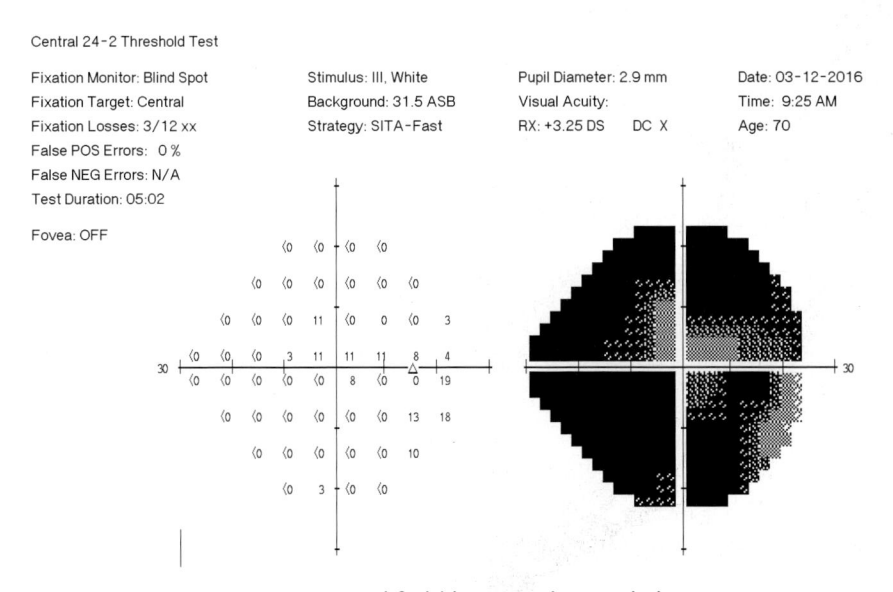

Central 24-2 Threshold Test

Fixation Monitor: Blind Spot
Fixation Target: Central
Fixation Losses: 3/12 xx
False POS Errors: 0 %
False NEG Errors: N/A
Test Duration: 05:02

Fovea: OFF

Stimulus: III, White
Background: 31.5 ASB
Strategy: SITA-Fast

Pupil Diameter: 2.9 mm
Visual Acuity:
RX: +3.25 DS   DC X

Date: 03-12-2016
Time: 9:25 AM
Age: 70

Fig. 5.2. Severe visual field loss in advanced glaucoma.

Optic Disc Cup (Open-Angle Glaucoma)

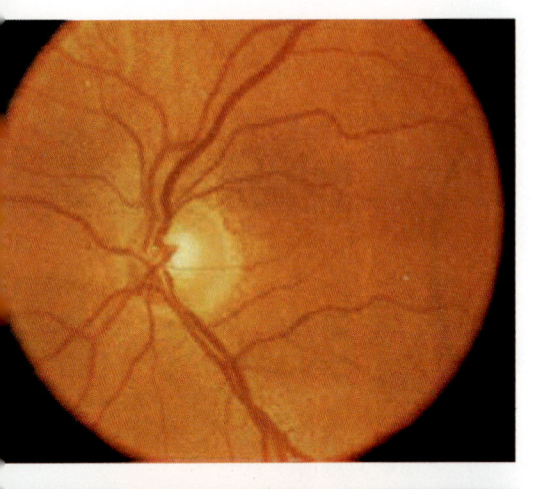

Fig. 5.3. Normal optic disc with cup–disc ratio 0.2.

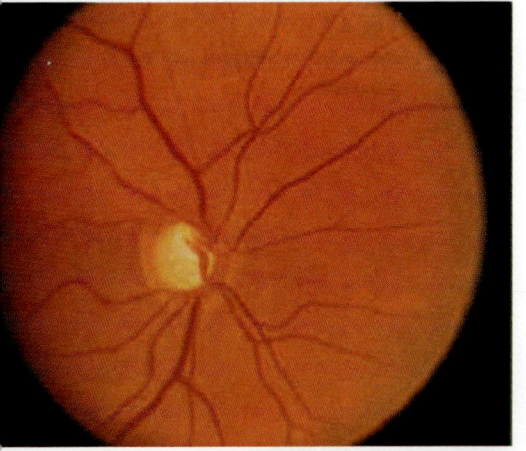

Fig. 5.4. Glaucomatous cup with cup–disc ratio 0.7 and early visual field defect.

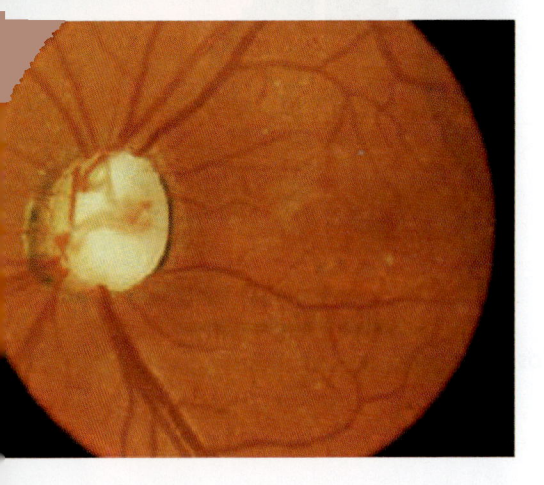

Fig. 5.5. Large advanced glaucomatous cup with cup–disc ratio 1.0 and optic atrophy. (Note the eye is blind.)

Closed-Angle Glaucoma

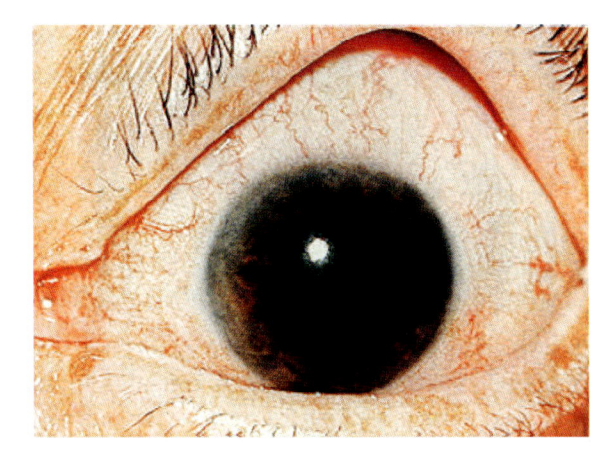

Fig. 5.6. Acute glaucoma presenting as a red eye with a fixed dilated pupil and corneal haze.

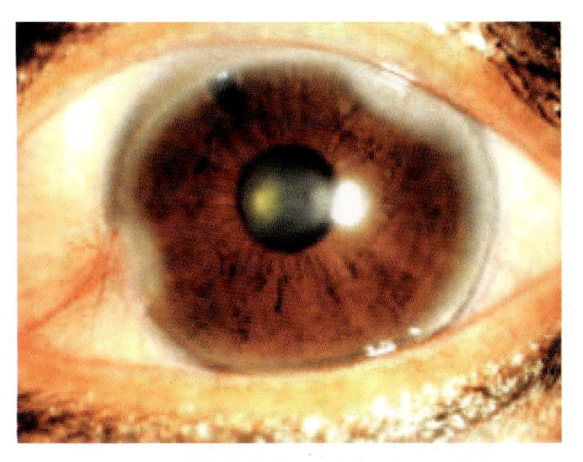

Fig. 5.7. Laser iridotomy seen at 11 o'clock reverses acute closed-angle glaucoma.

Secondary Glaucoma

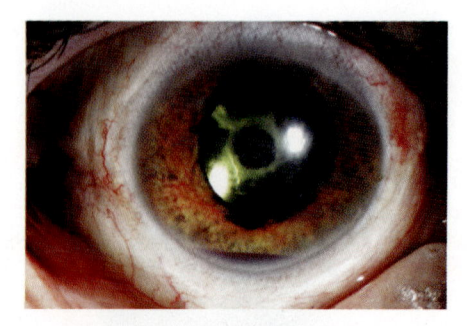

Fig. 5.8. Rubeosis iridis causing neovascular glaucoma. This can follow proliferative diabetic retinopathy or central retinal vein occlusion with retinal ischaemia. (Note the branching iris new vessels and also hyphaema.)

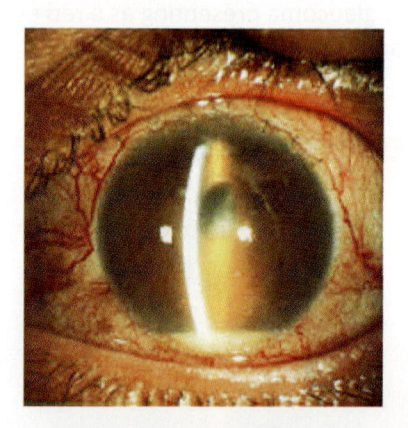

Fig. 5.9. Secondary glaucoma due to severe iridocyclitis. (Note the sterile hypopyon.)

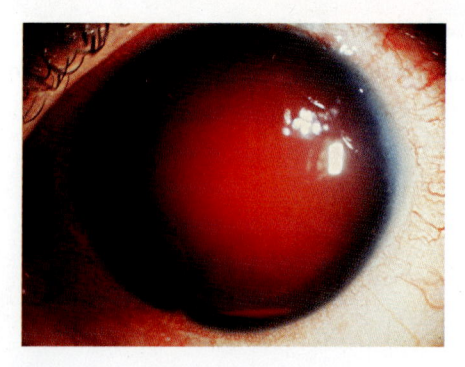

Fig. 5.10. Secondary glaucoma due to blunt trauma causing total hyphaema.

Operations

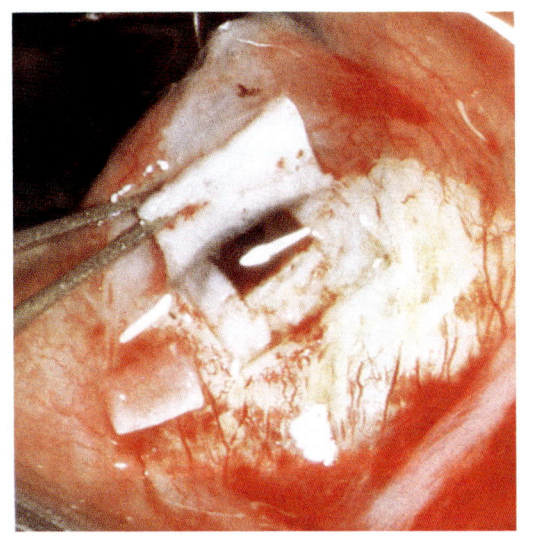

Fig. 5.11. Trabeculectomy, a commonly done filtrating operation for glaucoma.

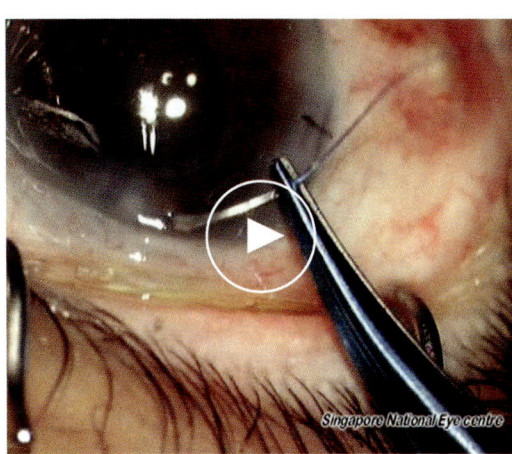

Video of trabeculectomy.

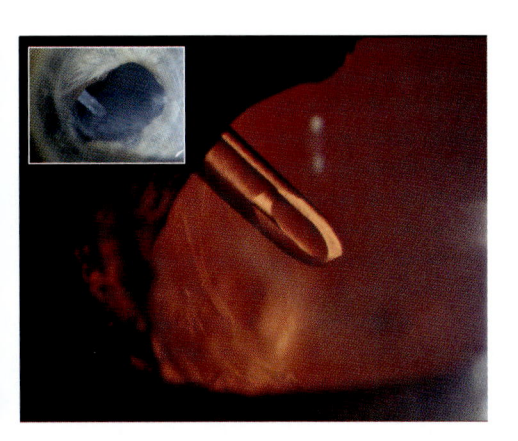

Fig. 5.12. Filtration Malteno tube inserted in a glaucomatous eye with an obliterated corneoscleral angle and subconjunctival scarring. Aqueous drains to a reservoir formed around a silicone implant on the scleral surface.

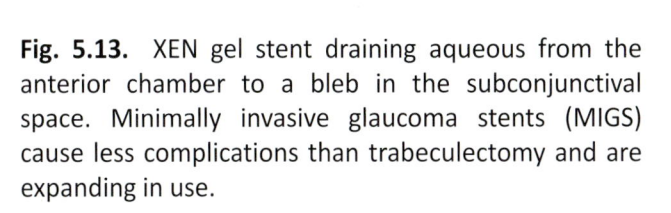

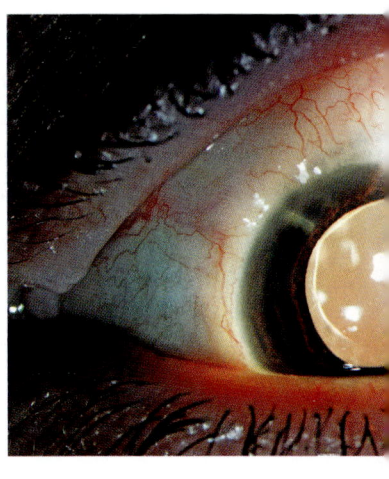

Fig. 5.13. XEN gel stent draining aqueous from the anterior chamber to a bleb in the subconjunctival space. Minimally invasive glaucoma stents (MIGS) cause less complications than trabeculectomy and are expanding in use.

6

UVEITIS: IRIS, CILIARY BODY AND CHOROID

UVEITIS AND DISEASES OF THE UVEAL TRACT

Inflammation of the uvea (uveitis or iritis) is an *important* cause of unilateral red eye and is sometimes related to systemic disease.

UVEITIS

Iridocyclitis (Iritis)

Iridocyclitis or iritis, inflammation of the iris and ciliary body, usually presents as a painful unilateral red eye. It must be differentiated from other common causes of a unilateral red eye, including acute closed-angle glaucoma, foreign body injury, keratitis and corneal ulcer.

The symptoms include photophobia, mild pain, blurred vision and watering. The pupil is small and slit-lamp examination shows flare (proteins) and cells in the anterior chamber, as well as deposits of white cells (keratic precipitates) on the posterior surface of the cornea. The inflamed iris may adhere to the anterior capsule of the lens (posterior synechia) or to the cornea at the filtration angle (peripheral anterior synechia). When the iridocyclitis is severe, secondary glaucoma and secondary cataract may result. Iridocyclitis tends to recur.

The cause is usually difficult to determine. Recurrent and severe iritis may be associated with joint diseases such as ankylosing spondylitis or Still's disease (juvenile rheumatoid arthritis), but rarely with sarcoidosis, syphilis, leprosy, tuberculosis or viral infection. There is a strong association with the HLA-B27 gene.

Cycloplegics such as atropine or homatropine are used to dilate the pupil and prevent posterior synechiae. They also relieve the pain. Steroid eye drops are critical for management, as they reduce the inflammation. Investigations should be carried out to exclude the known causes, especially in severe, bilateral or recurrent iridocyclitis.

Chorioretinitis

Inflammation of the choroid and retina, namely chorioretinitis, usually presents with painless visual blur. In the acute stage, if the inflammation is at the macula, the patient will present with visual loss. Lesions which are not at the macula may be silent and are found only when routine examination shows a chorioretinal scar. In pars planitis (chorioretinitis at the extreme fundal periphery), the condition may remain silent for many months or years and it manifests itself only when the vision is affected by vitreous opacities or macular oedema.

In the majority of cases, the cause is unknown. In some cases, the condition may be due to toxoplasmosis. Less commonly, it is associated with syphilis, tuberculosis, sarcoidosis, *Toxocara* worm infestation, histoplasmosis and AIDS.

Investigations to find the cause should be carried out. Treatment can be difficult. The use of systemic steroids may help, in addition to therapy for specific infections. Recurrences are common. In recalcitrant chorioretinitis cases, patients may need intravitreal injections of steroids (e.g. triamcinolone) and systemic immunosuppressive drugs (e.g. methotrexate, cyclosporine, cyclophosphamide, azathioprine). As the latter drugs have serious side effects, joint management of the patient with a physician or an immunologist is important.

AIDS

In HIV retinopathy, cotton wool spots in the fundi are the most common ocular lesions. They are ischaemic lesions, possibly caused by vasculitis and may be associated with flame-shaped haemorrhages. More severe vasculitis can lead to necrosis and haemorrhagic retinitis. Other ocular features of AIDS include neoplasms in the eyelid, conjunctiva or orbit such as Kaposi sarcoma, neuro-ophthalmic lesions and associated opportunistic infections.

Opportunistic Chorioretinitis

Opportunistic infectious organisms may be dormant until the patient is severely immunosuppressed with therapy or neoplastic diseases and then cause chorioretinitis or even retinal necrosis. The most common ocular opportunistic infection is cytomegalovirus (CMV) retinitis. This produces a characteristic picture of white retinal lesions associated with haemorrhage resembling "crumbled cheese and ketchup". Treatment includes the use of systemic or intravitreal antiviral agents, ganciclovir or foscarnet. Other opportunistic pathogens include *Toxoplasma gondii*, herpes simplex and zoster, *Candida albicans* and *Pneumocystis carinii*.

Tumours of the Uveal Tract

Benign naevus of the iris or choroid

A naevus is a flat, round, pigmented lesion of the iris or choroid. It rarely causes any visual disturbance and can be observed.

Iris melanoma

A malignant iris lesion is raised and vascularised. It is rare and unlikely to ever metastasise. Usually, it is easy to distinguish between a flat benign choroidal naevus and a raised iris melanoma. Treatment is considered if growth is observed. Radiation plaque therapy is preferable to radical surgical excision.

Malignant melanoma of the choroid and ciliary body

A pigmented lesion of the choroid, if thickened by more than 3 mm, is usually a malignant choroidal melanoma. It sometimes presents with retinal detachment, and occasionally with vitreous inflammation, haemorrhage or secondary glaucoma. Because of this, malignant melanoma should be excluded in unilateral blind eyes of uncertain aetiology. Over 90% of melanomas occur in Caucasians and the condition is rare in other races.

Diagnosis is usually made on clinical examination aided by B-scan ultrasound, colour imaging and fluorescein angiography. Choroidal and ciliary body melanomas have a serious risk overall of up to 50% for metastasis mainly to the liver and lungs. Prognosis depends on size, cell type and site. A ciliary body melanoma tends to be asymptomatic and hidden behind the iris until it is large.

The risk of metastatic spread may be investigated by fine needle biopsy, and this allows multigene array analysis for prognosis. Melanoma tissue with epithelioid cells or an absence (monosomy) of chromosome 3 has a higher risk of systemic spread. Detection of metastatic spread involves a chest X-ray, liver ultrasonography and a PET scan.

Enucleation of the eye is usually required for larger tumours. In selected patients with only one good eye left, or those with smaller tumours, scleral surface plaque or proton beam irradiation, photocoagulation or (rarely) local surgical excision may be performed. Small choroidal melanomas may be kept under observation without treatment, provided that they are regularly evaluated with B-scan ultrasonography and fundus photography for enlargement.

Choroidal metastastic tumours

Choroidal metastasis may result from a wide variety of cancers, including breast and lung cancer. It is not common and tends to occur in the clinical setting of advanced metastatic disease. It usually presents in the eye as flat multiple deposits at the posterior pole associated with an exudative retinal detachment. Treatment with radiotherapy may help to retain vision for the limited lifespan of the patient.

Uveitis

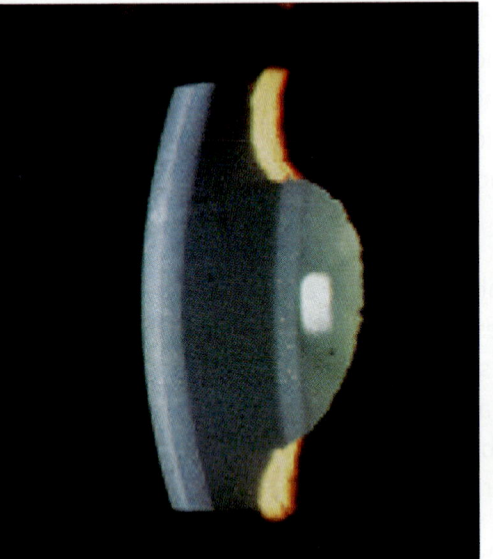

Fig. 6.1. Iridocyclitis presenting with flare in the anterior chamber.

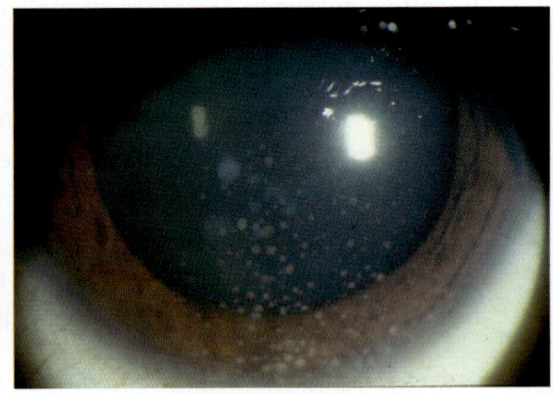

Fig. 6.2. Cellular deposits on corneal endothelium (keratic precipitates).

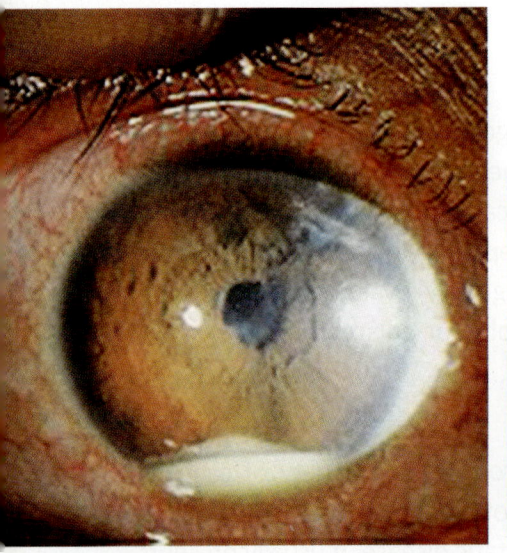

Fig. 6.3. Severe iritis associated with a sterile hypopyon.

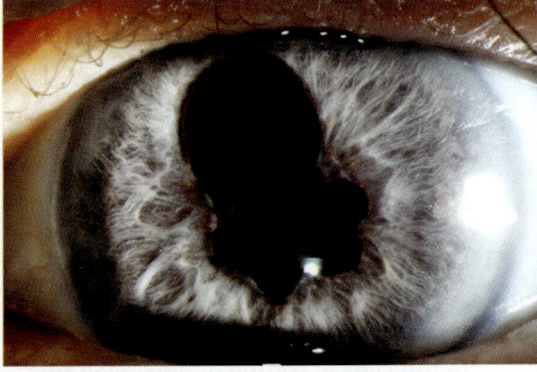

Fig. 6.4. Iridocyclitis with posterior synechiae.

Chorioretinitis

Fig. 6.5. Reactivated toxoplasmic chorioretinitis.

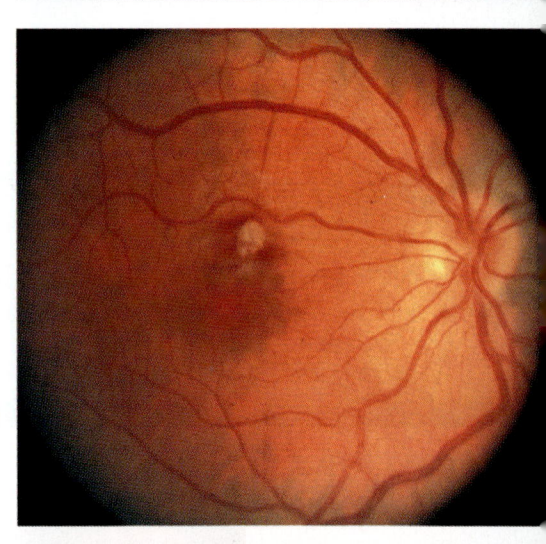

Fig. 6.6. Focal haemorrhagic lesion due to dengue fever vasculitis. Mosquito-borne dengue is a serious endemic disease in parts of Asia and Africa.

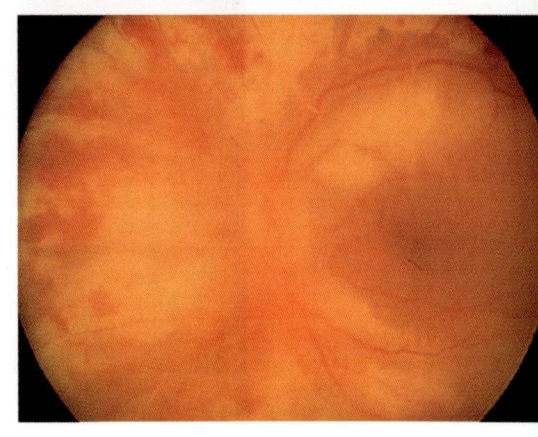

Fig. 6.7. Cytomegalovirus chorioretinitis in an immunocompromised patient with systemic lymphoma.

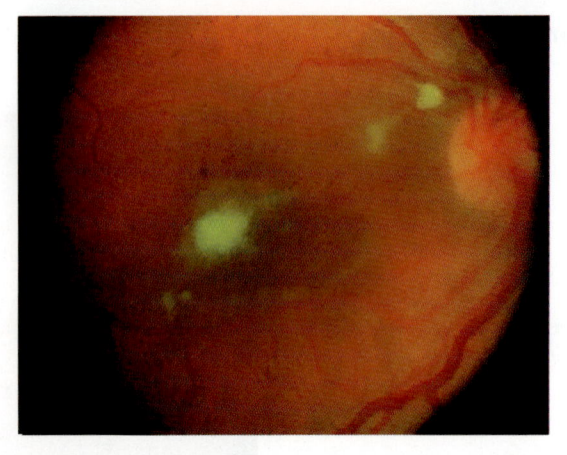

Fig. 6.8. Fungal chorioretinitis due to a contaminated needle in an intravenous drug user.

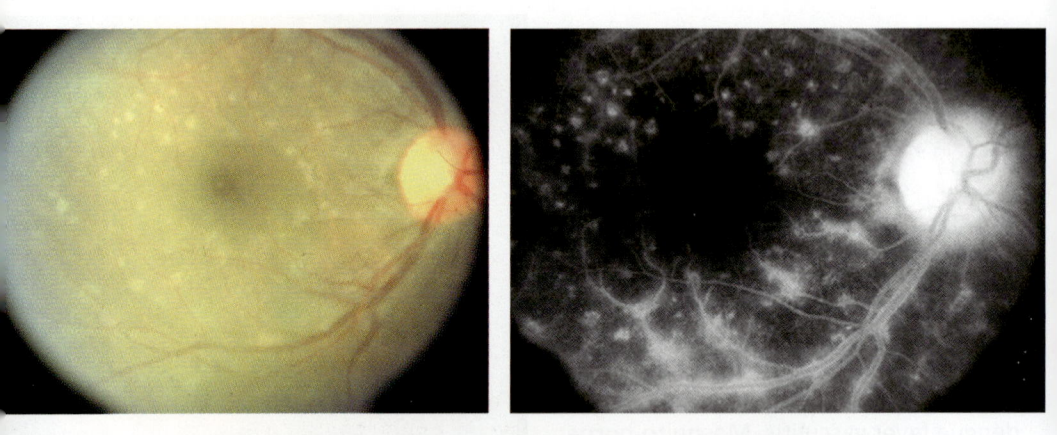

Fig. 6.9. Acute multifocal chorioretinitis due to stage 2 syphilis.

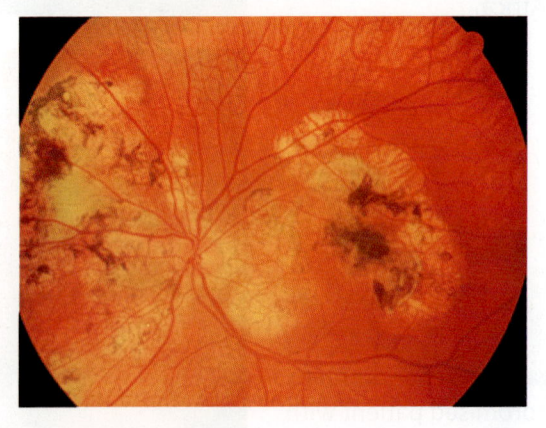

Fig. 6.10. Possible tuberculous chorioretinitis.

Many inflammatory ocular conditions, including uveitis and scleritis, are associated with focal tuberculous infection. However, it is unlikely that tuberculosis is a significant causative agent in most cases of chorioretinal scarring.

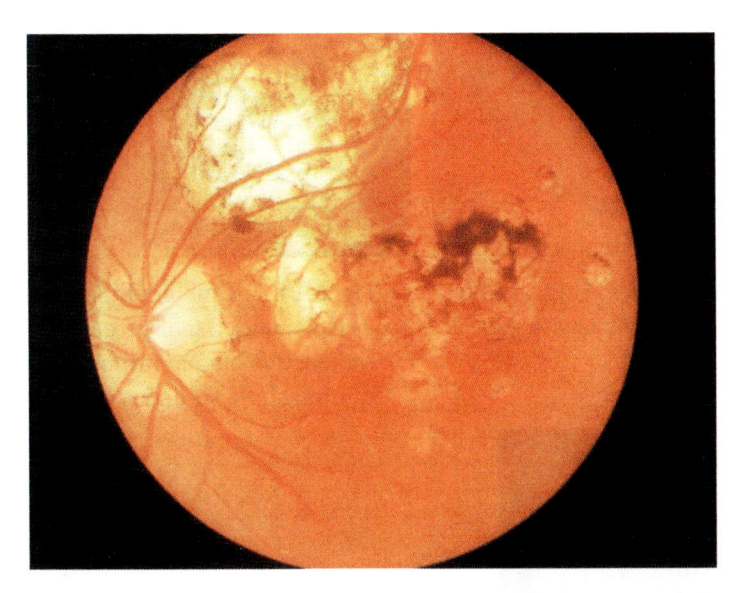

Fig. 6.11. Pigmented chorioretinal scars following chorioretinitis of unknown cause.

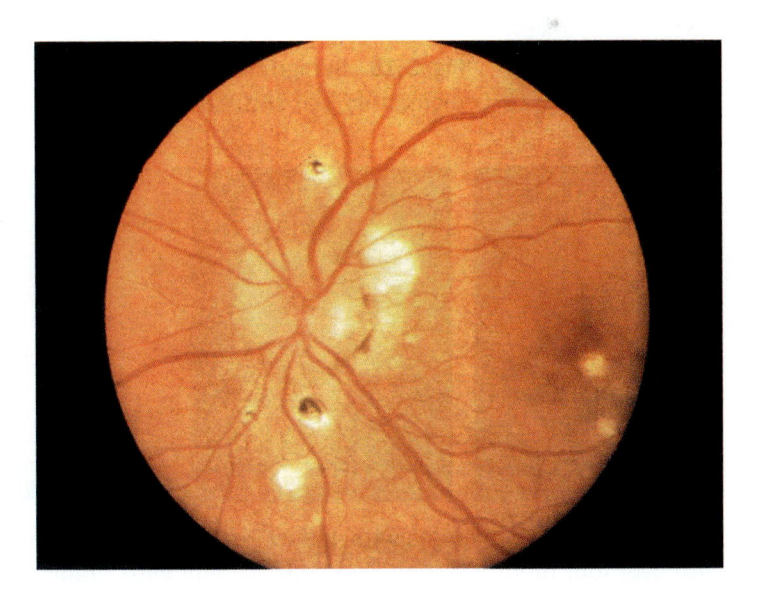

Fig. 6.12. Small, round chorioretinal scars from presumed histoplasmosis.

Pigmented Lesions of the Iris, Ciliary Body and Choroid

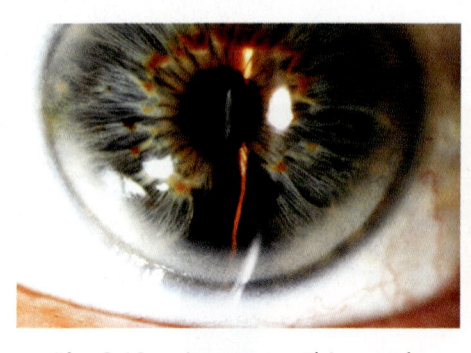

Fig. 6.13. Iris naevus. This may be followed without any treatment over many years.

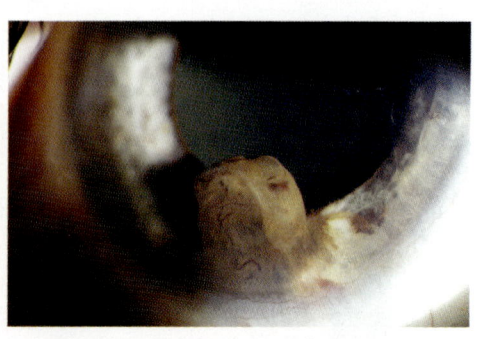

Fig. 6.14. Iris melanoma. Raised and vascularised. Usually treated with a surface radioactive plaque rather than excision. Risk of metastatic spread is very low.

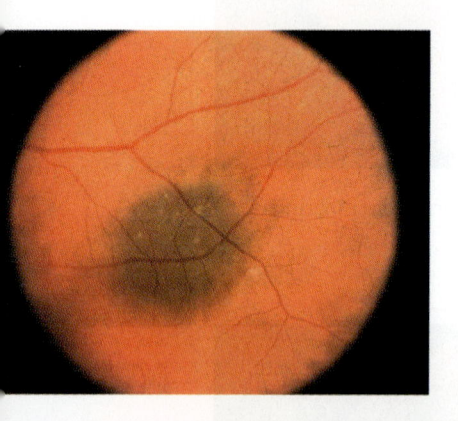

Fig. 6.15. Benign choroidal naevus — pigmented, flat and stationary.

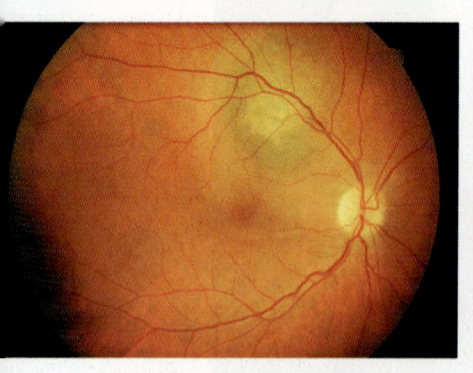

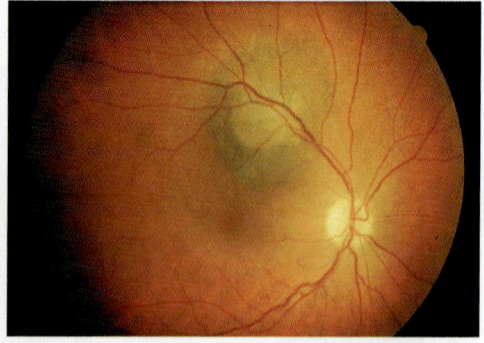

Fig. 6.16. Small, raised choroidal melanoma with surface orange pigment and documented growth over four months. Globe-sparing treatment with a radioactive scleral plaque (brachytherapy) may be indicated.

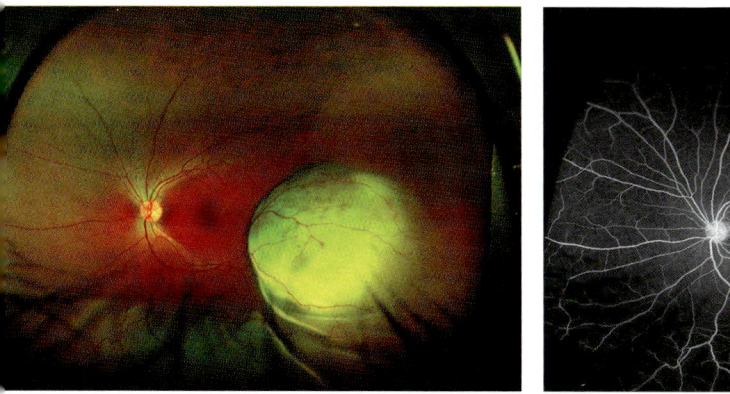

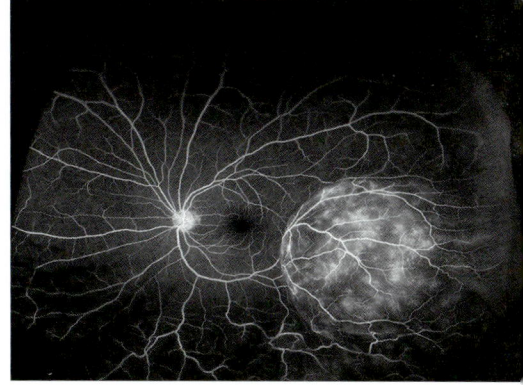

Fig. 6.17. Large, raised malignant choroidal melanoma. FA shows tumour vessels. Treatment is with radioactive plaque or enucleation.

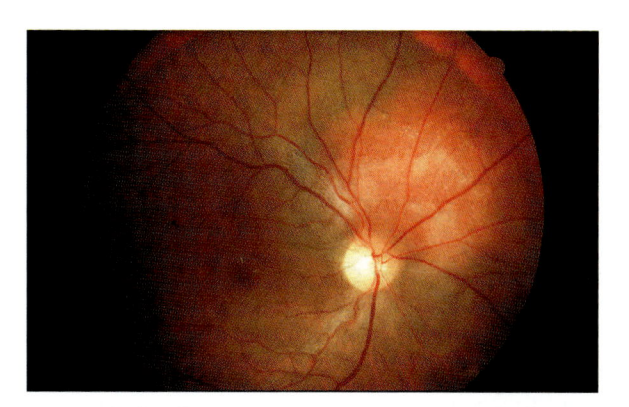

Fig. 6.18. Choroidal haemangioma. Raised, pink and prone to leakage of subretinal fluid. Haemangioma must be differentiated from apigmented malignant melanoma.

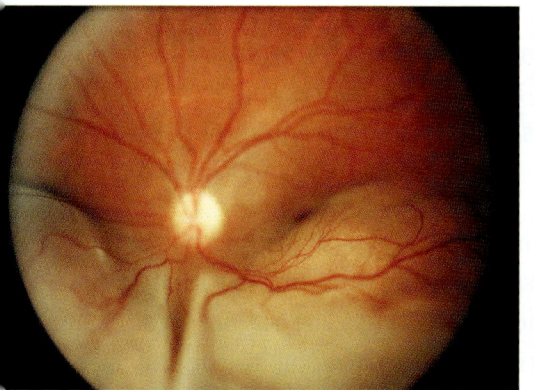

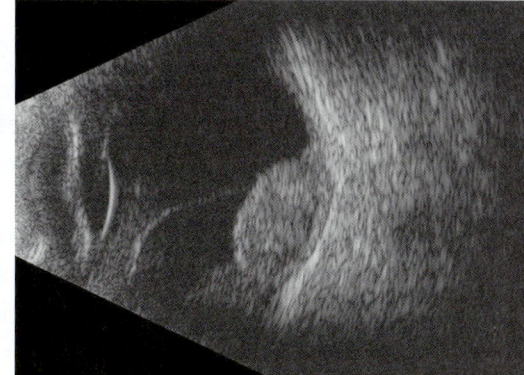

Fig. 6.19. Choroidal metastatic breast carcinoma presenting as retinal detachment with multilobulated subretinal masses.

7
RETINA AND VITREOUS

INTRODUCTION

Retinal disorders, including macular degeneration and diabetic retinopathy, account for almost half of all loss of vision in developed countries with ageing populations. Great advances in diagnostic and surgical instrumentation and in therapies, including anti-VEGF injections, have transformed the outlook for many retinal diseases.

RETINAL VASCULAR DISEASES

Central Retinal Artery Occlusion

In occlusion of the central retinal artery, the patient notices sudden visual loss in one eye and, within a few minutes, the eye may become totally blind. In complete obstruction of the central retinal artery, there is a dilated afferent pupil defect. The retinal arteries are constricted and look like thin threads, while the smaller vessels are scarcely visible. The fundus appears milky-white because of ischaemic retinal oedema. In contrast to this, there is a "cherry-red spot" at the macula where the retina is thin, allowing the red choroidal circulation to show through. Haemorrhages are not seen in central retinal artery occlusion unless the vein is also occluded.

After a few weeks, the retinal swelling subsides and the retina is thinned and regains its transparency, but the disc becomes pale because of atrophy of the optic nerve fibres. The retinal arterioles remain narrow. Visual prognosis is poor. Lowering the intraocular pressure soon after the onset (such as by aspirating aqueous) may give a slight chance of partial visual recovery.

The causes of central retinal artery occlusion include arteriosclerosis with or without hypertension and emboli from diseased heart valves or carotid atheroma. Emboli may also cause a Branch retinal artery occlusion. In elderly patients with central retinal artery occlusion, one must exclude giant cell temporal arteritis by performing a blood ESR and, if in doubt, by biopsy of the temporal artery. Failure to recognise this cause, which is controlled with high doses of systemic steroids, may lead to blindness in the fellow eye.

Central Retinal Vein Occlusion

Central retinal vein occlusion (CRVO) is less abrupt in presentation than occlusion of the central retinal artery and the loss of sight is not complete. Visual acuity may be 6/9 down to counting fingers. The predisposing causes are hypertension, diabetes mellitus, arteriosclerosis in the elderly, open-angle glaucoma and factors or conditions which increase coagulability or viscosity of the blood including genetic defects (e.g. factor V Leiden), macroglobulinaemia and the use of oral contraceptives.

Examination with the ophthalmoscope shows grossly tortuous and engorged retinal veins, especially near the optic disc. Very often, unilateral disc oedema is present. Scattered all over the retina, from the disc to the periphery, are blot haemorrhages of all shapes and sizes. These may be accompanied by soft exudates.

CRVO is sub-classified into ischaemic and non-ischaemic types. After a period of many weeks, the haemorrhages clear gradually and there may be little evidence of the occlusion, except for shunt vessels on the optic disc. Many patients, however, fail to re-establish venous drainage, and develop persistent macula oedema. Anti-vascular endothelial growth factor (anti-VEGF) antibodies injected into the vitreous can dramatically improve the vision. A few patients may benefit from creation of a laser venous shunt to bypass the blockage. Vision fails to be fully restored in the majority of the elderly but the prognosis for younger patients is much better in non-ischaemic CRVO.

Chronic ischaemic CRVO may also lead to neovascularisation of either the retina or the iris (rubeosis iridis). Vitreous haemorrhage may require vitrectomy. New iris vessels may obstruct drainage in the filtration angle and cause painful secondary neovascular glaucoma.

Panretinal laser photocoagulation is indicated to prevent both these secondary complications. If rubeosis iridis develops, medical therapy to lower the pressure, anti-VEGF injections into the vitreous, retinal laser and glaucoma surgery may all be required.

Ocular Ischaemic Syndrome

Poor ocular perfusion may occur with carotid stenosis. This presents with diffuse retinal haemorrhages and looks similar to a CRVO. Iris neovascularisation and secondary glaucoma may follow. Carotid ultrasonography confirms the diagnosis. Treatment includes lowering of intraocular pressure, anti-VEGF injections and panretinal laser. Endovascular carotid surgery may also be indicated.

Branch Retinal Vein Occlusion

Branch retinal vein occlusion occurs at an arteriovenous junction, where a vein is crossed by a sclerotic artery. The superior temporal vein is the branch most commonly affected. The main predisposing causes of branch retinal vein occlusion are long-standing hypertension, arteriosclerosis, diabetes and chronic glaucoma. The visual symptoms depend on the site of occlusion. The fundus shows a characteristic fan-shaped distribution of retinal haemorrhages which radiate from the site of obstruction. If the macula is involved, the patient will complain of blurred central vision. Macular oedema may persist after the haemorrhages are absorbed, and swelling disrupts the fovea, leading to visual loss. Moreover, vitreous haemorrhage from abnormal new vessels may later cause sudden visual loss.

After some months, there is re-establishment of local circulation around the site of the occlusion and the haemorrhages and exudates are absorbed, but vision recovers without treatment in less than half of the patients.

Anti-VEGF antibody injections are therefore used to dry out the macula and restore visual acuity. Intravitreal corticosteroid injections may help if unresponsive to anti-VEGF injections. Laser photocoagulation is also used to ablate the damaged capillary bed if macular oedema persists despite injections or when there is vitreous haemorrhage from secondary new vessel formation.

Other Retinal Vascular Conditions

Coats' disease

Usually unilateral and presenting in young males, Coats' disease is characterised by leaking telangiectatic capillaries and microaneurysms affecting areas of the peripheral retina and the macula. It may be treated with laser and anti-VEGF injections but may progress to extensive subretinal yellow exudation and sometimes secondary glaucoma and blindness.

Eales disease

Eales disease is another retinal vascular condition, sometimes associated with previous healed tuberculosis. It is considered to be a form of retinal vasculitis and presents with blurred vision in one or both eyes in young to middle-aged patients due to vitreous haemorrhage or macular involvement. Treatment is by laser to the leaking areas of the retina delineated by fluorescein angiography.

Retinal macroaneurysm

Associated with chronic hypertension, an isolated arterial macroaneurysm presents with loss of central vision due to leakage of serum or bleeding into the macula. It is treated with laser or anti-VEGF injections in the vitreous. It sometimes requires emergency vitrectomy, a tissue plasminogen activator and a gas bubble to remove or displace blood from the vitreous and under the macula.

Other retinal vascular conditions associated with retinal vasculitis include anaemia, blood dyscrasias and sickle cell haemoglobinopathy. These are covered in Chapter 8.

RHEGMATOGENOUS RETINAL DETACHMENT

Retinal detachment is the separation of the retinal neurosensory layer from the retinal pigment epithelium. It is caused by tears (holes) which are usually located at the peripheral areas of the retina. These tears occur when degenerate vitreous contracts with age or in a larger myopic eye and there also happens to be a local attachment point between retina and vitreous. Vitreous traction then tears the thin peripheral retina.

Retinal detachment is most common in patients with degenerative (high) myopia, in the elderly, in patients after cataract surgery and as a result of ocular injuries.

The symptoms of a retinal tear include seeing multiple floaters of recent onset and flashes of light. Vitreous floaters have been described by patients as dots, flies or cobwebs in their field of vision. However, if the patient has seen a single floater for many months, it is usually harmless and due to minor degeneration of the vitreous gel.

On the other hand, a large number of floaters appearing suddenly together with flashes of light requires retinal assessment by an ophthalmologist. These symptoms signal a separation of the vitreous body from the retina (posterior vitreous detachment), and a retinal tear must be excluded. Retinal traction may cause vitreous haemorrhage or a tear and lead to detachment of the retina from the pigment epithelium, resulting in sudden visual loss.

With the development of retinal detachment there is loss of the peripheral visual field. The typical symptom described is that of a curtain obstructing part of the vision. If the macula is affected, there will be loss of central vision. Ophthalmoscopy shows loss of the red reflex with areas of detached retina appearing grey and undulating. Diagnosis is confirmed by an ophthalmologist, by examining the retina with full dilatation of the pupils using an indirect ophthalmoscope with scleral indentation.

Retinal detachment is an ocular emergency. The spread of the subretinal fluid due to gravity may detach the macula, leading to permanent loss of central vision. Surgery must be carried out as soon as possible and preferably on the same day.

Retinal detachment surgery consists of three components: eliminating the vitreous traction, draining of subretinal fluid to flatten the retina and sealing the retinal tears.

It is important to find all the retinal tears (holes), which must be sealed with adhesive scars produced by laser photocoagulation or external cryoapplications. Laser causes less inflammation than cryotherapy and has largely replaced it. Intravitreal surgery (vitrectomy, internal drainage of subretinal fluid, gas–fluid exchange of the vitreous cavity and laser) has become the preferred method of reattaching the retina. Scleral buckling with silicone material is also frequently used to push the wall of the sclera inwards to close the tear and permanently reduce the vitreous traction. The two methods are used together in complex cases. The success rate with one operation is over 90% but a few patients require more than one.

Predetachment changes, including retinal holes and lattice degeneration, are sometimes found in the other eye, which should also be thoroughly examined with the indirect ophthalmoscope. If retinal tears are found, they should be sealed with laser.

Exudative and Traction Retinal Detachment

Less commonly, retinal detachment is not due to a retinal tear but to exudation of fluid into the subretinal space, as in malignant choroidal tumours, severe uveitis or toxaemia of pregnancy.

Another cause of retinal detachment is traction from scar tissue. This can occur in proliferative diabetic retinopathy, penetrating injury, retinopathy of prematurity or after a rhegmatogenous retinal detachment (proliferative vitreoretinopathy). Contracting scar tissue pulls the neurosensory retina away from the retinal pigment epithelium in the absence of a retinal tear. Vitrectomy is required to relieve the traction along with an encircling scleral buckle.

MACULAR DISEASES

Macular diseases are common and may result in a disabling loss of central vision. Loss of visual acuity can be classified as legal blindness even though peripheral vision remains.

Chronic macular diseases which cause gradual loss of central vision include dry age-related macular degeneration, diabetic maculopathy, degenerative high myopia, and macular dystrophy in young people. Acute macular conditions include exudative or wet macular degeneration, central serous retinopathy, macular hole and macular vein occlusions.

Diffuse retinal conditions may also affect the macula and include retinal vascular occlusions, diabetic retinopathy and retinal detachment.

In the past, many macular diseases were untreatable. A better understanding of the pathophysiology of these conditions, OCT and a wide range of new treatment modalities, especially anti-VEGF injections, have transformed the outlook for macular diseases.

Macular Dystrophies

A spectrum of hereditary macular dystrophies occur in the young. Macular dystrophy is bilateral and symmetrical, and causes gradual painless loss of vision. A variety of clinical entities exist with different underlying genetic defects, many of which have now been identified. Macular dystrophies include Stargardt macular dystrophy, cone dystrophy, vitelliform dystrophy, pseudoxanthoma elasticum and macular telangiectasia type 2.

Although there is no proven effective treatment, rapid advances in gene replacement therapy and stem cell biology give hope for the future. In the meantime documentation of visual function, fields, retinal imaging, electrophysiology and gene analysis allow precise diagnosis. Visual aids and genetic and occupational counselling are very important.

Age-related Macular Degeneration

Age-related macular degeneration (AMD) is a bilateral degeneration of the macula which presents in or after the sixth decade. It causes loss of central vision. It accounts for over 40% of legal blindness in Caucasians (less than 6/60 visual acuity) and although less prevalent in other races the incidence is increasing in all ageing populations. Besides age, environmental risk factors include cigarette smoking and a high saturated fat diet lacking in fresh vegetables.

AMD has a significant genetic component which is often dominantly transmitted. Variants of the complement factor H gene, along with other gene variations involved in the alternative complement pathway, are associated with up to 50% of AMD cases.

A patient with AMD usually complains of increasing blurring or distortion of central vision. One letter or word may appear at a different level from its neighbour or there may be missing letters or words. The ophthalmoscopic picture varies. In the early stages of AMD, the macula usually has fine pigmentary clumps and patches of atrophy. Classically, yellow–white round spots called drusen are seen. They are waste deposits from the receptor outer segments which accumulate beneath the retinal pigment epithelium. Drusen by themselves do not usually cause significant visual loss, especially if they are few in number and are sharply demarcated (hard drusen). Large and indistinct drusen (soft drusen) or confluent drusen are frequently associated with progression to later stages of macular degeneration.

Treatment for early AMD involves a low saturated fat diet with lots of green leafy vegetables, fish and nuts. Dietary supplements of antioxidants (e.g. vitamins C and E, zinc and β-carotene) may slow the progression of early-to-late stages of AMD.

Progressive AMD can be classified as "dry" or "wet".

In dry AMD, there is slow progressive degeneration of the central retina, resulting in patches of atrophy called geographic atrophy. Diet and antioxidants slow the progression. Trials of several agents that may modulate the alternative complement pathway are under way.

In wet AMD, vision suddenly becomes distorted or blurred because of subretinal leakage of fluid or blood from a localised new vessel growth from the choroid. If untreated, this leads to disciform subretinal scarring and permanent loss of vision.

In cases of sudden visual loss, urgent OCT and fluorescein angiography should be carried out. Choroidal neovascularisation is treated with a series of intravitreal injections of anti-VEGF agents that reverse the fluid leak and retard the growth of the new vessel (ranibizumab, aflibercept or bevacizumab).

Photodynamic therapy is the activation of a systemically administered photosensitive drug, verteporfin, by low-intensity laser. It has been used for wet AMD in the past but is now reserved for a subvariant called polypoidal choroidopathy. This is very important in Asian populations, where it accounts for up to 40% of cases. The choroidal polyps are diagnosed by indocyanine green angiography.

For late-stage wet AMD with advanced subretinal scar tissue, surgical transposition of the macula and retinal pigment epithelial transplants derived from stem cells have been shown to be feasible but are not clinically practical.

It is important to emphasise to patients with macular degeneration that they will not go totally blind from the condition as peripheral vision will not be affected. Some patients benefit from the use of strong glasses and a variety of visual aids for distant and near vision. These include magnifying lenses and special telescopic spectacles. Modern e-readers and smartphones are also adaptable to the requirements of low vision.

Central Serous Retinopathy (Central Serous Choroidopathy)

Central serous retinopathy (CSR) is common in males from 20 to 50 years of age. It occurs spontaneously and is characterised by fluid leaking from the choroidal capillaries through the pigment epithelium and subsequently accumulating under the macula. The aetiology is unknown.

The patient complains of recent disturbance of central vision which is generally described as a dulling, darkening or blurring of vision. In most cases, there is micropsia (objects appearing smaller). Ophthalmoscopically, the macula shows a characteristic round swelling with a ring reflex at its border. Diagnosis is confirmed by OCT and fluorescein or ICG angiography, which shows a leaking defect in the retinal pigment epithelium and thickening of the choroid underneath.

CSR is usually self-limiting and benign. It is made worse by systemic steroid therapy. If severe or if it persists for many months, laser photocoagulation is used to seal the leak. Recurrences are common. A minority of patients have widespread pigment epithelial disturbances. This atypical subgroup have a less favourable prognosis and their condition is often bilateral. Photodynamic therapy with a reduced dose of verteporfin is used in refractory cases.

Degenerative (High) Myopia

Degenerative myopia is often familial and is characterised by a progressive increase in the axial length of the eye from the time of adolescence which may lead to chorioretinal atrophy at the posterior pole. This causes slow progressive loss of central vision. A common complication is a choroidal new vessel which may bleed (Fuchs' macular haemorrhage). Other complications include macular schisis (splitting), macular hole and retinal detachment.

Direct ophthalmoscopy is difficult, owing to the high refractive error. The view is improved by examining the fundus through the patient's glasses or contact lenses. The disc shows a typical crescent or ring of chorioretinal atrophy surrounding its margin.

No treatment is available to change the progress of myopic macular degeneration. Vocational guidance may be useful prior to the loss of central vision. The rate of deterioration is unpredictable.

Epiretinal Membrane (Premacular Fibrosis)

Older patients experience spontaneous posterior vitreous detachment very commonly. This may be followed by growth and contraction of a thin membrane across the macula. Also, the normal internal limiting membrane on the macular surface may contract and cause retinal wrinkles or striae. The patient may experience distortion, ghosting, blurred vision and headache when reading.

An OCT scan confirms the diagnosis. Epiretinal membrane can be peeled after vitrectomy. The prognosis is then good but vitrectomy is likely to accelerate cataract, requiring a second surgery.

Macular Hole

Another not uncommon result of vitreous traction is the formation of a central macular hole. Those at risk have a focal adhesion of the vitreous to the foveal area, which then pulls out a tissue disc of the perifoveal retina. Vision drops rapidly to 10–20% of normal.

OCT shows a full-thickness central hole in the macula. Surgery comprises vitrectomy, detachment of the surrounding vitreous, staining and peeling of the internal limiting membrane and gas–fluid exchange. The hole then closes and most of the vision is restored in 95% of cases.

Generalised Hereditary Retinal Dystrophies

Retinitis pigmentosa

Retinitis pigmentosa is a panretinal dystrophy characterised by defective night vision and progressive loss of the peripheral visual field. The hereditary pattern may be recessive, dominant or x-linked. Onset of night blindness and mid-peripheral field loss starts in the first or second decade of life. The vision usually deteriorates to low levels by the fifth or sixth decade. The ophthalmoscopic signs include proliferation of retinal pigment with a characteristic dark-brown–black "bone spicules" appearance, a waxy yellow optic disc and attenuated retinal vessels.

It is important to study the family history in this condition and to look for known gene defects in order to allow genetic counselling. Electroretinography is abnormal before ophthalmoscopic signs develop in children. Progression is best followed by periodic Goldmann visual field examination. Retinitis pigmentosa is sometimes associated with a variety of rare systemic abnormalities and also deafness (Usher syndrome), cataract and glaucoma. Recent research gives hope for a treatment and includes gene therapy, stem cell implants and an implantable array of electrodes that stimulate adjacent ganglion cells in response to digitised video images (bionic eye).

Other general retinal dystrophies include juvenile retinoschisis and choroideraemia. Both are X-linked, so only males are affected. Progress for treatment with gene therapy is promising.

VITREOUS CONDITIONS

Degeneration of the vitreous occurs as a result of age and in high myopia. The vitreous becomes more fluid and may spontaneously detach itself from the retina. Vitreous detachment is associated with flashes and floaters. A retinal tear must always be excluded. Floaters are a particularly common ocular complaint and are usually harmless. A few patients are so bothered by them that laser vitreolysis can be used to disintegrate them.

Other forms of vitreous degeneration which are sometimes present but harmless are white deposits (asteroid hyalosis and synchisis scintillans). If the vitreous opacities are concentrated enough to decrease vision, then vitrectomy is curative.

Vitreous Haemorrhage

This is a frequent cause of sudden visual loss. It is due to trauma, posterior vitreous detachment, retinal tear or abnormal blood vessels, especially from proliferative diabetic retinopathy, CRVO or haemorrhagic AMD. The blood may be absorbed over many months, but if the condition is treated conservatively, B-scan ultrasonography is done regularly to exclude retinal detachment. Vitrectomy has become a safe predictable procedure and it is the usual practice to operate early if the blood is not quickly absorbed or if a retinal tear or progressing diabetic neovascularisation cannot be excluded.

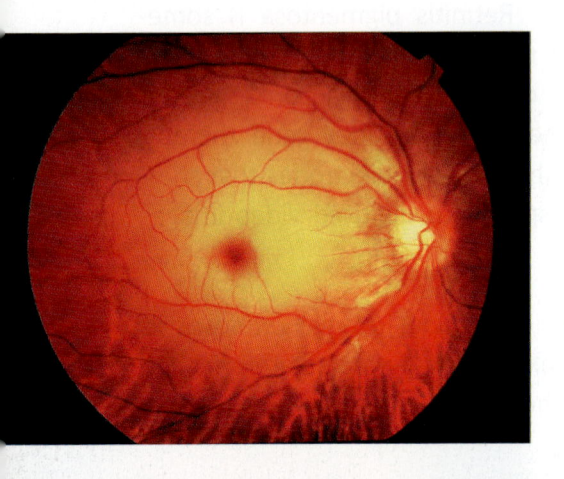

Fig. 7.1. Acute central retinal artery occlusion showing a cherry-red spot surrounded by white retinal oedema. The retinal vessels are narrow. The eye is blind.

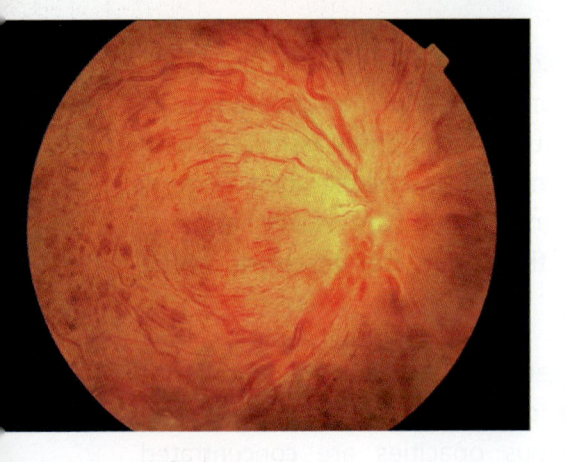

Fig. 7.2. Central retinal vein occlusion showing multiple flame-shaped haemorrhages with macular and optic disc oedema. Visual acuity: Count fingers to 6/9

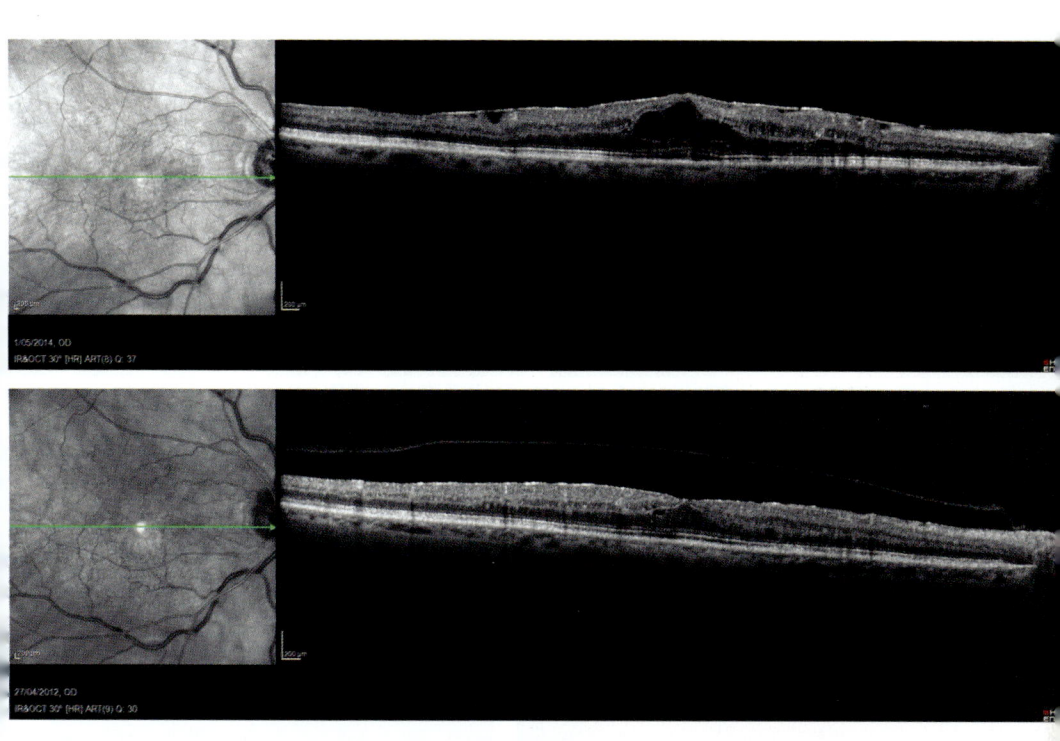

Fig. 7.3. Central retinal vein occlusion given 15 bevacizumab injections over three years. Macular oedema finally resolved. Vision improved from 6/24 to 6/9.

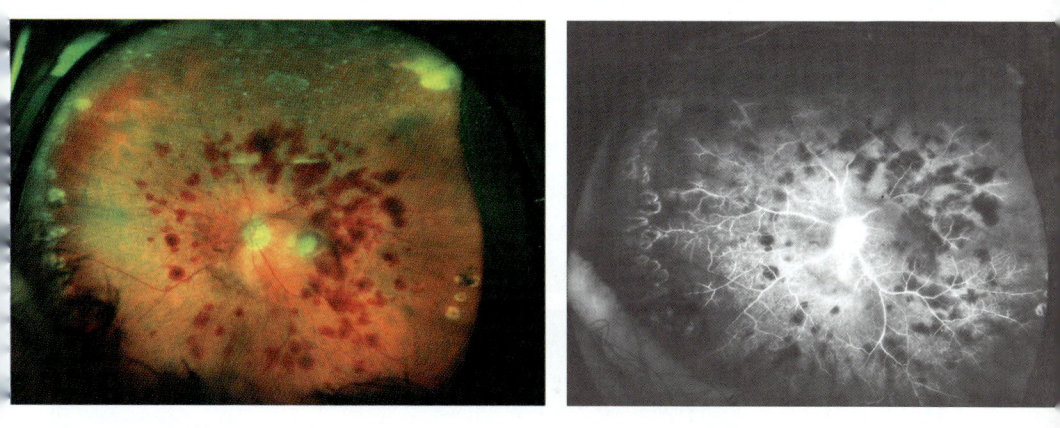

Fig. 7.4. Ocular ischaemic syndrome associated with carotid stenosis and generalised cardiovascular disease.

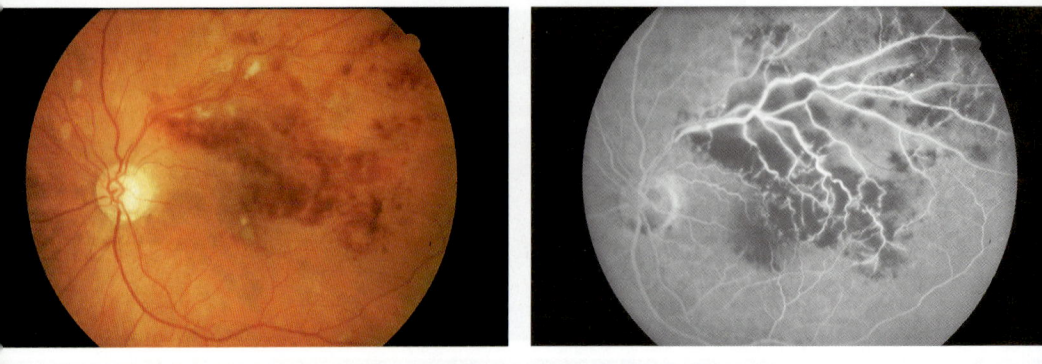

Fig. 7.5. Branch occlusion of superior temporal retinal vein causing flame-shaped retinal haemorrhages.

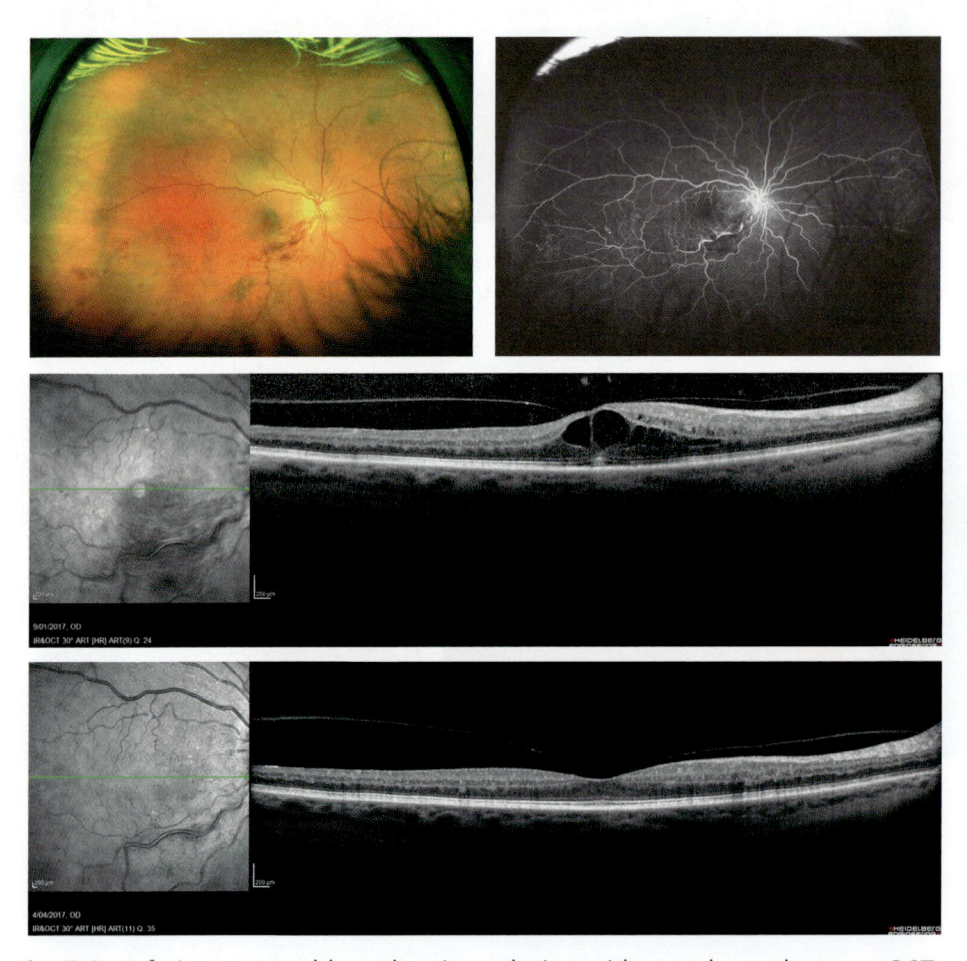

Fig. 7.6. Inferior temporal branch vein occlusion with macular oedema on OCT and response after two bevacizumab injections. VA improved from 6/18 to 6/4.5.

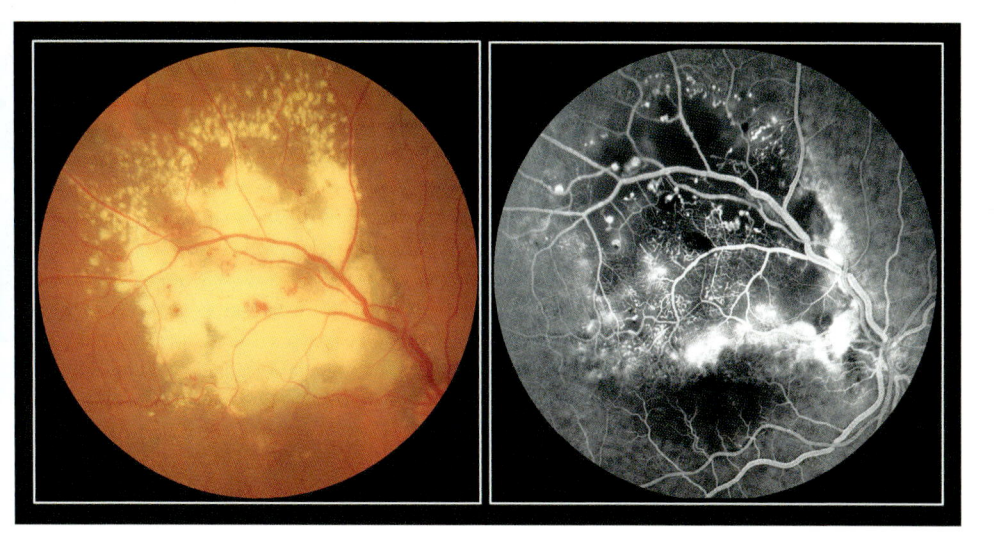

Fig. 7.7. Coats' disease showing widespread retinal microaneurysms and extensive subretinal exudate.

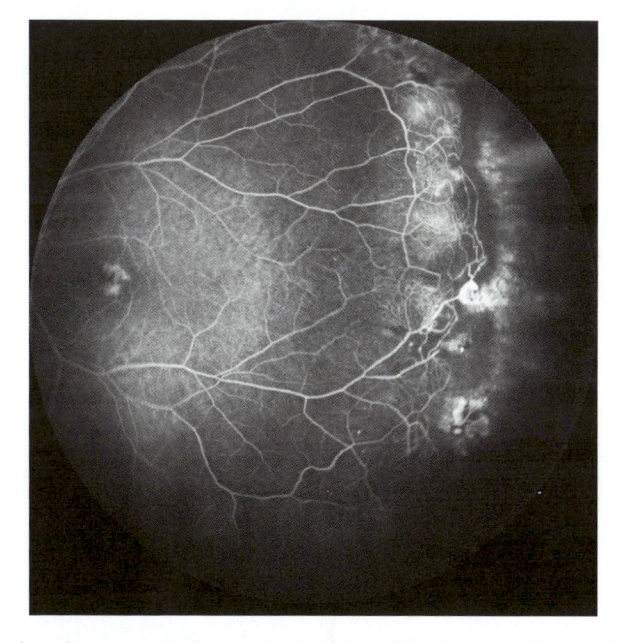

Fig. 7.8. Eales disease. FA showing peripheral leakage and macular oedema from abnormal retinal vessels.

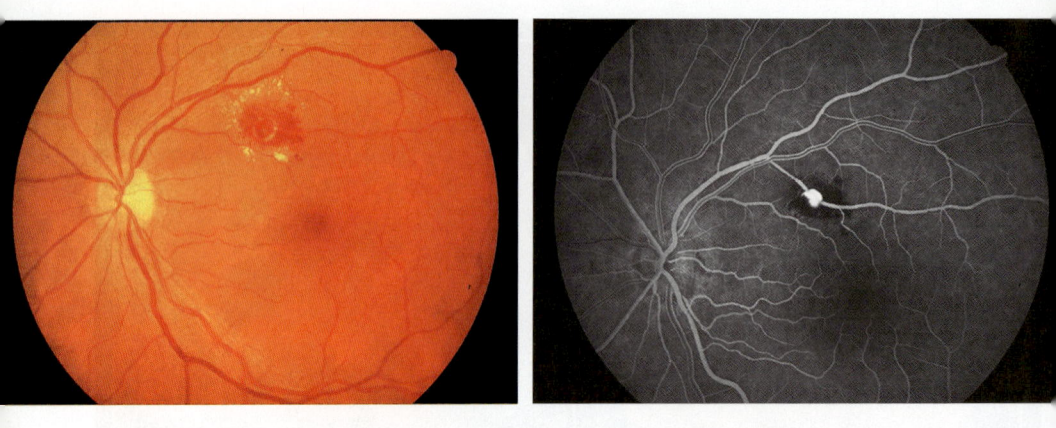

Fig. 7.9. Retinal arteriolar macroaneurysm with surrounding leakage of blood. Laser or anti-VEGF injections can close it and prevent macular haemorrhage.

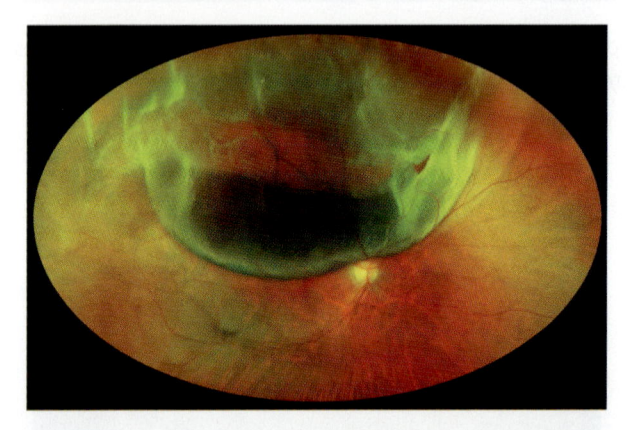

Fig. 7.10. Ballooning superior temporal retinal detachment. (Note the retinal tear at 2 o'clock.) Urgent surgery is required.

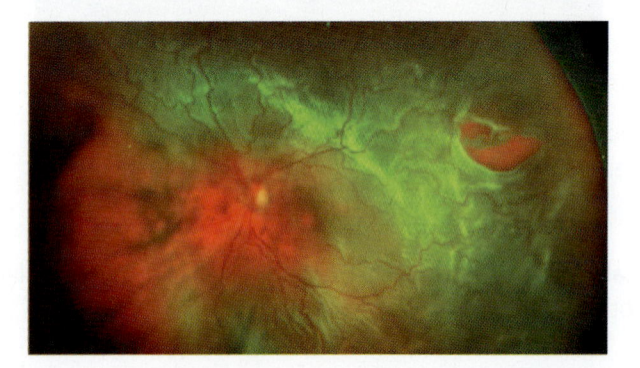

Fig. 7.11. Retinal detachment with a large tear, macula involvement and signs of early scar tissue formation (proliferative vitreoretinopathy).

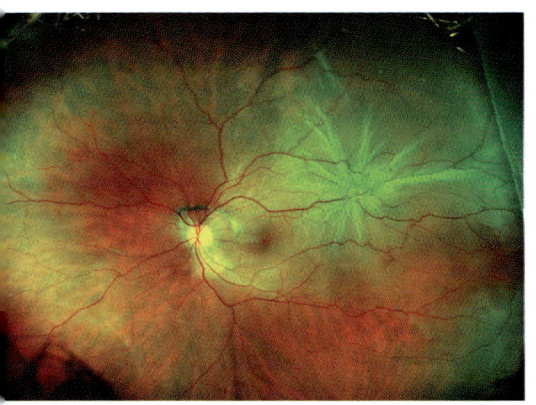

Fig. 7.12. Localised retinal detachment involving macula with a fixed star-shaped epiretinal fold. This requires peeling of the retinal surface at the time of vitrectomy.

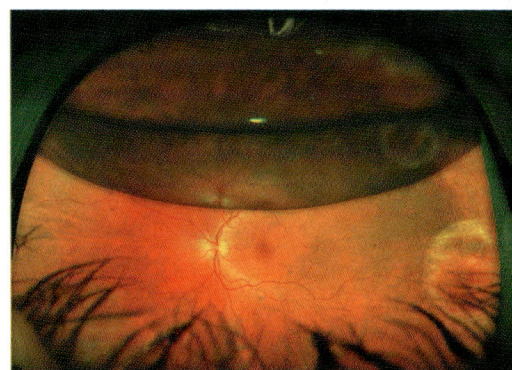

Fig. 7.13. Reattached retina following vitrectomy, gas–fluid exchange and laser to seal the tear. (Note the gas bubble above, partly reabsorbed.)

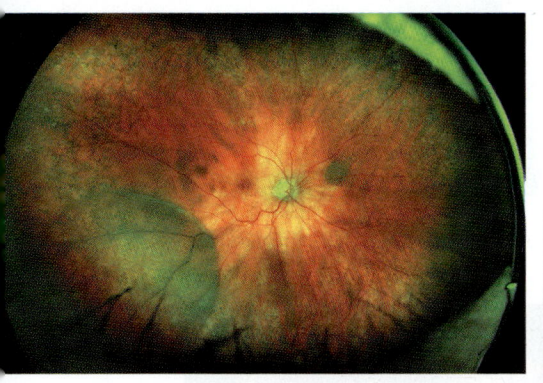

Fig. 7.14. Ballooning adult retinoschisis in the inferotemporal quadrant. This may be mistaken for retinal detachment.

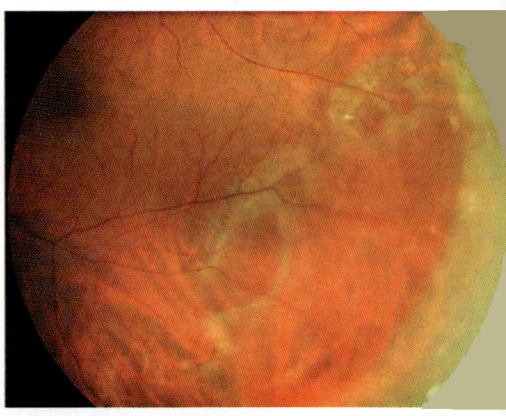

Fig. 7.15. Adult retinoschisis with outer layer retinal breaks. Laser or cryotherapy can prevent retinal detachment but no treatment is indicated in the absence of outer retinal breaks.

Vitreoretinal Surgical Techniques

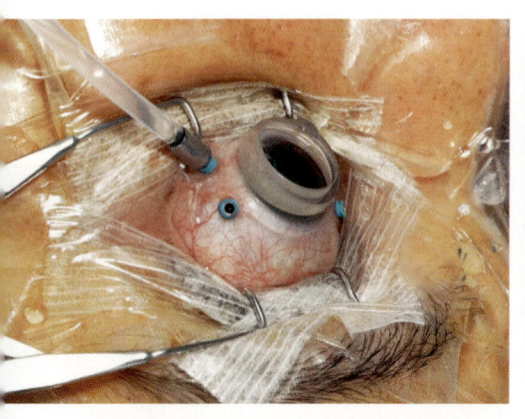

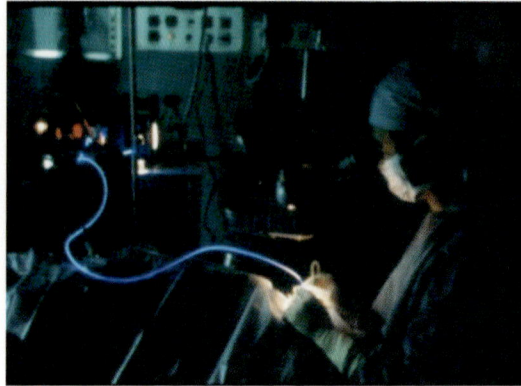

Fig. 7.16. Vitrectomy entry ports and contact lens. Surgery under fibre-optic illumination.

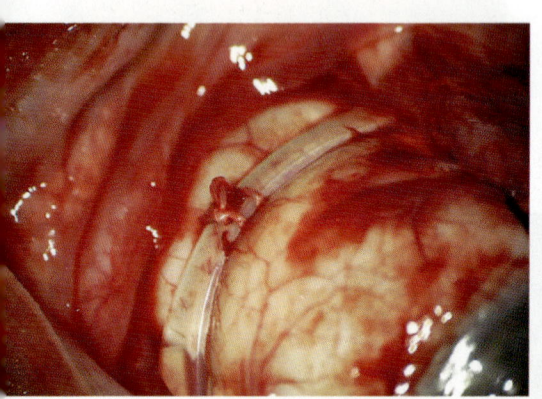

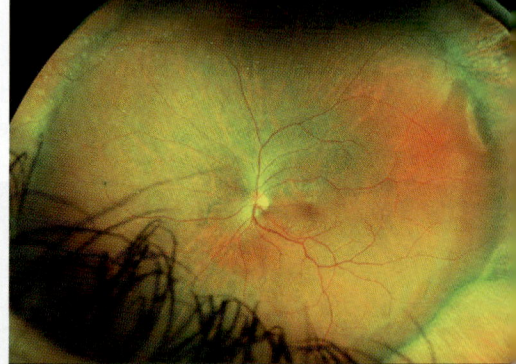

Fig. 7.17. Encircling scleral band. Indenting scleral buckle.

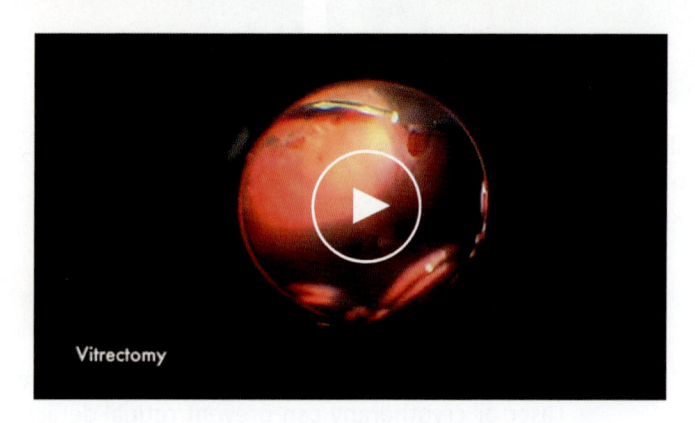

Video of vitrectomy for retinal detachment.

Macular Dystrophies

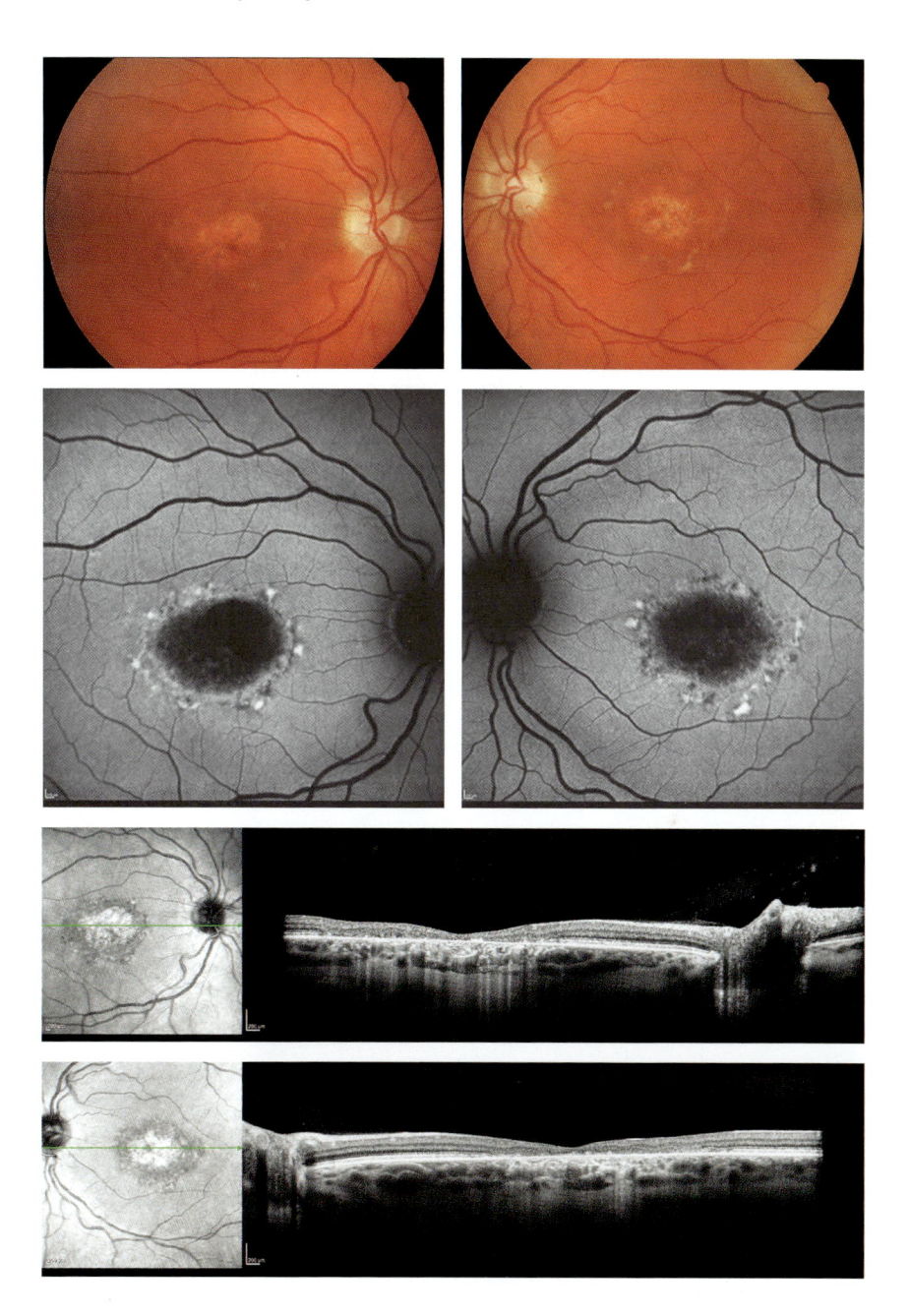

Fig. 7.18. Stargardt macular dystrophy. (Note the autofluorescence of the yellow spots around a patch of central macular atrophic thinning on the OCT.)

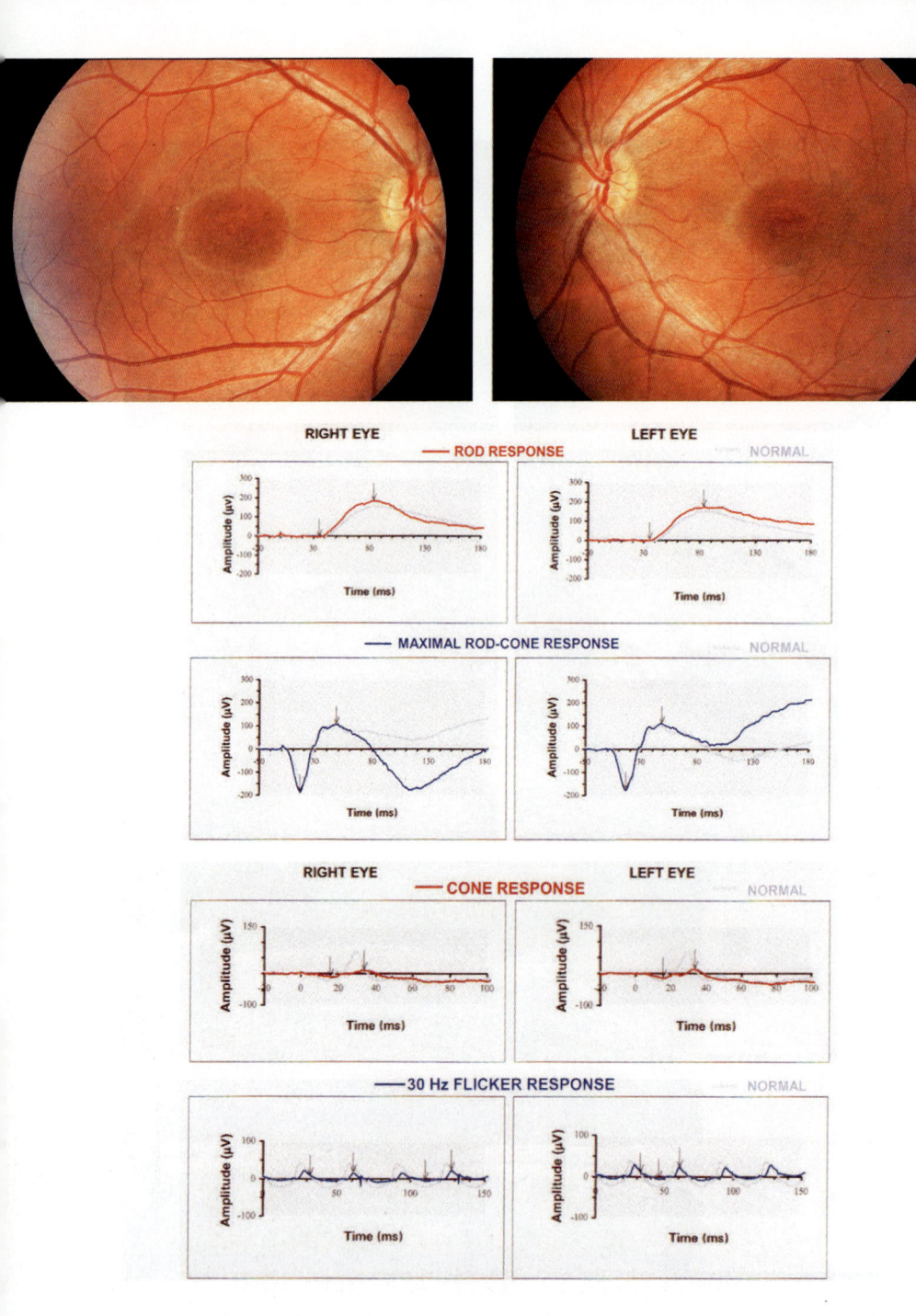

Fig. 7.19. Cone dystrophy. Symmetry in the two eyes, poor vision in bright light and poor colour vision. The electroretinogram cone response is flat, while the rod response is reasonable.

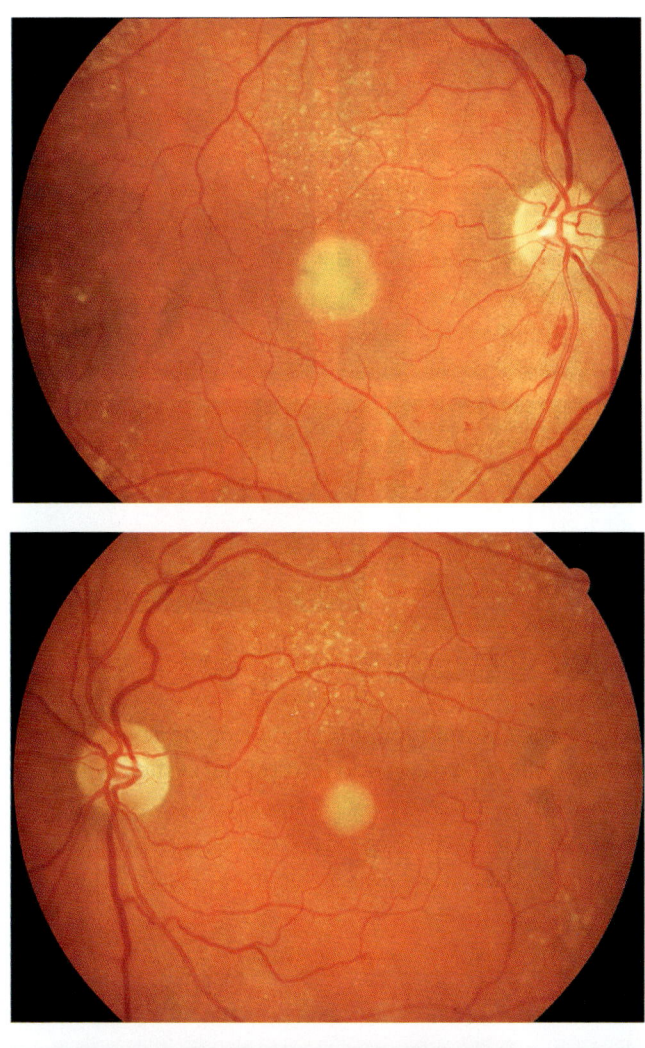

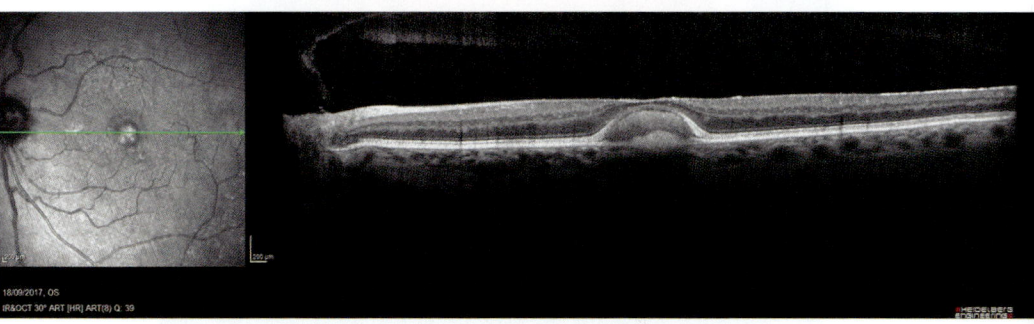

Fig. 7.20. Vitelliform macular dystrophy (Best disease) causes a yellow deposit at the macula.

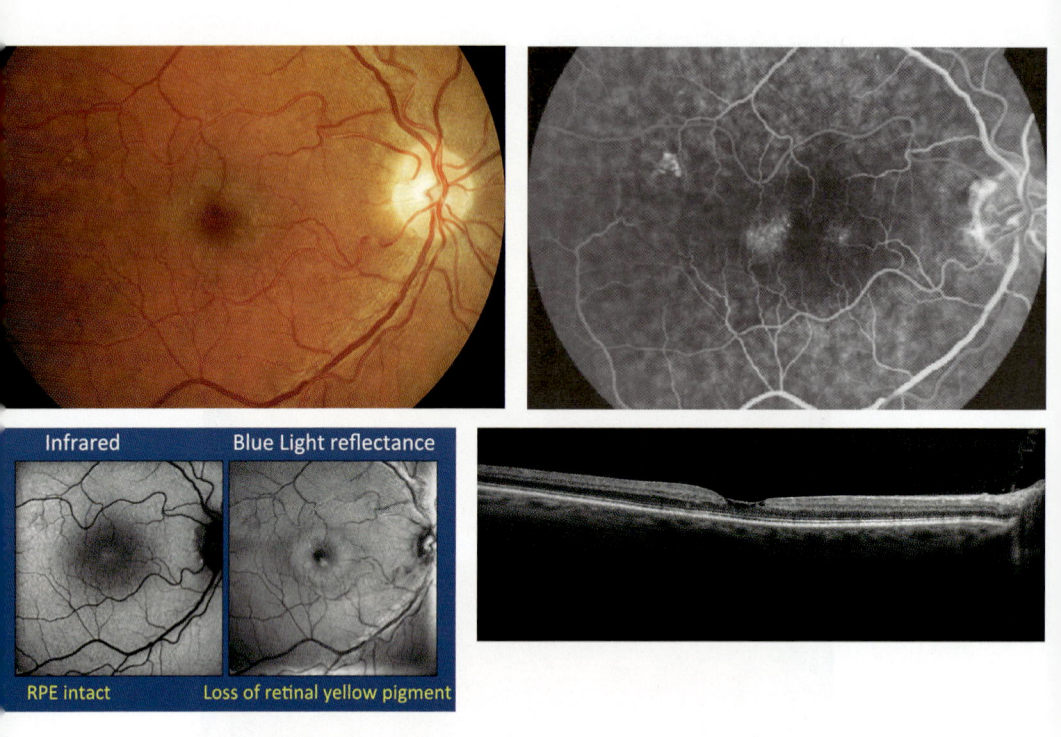

Fig. 7.21. Macular telangiectasia type 2. Cloudy ring on colour, temporal leakage on FA, loss of xanthophyll yellow pigment and intraretinal cystic cavitation on OCT.

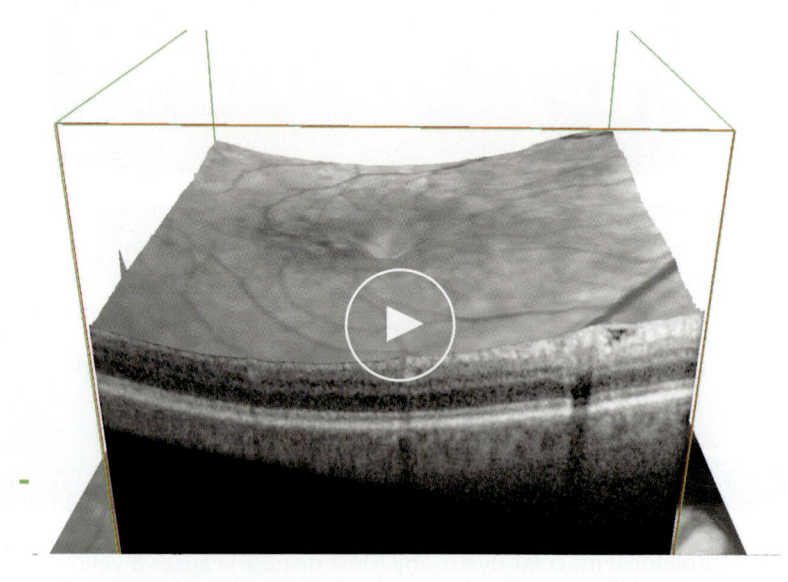

OCT video: Macular telangiectasia type 2 showing an intraretinal cyst and a break in the photoreceptor layer.

Age-Related Macular Degeneration (AMD)

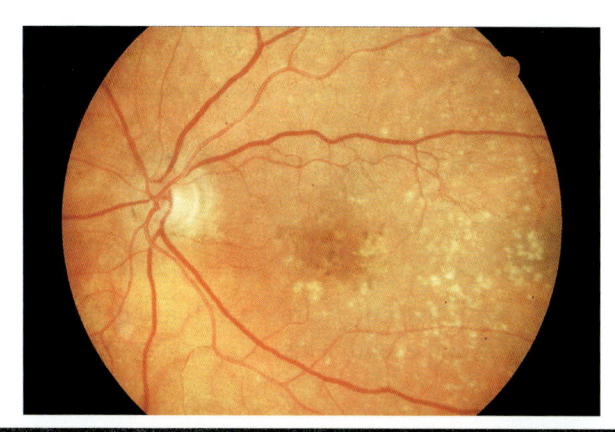

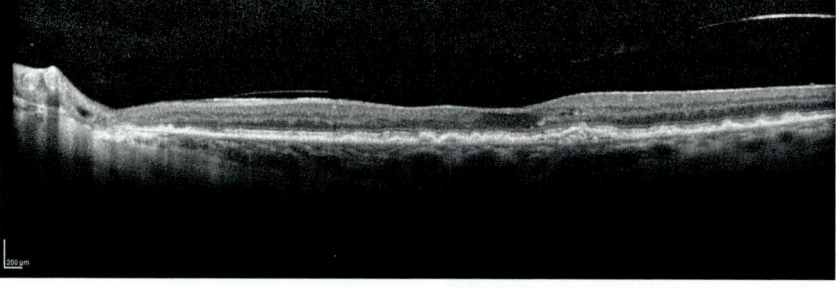

Fig. 7.22. Widespread small drusen with early pigment clumps in the perifoveal area. Vision remains 6/9, with the receptor cell line on OCT still intact under the fovea.

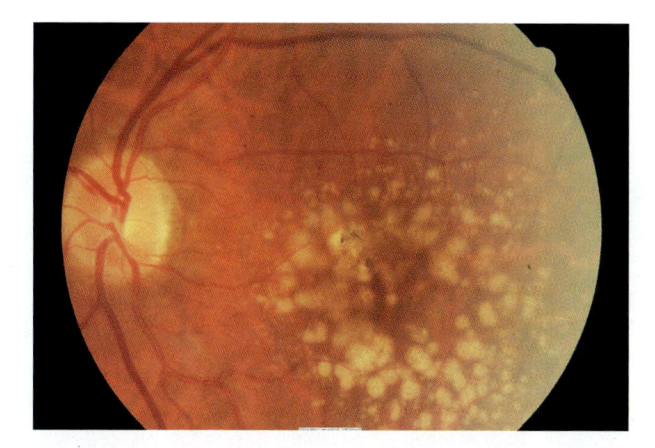

Fig. 7.23. Widespread large soft drusen with a high risk of progressive vision loss. Antioxidant vitamins, zinc and green leafy vegetables in the diet may slow progression.

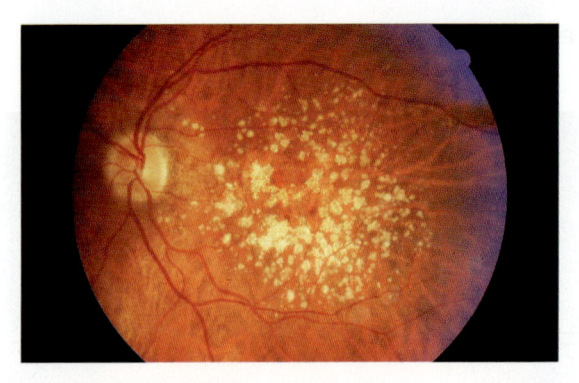

Fig. 7.24. Extensive hard drusen of the macula. These deposits under the RPE lead to pigment clumping and eventual loss of overlying retinal receptor cells.

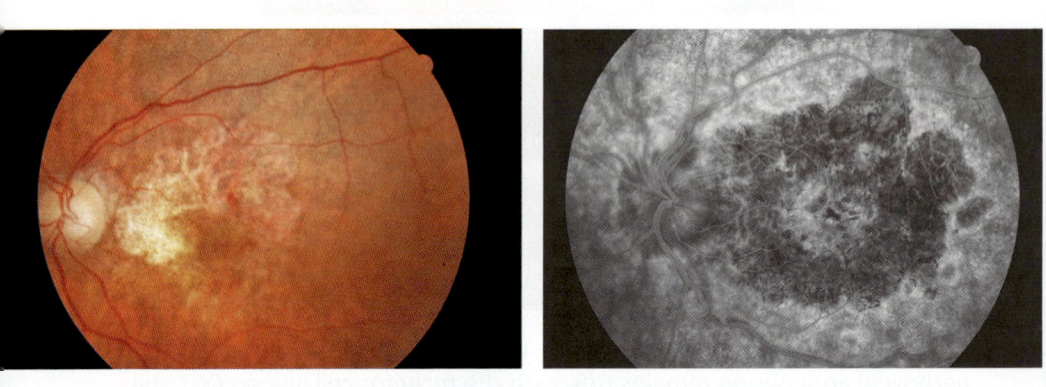

Fig. 7.25. Advanced dry macular degeneration with loss of all central vision due to geographic choroioretinal atrophy.

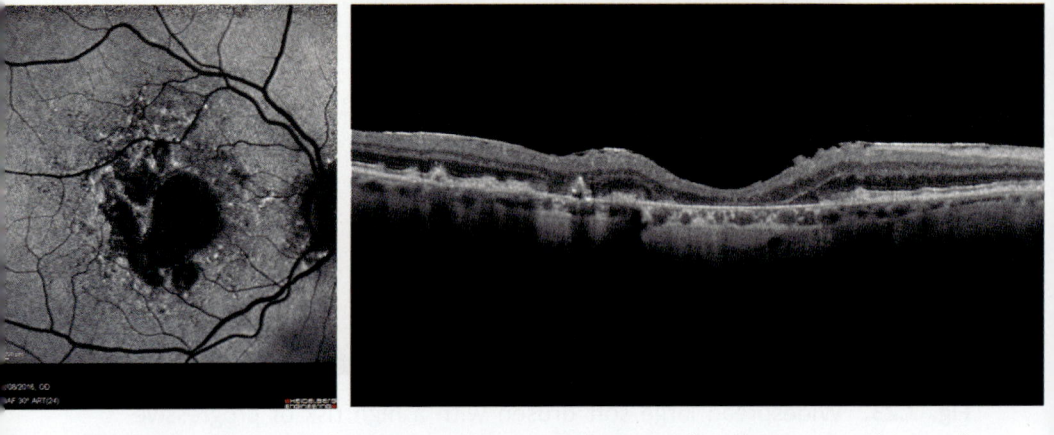

Fig. 7.26. Advanced dry AMD with geographic atrophy. There is total loss of the receptor layers on OCT in the central macular area.

Wet forms of AMD

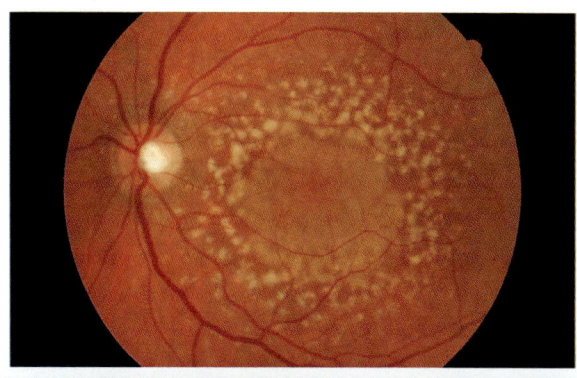

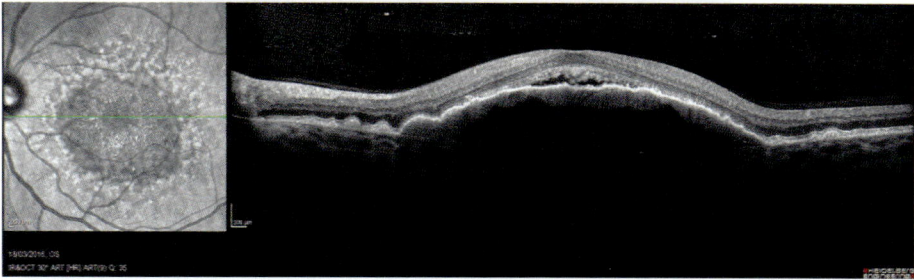

Fig. 7.27. Detachment of the retinal pigment layer (RPE) on OCT with drusen. RPE detachment is often associated with a sub-RPE new vessel.

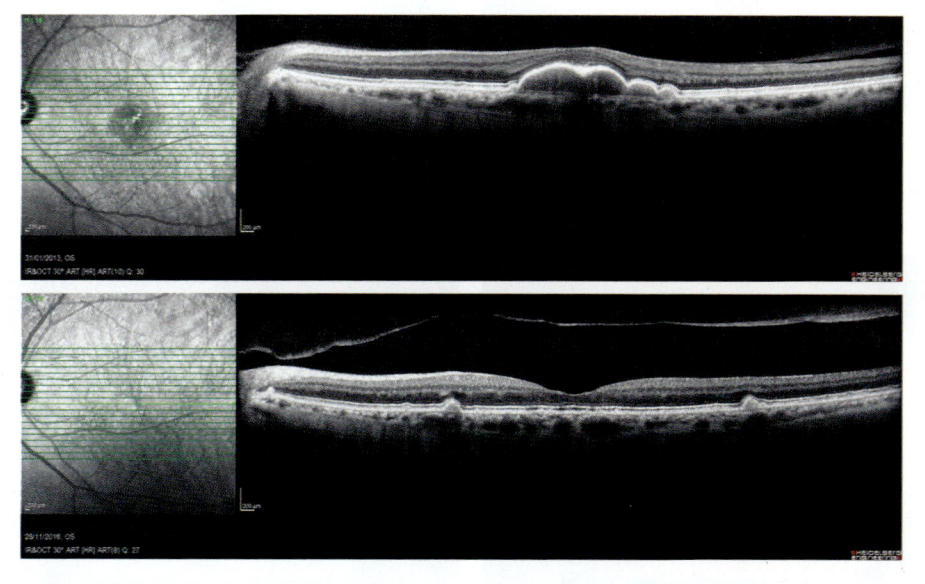

Fig. 7.28. RPE detachment showing a favourable response to a series of aflibercept injections.

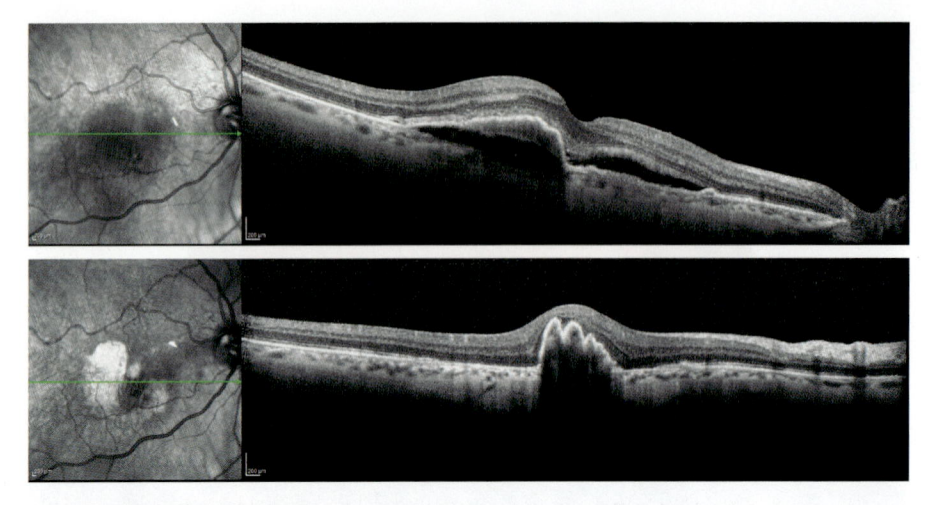

Fig. 7.29. Retinal pigment epithelial rip in wet AMD after four anti-VEGF injections, causing further loss of vision.

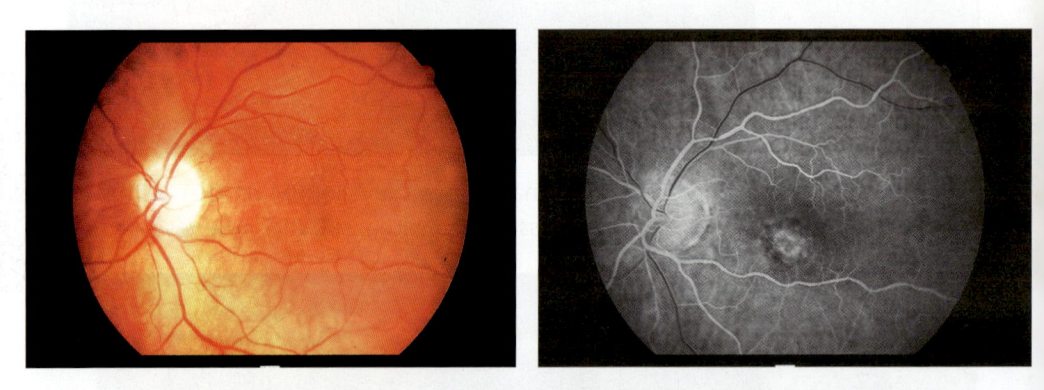

Fig. 7.30. Early choroidal new vessel (CNV) leaking fluorescein under the macula. Urgent referral is required for anti-VEGF injection therapy.

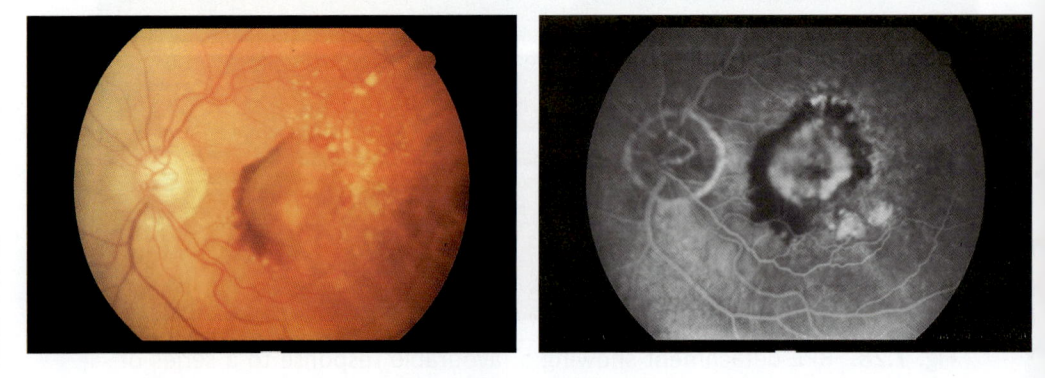

Fig. 7.31. More established CNV still amenable to injection therapy.

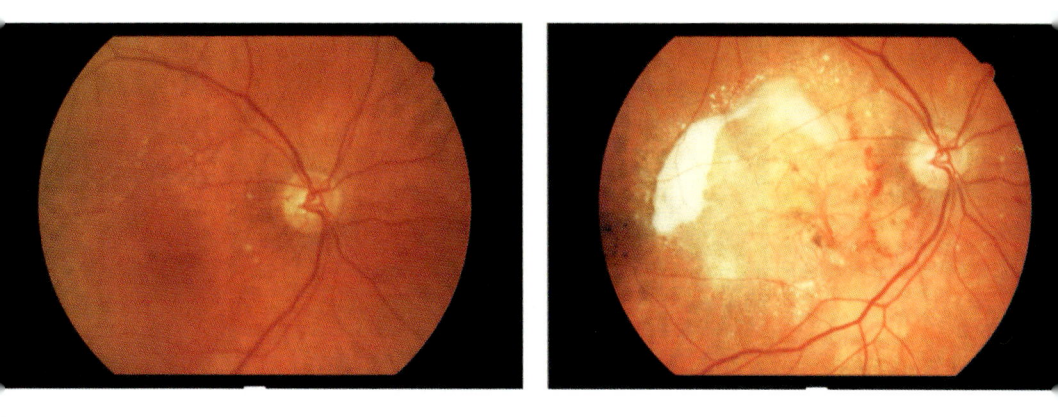

Fig. 7.32. Progression of wet AMD to an advanced disciform macular scar over three years.

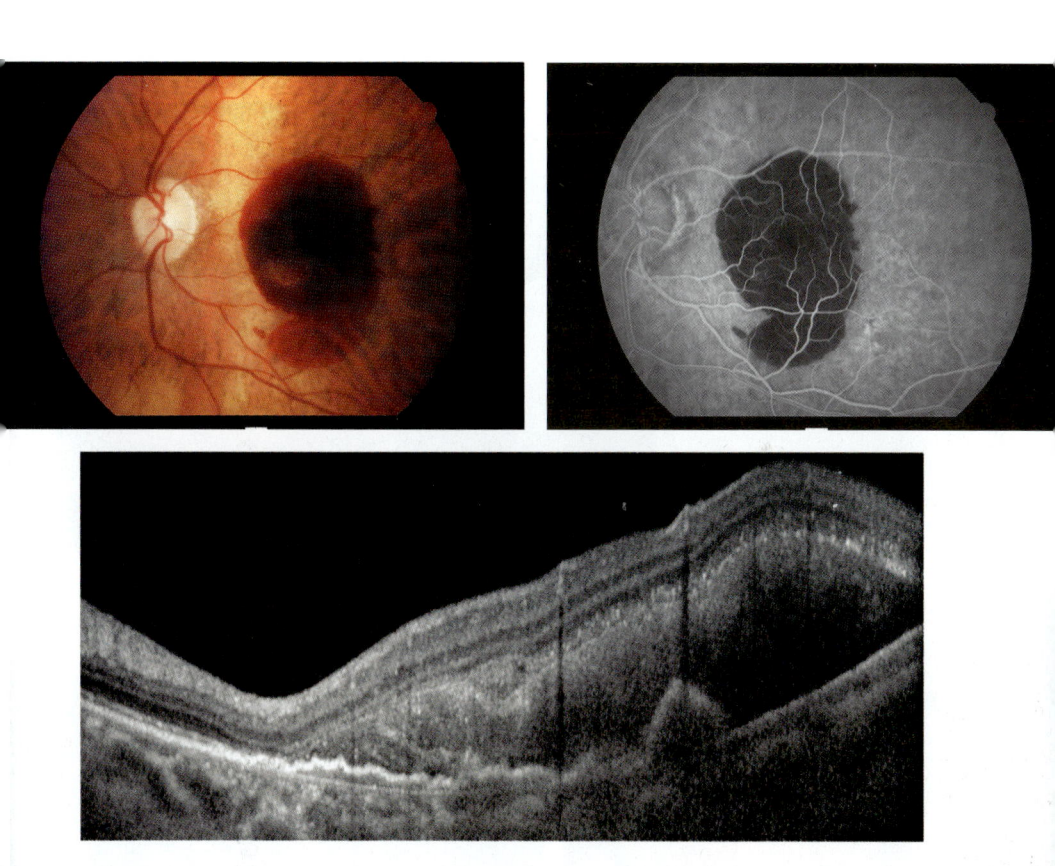

Fig. 7.33. AMD with a large subretinal haemorrhage. FFA shows choroidal haemorrhage posterior to retinal vessels and deep to the retina on OCT. Treatment with a gas bubble in the vitreous to displace the blood from the macula or vitrectomy and thrombolysis with tissue plasminogen activator may restore some vision.

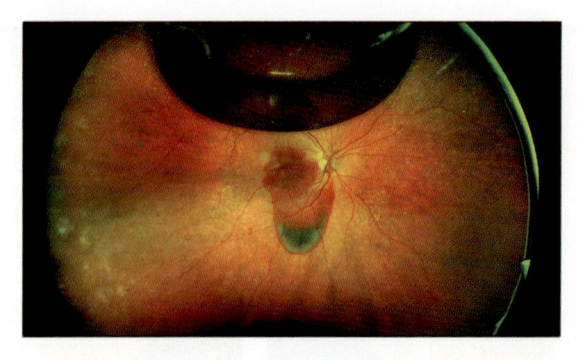

Fig. 7.34. Gas bubble injected into the vitreous has displaced most of a submacular haemorrhage inferiorly, improving vision from counting fingers to 6/24.

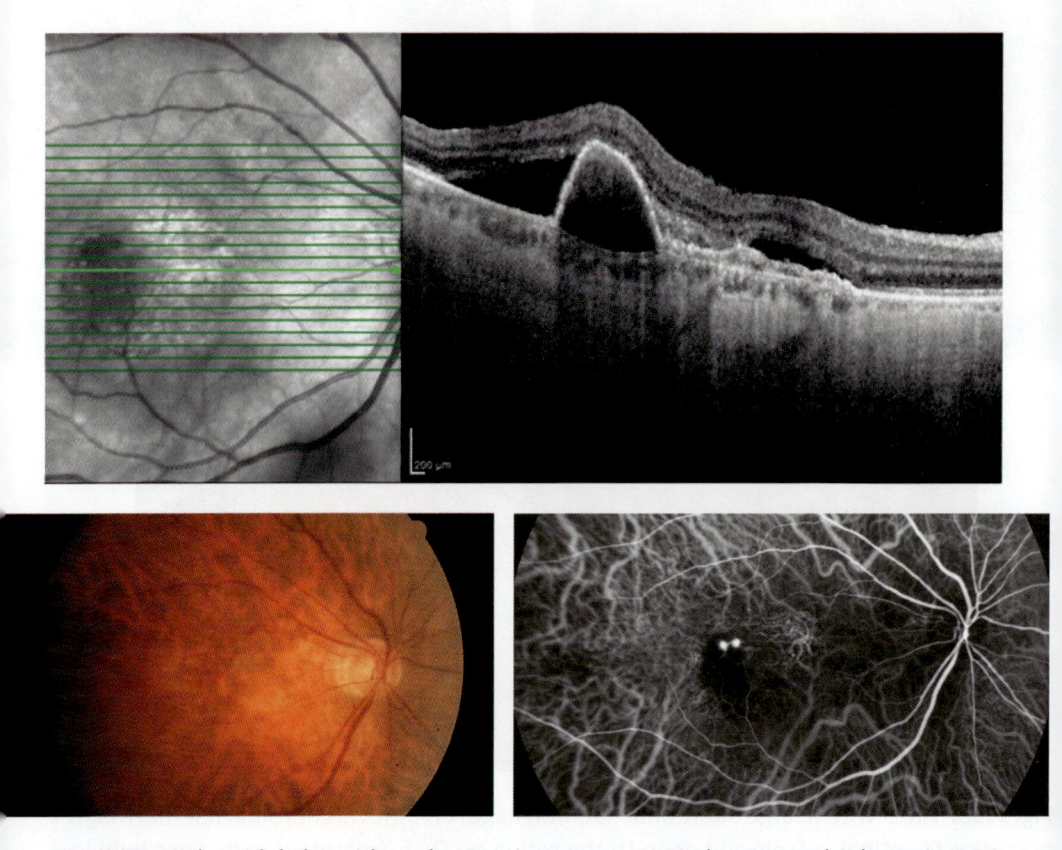

Fig. 7.35. Polypoidal choroidopathy. Persistent wet AMD despite multiple anti-VEGF injections over two years. ICG angiography shows two choroidal polyps under the RPE detachment seen on OCT. These were closed by photodynamic therapy with intravenous verteporfin.

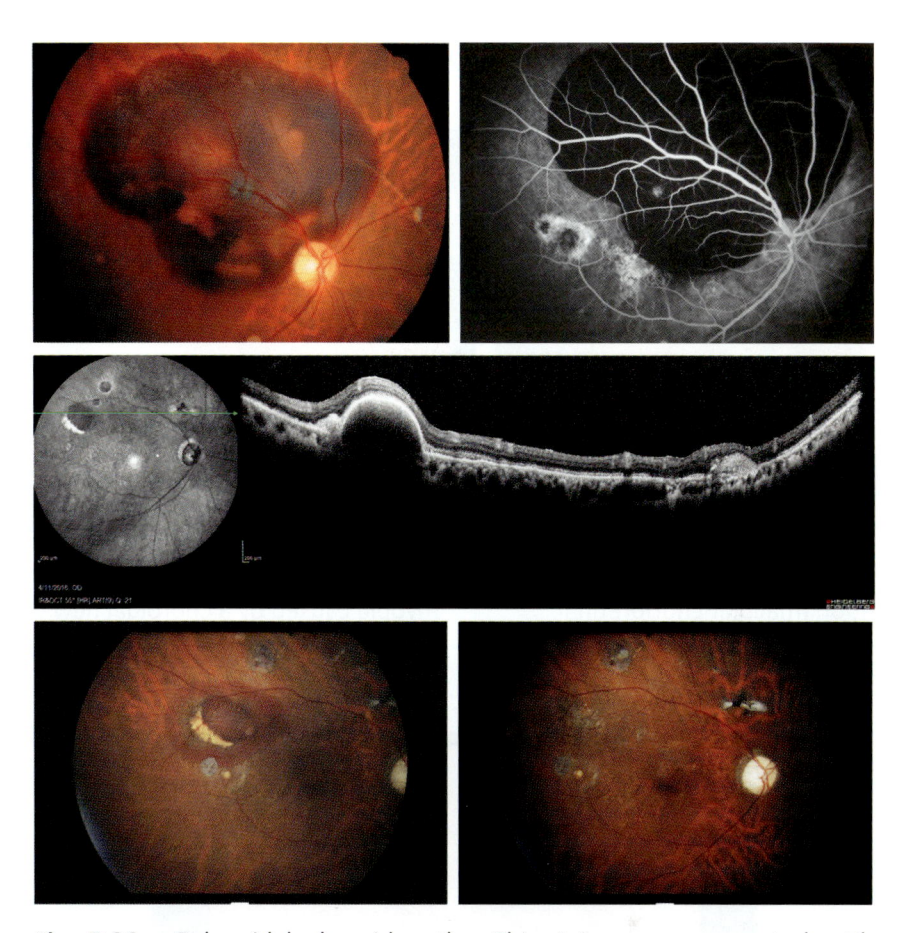

Fig. 7.36. Polypoidal choroidopathy. This Asian man presented with sudden vision loss due to subretinal haemorrhage. He was treated by vitrectomy and tissue plasminogen activator. A recurrent choroidal polyp two years later, shown on ICG angiography and OCT, was treated with photodynamic laser after intravenous verteporfin as well as anti-VEGF intravitreal injections.

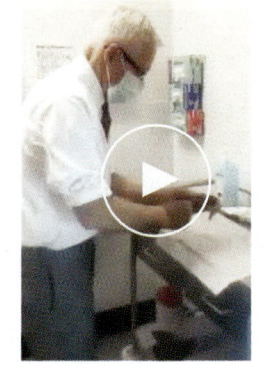

Video of intravitreal injection with anti-VEGF.

Myopic macular degeneration

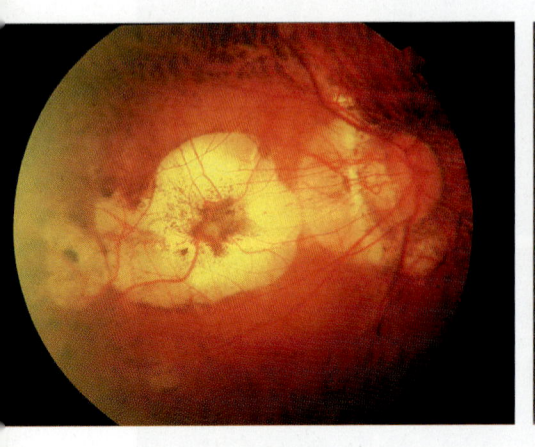

Fig. 7.37. Myopic macular degeneration (macular chorioretinal atrophy from high myopia).

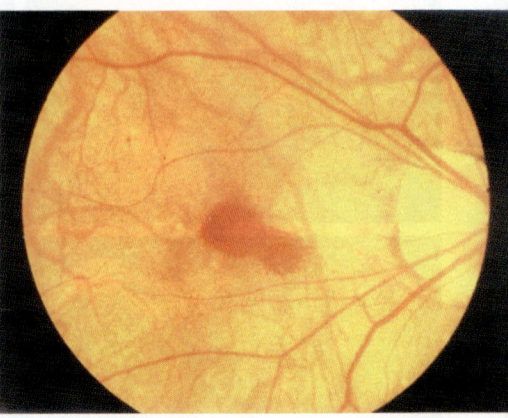

Fig. 7.38. Macular haemorrhage in high myopia caused by a choroidal new vessel. This needs anti-VEGF injection therapy.

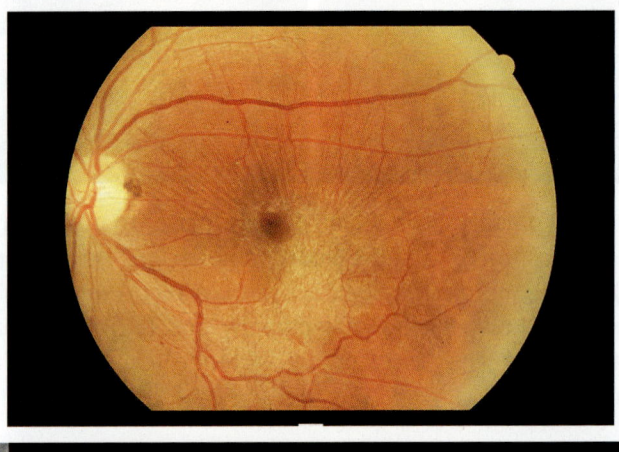

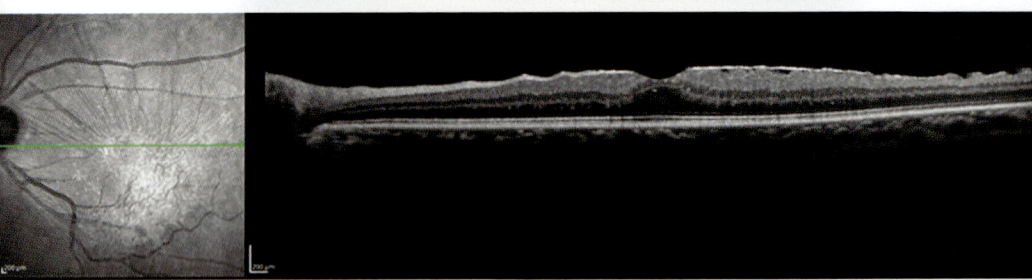

Fig. 7.39. Epiretinal membrane (premacular fibrosis). This causes distorted and blurred vision and may be peeled off during vitrectomy.

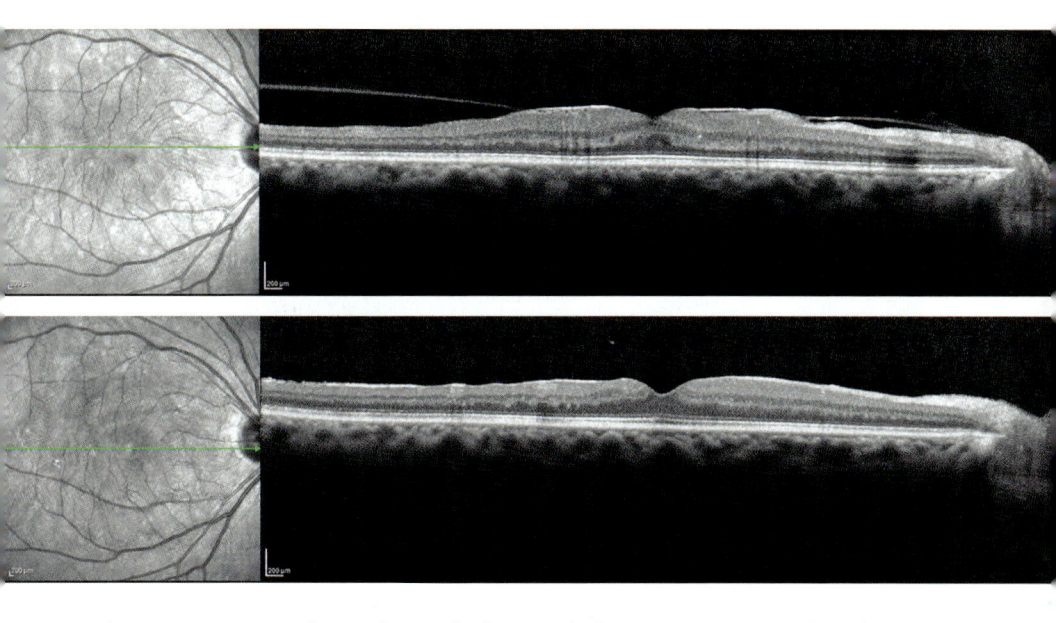

Fig. 7.40. Epiretinal membrane before and after vitrectomy and peeling.

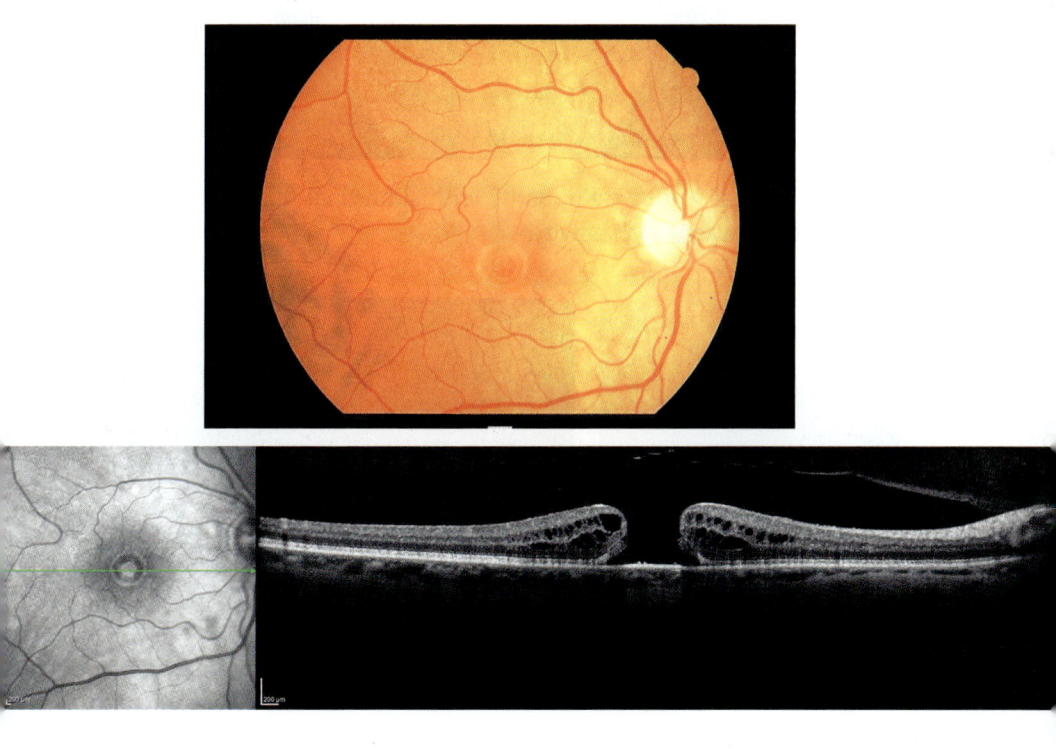

Fig. 7.41. Macular hole with OCT appearance.

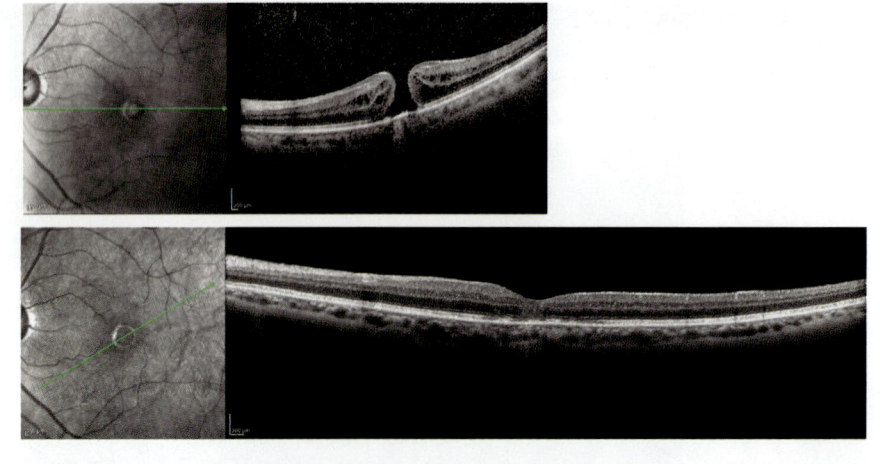

Fig. 7.42. Macular hole healed two weeks after vitrectomy, removal of the internal limiting membrane and gas exchange of the vitreous fluid.

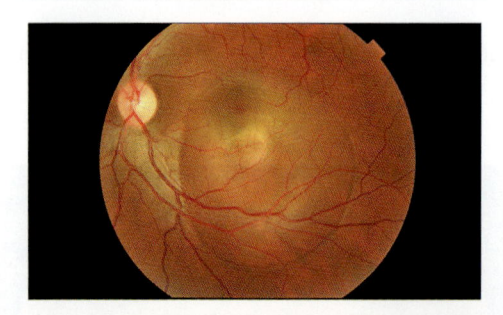

Fig. 7.43. Central serous retinopathy with subretinal fluid at the macula extending downwards with gravity.

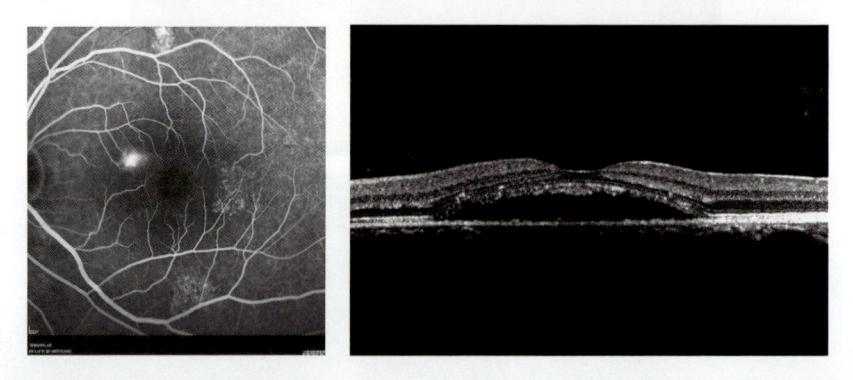

Fig. 7.44. Central serous chorioretinopathy showing a focal leak on FFA and subretinal fluid at the macula on OCT. The leak can be treated with focal laser if not healed after three months, providing that it is not too close to the fovea. Most cases heal without treatment.

Generalised Hereditary Retinal Dystrophies

Retinitis pigmentosa

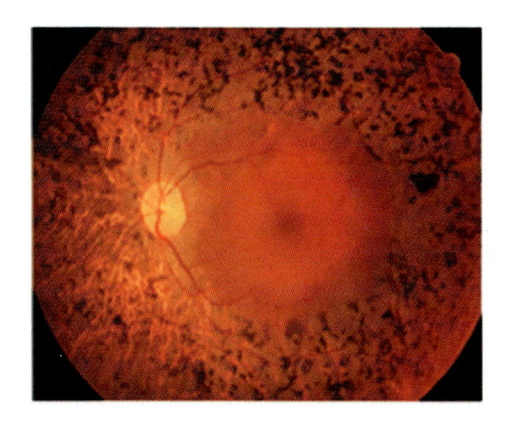

Fig. 7.45. Retinitis pigmentosa with peripheral pigment and retention of central 30° of the visual field.

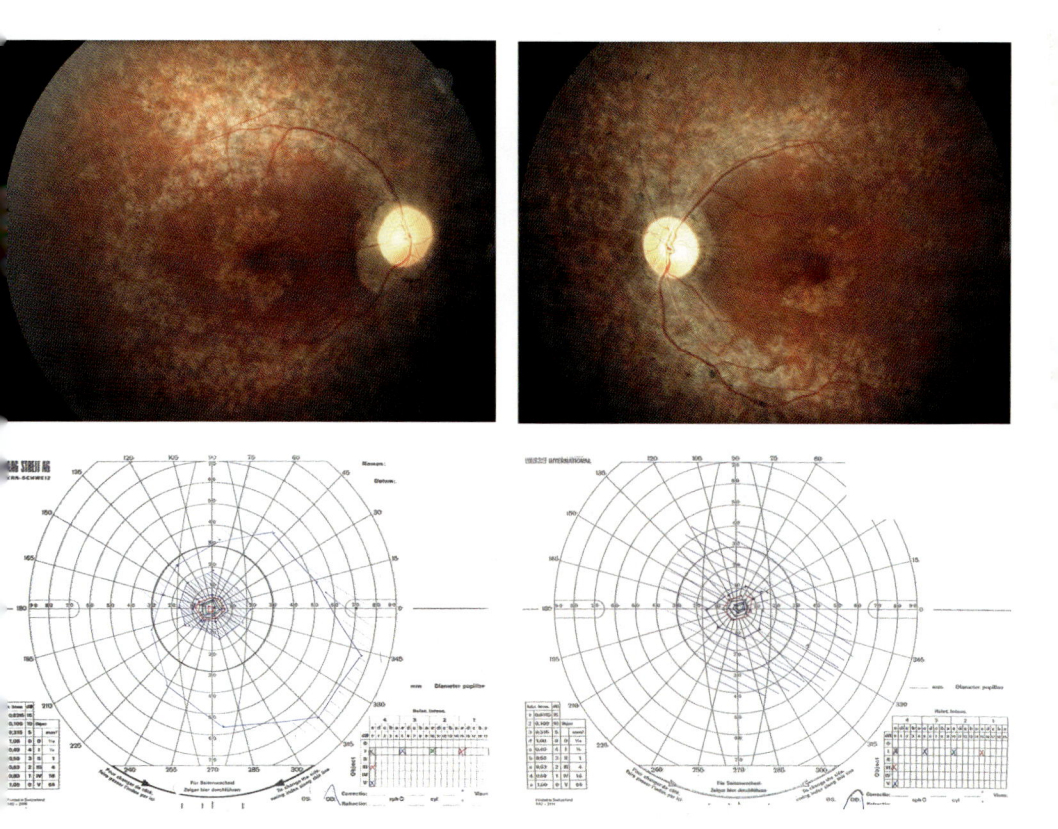

Fig. 7.46. Advanced retinitis pigmentosa with diffuse peripheral pigment clumping, pale optic discs and narrowed retinal blood vessels. Perimetry shows advanced visual field constriction.

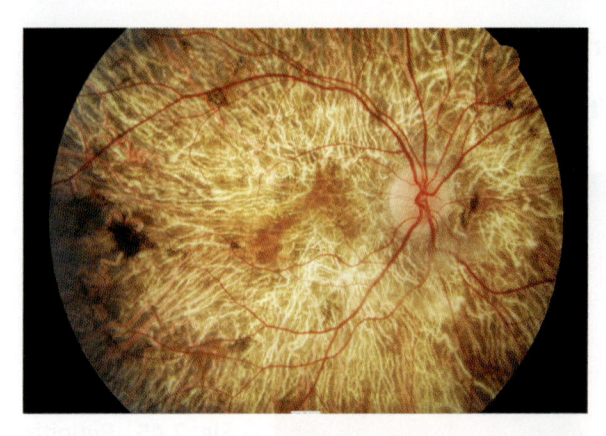

Fig. 7.47. X-linked choroideraemia. There is diffuse atrophy of the choroid and overlying retina, with a surviving island allowing some retention of central vision. Clinical trials of gene therapy show promise.

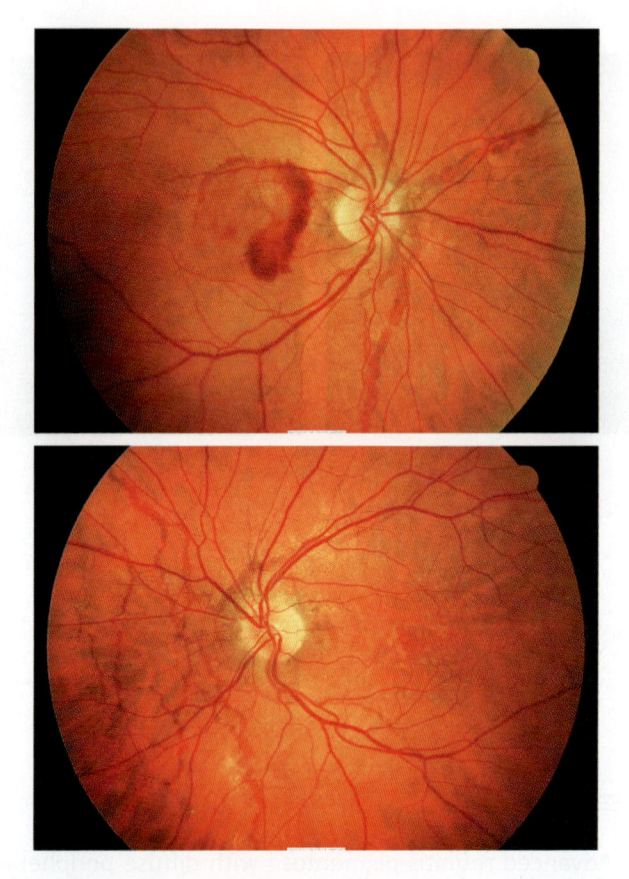

Fig. 7.48. Pseudoxanthoma elasticum with angioid streaks and a choroidal neovascular membrane in the right eye.

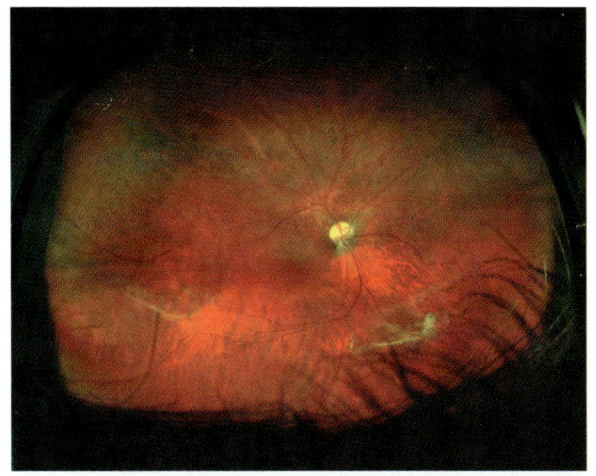

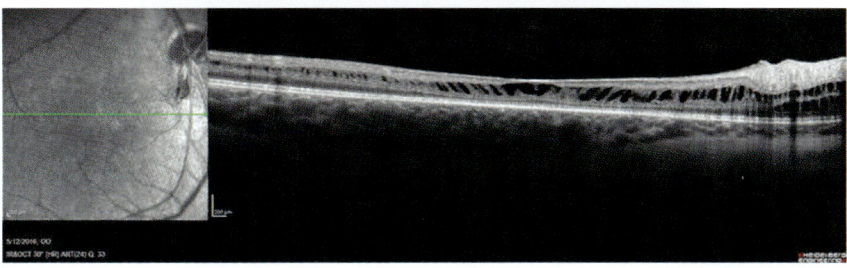

Fig. 7.49. X-linked juvenile retinoschisis with inferior and macular retinal splitting on OCT.

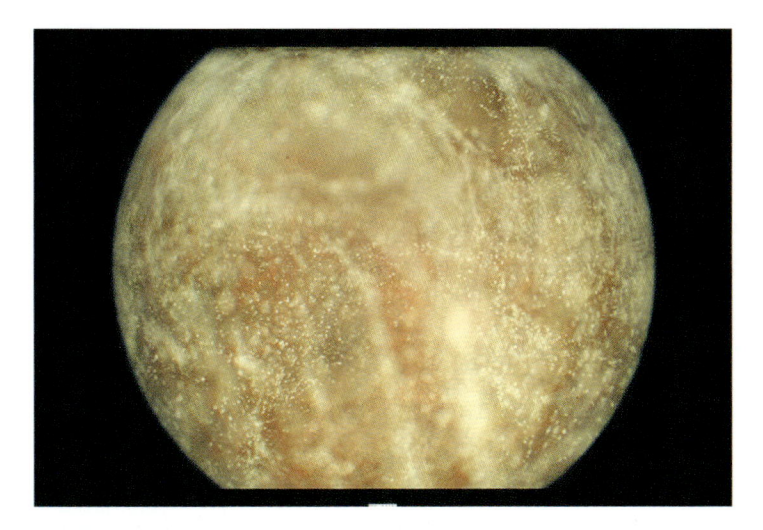

Fig. 7.50. Asteroid hyalosis. These vitreous opacities may prevent an ophthalmoscopic view of the retina but often have little effect on vision.

8
DIABETIC RETINOPATHY AND THE EYE IN SYSTEMIC DISEASES

INTRODUCTION

Many systemic diseases have ocular manifestations. The most important of these is diabetic retinopathy. Laser photocoagulation and anti-VEGF injections that prevent vessel growth and leakage protect against blindness in the majority of patients if treatment is started early.

Other systemic conditions affecting the eye include hypertension, thyroid and rheumatoid diseases. In some developing countries, keratomalacia (vitamin A deficiency) and onchocerciasis (filarial worm infection) are major causes of blindness.

DIABETES MELLITUS

Diabetes can cause a variety of ocular complications, of which the most important is diabetic retinopathy.

Refractive Changes

Blurring of vision in a diabetic patient is sometimes the result of refractive changes in the eye due to fluctuation in blood sugar levels. This occurs commonly when patients commence treatment. The patient should be assured that the refractive changes will stop once the blood glucose level is stabilised.

Extraocular Muscle Paralysis

Diabetes sometimes affects the third or sixth cranial nerve. A third cranial nerve lesion due to diabetes may be associated with a unilateral headache. The pupil is usually not affected. A painful third nerve palsy may also occur with a cerebral aneurysm which is life-threatening. Diabetic third and sixth nerve palsies usually resolve spontaneously within three months.

Pupil and Iris Abnormalities

Diabetic pupils may respond sluggishly to light or fail to dilate with mydriatic eye drops. Neovascularisation of the iris may develop (rubeosis iridis) in some patients with severe ischaemic or proliferative diabetic retinopathy, leading to neovascular glaucoma and blindness if untreated. Anti-VEGF injections, retinal laser and glaucoma surgery are required.

Cataract

Cataract develops more often in a person with diabetes and at a younger age. It may develop rapidly as a dense fluffy white cataract in a young diabetic person with severe uncontrolled diabetes but usually presents with cortical spoke-like opacities.

Ischaemic Optic Neuropathy

Ischaemic optic neuropathy in diabetics is an uncommon but serious cause of visual loss. It may present with an altitudinal hemianopia or loss of the whole visual field. There is no satisfactory treatment and the prognosis is poor.

DIABETIC RETINOPATHY

The most important ocular manifestation of diabetes is diabetic retinopathy. It is a major cause of blindness globally. It affects about 20–30% of people with diabetes.

Diabetic retinopathy develops because of local microvascular leakage and retinal ischaemia. The development is related to the duration of the disease (i.e. the length of time for which the patient has diabetes). Other contributing factors are poor hyperglycaemic control, hypertension, hyperlipidaemia and smoking. In recent years, with better medical treatment, people with diabetes have lived longer and the cumulative prevalence of diabetic retinopathy has increased.

Classification of Diabetic Retinopathy

1. Non-proliferative diabetic retinopathy
2. Proliferative diabetic retinopathy
3. Diabetic maculopathy (macular oedema)

Non-proliferative or background diabetic retinopathy

The classic signs include characteristic red spots, retinal microaneurysms or round dot haemorrhages, and hard exudates. The hard exudates appear as small, yellow, well-defined deposits. These are usually multiple and scattered. They may become more extensive later and form large confluent patches.

Mild non-proliferative diabetic retinopathy consists of a few microaneurysms.

Mild diabetic retinopathy may progress slowly over the years. The majority of the patients do not lose their central vision.

As the disease progresses to the moderate stage, more extensive microaneurysms, haemorrhages and hard exudates appear.

In severe non-proliferative retinopathy (preproliferative diabetic retinopathy), vascular obstructive changes are seen. These obstructive features include cotton wool spots (soft exudates), larger blot haemorrhages, dilated or segmented veins and venous loops. These changes indicate more severe ischaemic retinal damage, and fluorescein angiography shows patchy loss of the capillary circulation.

Proliferative diabetic retinopathy

The most severe type of diabetic retinopathy is known as proliferative diabetic retinopathy, which occurs in about 10% of patients with diabetic retinopathy. This must be recognised early, as severe visual loss and blindness can ensue rapidly.

The classic sign of proliferative retinopathy is the appearance of new blood vessels which grow on the retinal surface and at the optic disc. They are fragile and tend to bleed into the vitreous. In the late stage, fibrous scar tissue formation may lead to traction retinal detachment and blindness.

Diabetic macular oedema (maculopathy)

A major cause of visual impairment in people with diabetes is the development of retinopathic changes in the macula, a condition known as diabetic macular oedema (maculopathy). Diabetic macular oedema can develop at any stage of diabetic retinopathy but is more common in patients at the more severe stages. Depending on the amount of haemorrhage and exudate, the degree of oedema and capillary loss at the macula, vision loss can be severe.

Prognosis

The visual prognosis depends on the type and severity of the retinopathy. Most patients with mild non-proliferative diabetic retinopathy do not develop visual loss. In patients with ischaemic signs, diabetic macular oedema or proliferative diabetic retinopathy, the visual outlook is worse. The presence of diabetic retinopathy, especially proliferative diabetic retinopathy, usually reflects the general state of the vascular health of the patients, and they may have renal disease, ischaemic cardiac and cerebral complications, ischaemic foot ulcers or peripheral neuropathy.

Management

Screening of diabetic retinopathy

As the early retinal changes can be easily missed, the fundus of all persons with diabetes should be regularly examined, with the pupils dilated. With advances in digital retinal photography, diabetic retinopathy screening may include routine colour fundus photography and review with intelligent software or via telemedicine. All diabetics should have a retinal screen every one to two years.

Systemic management

All diabetics without fundal changes require strict metabolic control and dietary advice to delay or prevent the development of vision loss from diabetic retinopathy and other complications. Patients already with diabetic retinopathy require an expert analysis of their diet and lifestyle, as well as improved metabolic control. The three most important risk factors to control are blood glucose levels, blood pressure and lipid levels. Adequate control of these risk factors may prevent deterioration of the retinopathy. The presence of retinopathy should be regarded as a warning that the control of these risk factors may have been sub-optimal over an extended period of time.

Ocular management

Ophthalmic assessment should include colour fundus photography and assessment of maculopathy using optical coherence tomography (OCT). Fluorescein angiography is important for evaluating the ocular circulation and extent of retinal involvement.

Laser photocoagulation and anti-VEGF intravitreal injections can prevent severe vision loss in over 90% of eyes with diabetic retinopathy, providing that treatment starts before it becomes irreversible.

Laser Photocoagulation

A laser photocoagulator produces an intense green light (argon laser or frequency-doubled YAG) which is focused on the retinal pigment epithelium, where the absorbed light is converted to heat. The resulting small chorioretinal burns coagulate ischaemic retinal tissue and reduce hypoxia-induced VEGF production.

Laser photocoagulation is effective in preventing blindness due to diabetic retinopathy. It can be carried out in the presence of diabetic retinal oedema that does not involve the fovea, or severe non-proliferative and proliferative diabetic retinopathy. In severe non-proliferative and proliferative diabetic retinopathy, more extensive photocoagulation (known as panretinal photocoagulation) is necessary in order to prevent vitreous haemorrhage and traction retinal detachment.

Anti-Vascular Endothelial Growth Factor (VEGF) Therapy

When diabetic retinal oedema involves the central macular area and there is vision loss, intravitreal injection of anti-VEGF agents (aflibercept, ranibizumab or bevacizumab) have been shown to achieve better visual outcomes than with laser alone. Intravitreal injections are given monthly until the macula is dry and then at increasing intervals. Each eye may require up to 12 injections over 2 years, as well as supplementary peripheral laser.

Anti-VEGF injections are also used for proliferative diabetic retinopathy, especially with vitreous haemorrhage in the absence of scar tissue traction. Laser PRP is then usually also required to prevent recurrence.

Diabetic Vitrectomy

Diabetic vitrectomy is indicated for non-clearing or recurrent vitreous haemorrhage, or for tractional retinal detachment. It is usually combined with retinal laser and anti-VEGF injection.

HYPERTENSION

Hypertension primarily affects the retinal arterioles. In young patients, the reaction of arterioles to moderately raised blood pressure is constriction. The ophthalmic signs are either diffuse or focal narrowing, or constriction of the arterioles.

In middle-aged patients, however, the walls of the arterioles become hardened and thickened (arteriosclerosis) and are unable to constrict. The thickened walls show a widening of the normal light reflex. As the thickening of the wall progresses, it gives a copper appearance to the blood column (copper wiring) and then a white appearance (silver wiring). At the arteriovenous crossings, the thickened arteriolar walls displace and constrict the veins (arteriovenous nipping). These changes are common in middle-aged patients with chronic hypertension. They may lead to a branch retinal vein occlusion.

In more severe hypertension, the arteriolar wall is damaged by necrosis, leading to leakage, and classic signs include flame-shaped haemorrhages and cotton wool spots caused by microinfarcts of the retina. Sometimes retinal oedema is present. Chronic retinal oedema at the macula results in hard exudates radiating from the macula (macular star). Finally, optic disc swelling (papilloedema) may develop. When this happens, the patient has malignant hypertension. Vision is usually normal except when there is associated macular involvement.

Hypertensive Retinopathy

Many attempts have been made to classify hypertensive retinopathy, and a simplified version of the Keith–Wagner classification is described below.

Mild hypertensive retinopathy

In young patients with mild hypertension, minimum narrowing and constriction and irregularity of the arterioles are found. In older hypertensives, however, there is often no arteriolar constriction but a widening of the light reflex of the arterioles because of the thickened sclerotic arteriolar wall. The retinal veins at the arteriovenous crossings appear constricted and are described ophthalmoscopically as arteriovenous nipping.

Moderate hypertensive retinopathy

At this stage, superficial flame-shaped haemorrhages appear near the disc with cotton wool spots. The retina is oedematous. Occasionally, small hard exudates may also appear.

Malignant or accelerated hypertensive retinopathy

Papilloedema is an ominous sign of malignant hypertension. When retinal oedema is substantial and prolonged, small hard exudates collect together and radiate from the macula in a characteristic star-shaped formation.

Significance

The significance of hypertensive retinopathy is that the retinal signs reflect the severity of the hypertension and the state of the arterioles elsewhere in the body. Patients with hypertensive retinopathy are at a higher risk for stroke, congestive heart failure and cardiovascular death. Thus, good blood pressure control is indicated in these patients. Furthermore, when the fundal changes are reversed, it serves as a good indication of the control of the hypertension.

Pre-Eclamptic Hypertension

In pre-eclamptic toxaemia or hypertension of pregnancy, there is a marked spasm of the arterioles as they are not sclerotic in young patients. All the more severe signs of hypertension may be superimposed. The condition is frequently associated with bilateral exudative inferior retinal detachment.

OTHER VASCULAR RETINOPATHIES

Severe anaemia is frequently associated with retinopathy that includes flame-shaped haemorrhages and cotton wool spots. The retinopathy has no unique features and is common in other conditions where there is an associated platelet deficiency, such as in pernicious anaemia and leukaemia.

Hyperviscosity retinopathy occurs in any condition which increases the blood viscosity, such as hyperglobulinaemia, multiple myeloma and polycythaemia vera. The retinal veins are engorged and are associated with retinal haemorrhages, cotton wool spots and oedema. The fundus appearance is very similar to that found in central retinal vein occlusion.

Sickle cell anaemia is a hereditary condition (SS or SC haemoglobin) common in African populations. Thalassaemia is another hereditary haemoglobinopathy, with retinal manifestations if homozygous. Occlusion of small vessels in the retinal periphery and ischaemia lead to capillary non-perfusion, neovascularisation, haemorrhages and fibrovascular proliferation. This may give a characteristic sea fan appearance. Localised peripheral chorioretinal scars are also characteristic of the condition. Vision may be lost from vitreous haemorrhage or traction retinal detachment but this may be prevented with laser photocoagulation.

Eales disease. Peripheral retinal vasculitis with vitreous haemorrhage (Eales disease) is characterised by recurrent vitreous haemorrhages associated with abnormalities of the peripheral retinal veins. This condition occurs particularly in young adult males who are otherwise well. The cause is unknown but has been thought to be due to sensitisation to tuberculosis. Photocoagulation or cryotherapy of the abnormal retinal vessels can prevent recurrent vitreous haemorrhage. Blindness from vitreous haemorrhage can be reversed in many cases by vitrectomy.

THYROID DISEASE

Hyperthyroidism (Graves' Disease)

Hyperthyroidism is associated with lid retraction and lid lag, and sometimes with proptosis and exophthalmos. The eyelid signs may be unilateral or bilateral. Bilateral lid retraction gives a typical staring appearance. Other signs of thyrotoxicosis include poor convergence and infrequent blinking.

Thyroid eye disease and exophthalmos

Thyroid eye disease may develop with or without hyperthyroidism, or following treatment for hyperthyroidism. The ocular signs are exophthalmos with oedema of the lids and conjunctiva. Sometimes there is restriction of ocular movement, particularly for elevation. As a result, the patient is unable to look upwards. Although the exophthalmos is usually bilateral, it can be unilateral. A CT scan is useful for diagnosis. It helps to differentiate a unilateral exophthalmos from that of a retrobulbar space-occupying lesion (e.g. orbital tumour) and it usually shows typical thickened extraocular muscles.

Complications

Severe thyroid exophthalmos may lead to difficulty in closing the eyelids, a condition known as lagophthalmos. This may cause exposure keratitis with corneal dryness, ulceration and infection. The increased intraorbital pressure due to infiltrative tissue may also cause glaucoma and damage the optic nerve.

Treatment

Hyperthyroidism should be treated. High doses of oral steroids may control the progressive exophthalmos. Surgery may be necessary to protect the cornea or to decompress the orbit. Surgical correction of diplopia is often necessary after the disease has burnt itself out.

AIDS (Acquired Immunodeficiency Syndrome)

See Chapter 6, page 100.

INFECTION AND MALNUTRITION

In developing countries, infection and nutritional diseases including onchocerciasis and keratomalacia are major causes of blindness. Their eradication depends on dealing with the problems of poverty and poor living conditions, diet and health education at the community level with the help of thousands of paramedics.

Keratomalacia (Vitamin A Deficiency)

Keratomalacia is an acute condition of the cornea due to vitamin A deficiency in the child. It is frequently precipitated by a gastrointestinal upset. It starts with xerosis (dryness of the conjunctiva) and may lead to melting and perforation of the cornea (keratomalacia). It has been estimated that a quarter of a million children in the world are blinded annually by this condition. This tragedy is now mitigated with better vitamin A supplementation in the diet (e.g. vitamin A-fortified rice).

Onchocerciasis (River Blindness)

This major blinding condition is due to invasion by microfilariae resulting from the bite of the jinja fly, which is common in parts of West Africa. The eye complications include iritis, secondary glaucoma, cataract and vitreoretinal damage. Blindness is common in the affected communities. The condition is prevented by the elimination of the vector fly. This is unfortunately not always possible. Treatment of the established condition with antihelminthic drugs or surgery does not restore vision. The drug ivermectin, which is donated by Merck, Sharp and Dohme has helped control this disease in many African countries.

Leprosy

This chronic bacterial infection of the skin and peripheral nerves affects the eye in 30% of the cases but most of the ocular complications are not serious. The facial nerve may be involved, resulting in paralysis of the orbicularis oculi muscle, ectropion and lagophthalmos, leading to exposure keratitis. There may also be madarosis (loss of eyebrows and eyelashes). Keratitis and anterior uveitis are uncommon.

Syphilis

This sexually transmitted infection may affect the eye at all stages of the disease. At the primary stage, the lesion rarely occurs on the eyelid or conjunctiva. At the secondary stage, it may cause uveitis. Optic atrophy occurs as a complication of tertiary syphilis. In congenital syphilis, bilateral interstitial keratitis and chorioretinal scars may develop.

Tuberculosis

Many inflammatory ocular conditions, including scleritis, uveitis and chorioretinitis, are said to be associated with a focal tuberculous infection. However, it is difficult to interpret the significance of positive tuberculous serology and Mantoux skin test in the absence of chest X-ray abnormalities because of the high frequency of positive tests and cross sensitivity to bovine tuberculosis in many developing countries.

RHEUMATOID ARTHRITIS

Rheumatoid arthritis can affect the eyes in several ways. It may cause persistent irritation and redness on account of dry eyes. Episcleritis is also a common cause of localised redness of the eyes in rheumatoid patients. Scleritis may be localised, nodular or diffuse. If it is severe, there is necrosis of the sclera, known as scleromalacia.

Treatment of rheumatoid arthritis may cause eye problems too. Long-term chloroquine use can cause maculopathy and serious visual loss, as well as minor corneal deposits. Cataract may develop with long-term systemic steroid therapy. Systemic immunosuppressive drugs (e.g. methotrexate) may be required in these cases to reduce steroid dependence.

MUCOCUTANEOUS DISEASES

Acne Rosacea

This may cause chronic conjunctivitis or blepharitis, which requires management with ocular lubricants and oral doxycycline. Severe bilateral superficial keratitis with corneal vascularisation may result in a central corneal opacity with loss of vision. Treatment then involves the use of steroid eye drops. Acne rosacea is more common among Caucasians.

Stevens–Johnson Syndrome

This is an acute inflammatory eruption of the skin and mucous membranes. It is sometimes caused by a severe reaction to a drug. The patient requires intensive care management of fluid balance in the acute stage. The most common ocular manifestation is severe keratoconjunctivitis, which may result in corneal vascularisation and scarring with dry eyes and corneal opacity. Treatment with artificial tears, contact lenses and oculoplastic surgical procedures may help but some patients become blind. Dramatic surgical recovery of vision has been achieved with an osteo-odonto-keratoprosthesis in a number of these blind patients.

Ear, Nose and Throat Conditions

Infection of the paranasal sinuses may lead to orbital cellulitis. This condition requires systemic antibiotics and sometimes surgical drainage of an orbital abscess localised by CT scan.

Occasionally, unilateral proptosis develops from a mucocele of a periorbital air sinus or from infiltration of the orbit by nasopharyngeal carcinoma, a common condition in the Chinese.

DIABETIC RETINOPATHY

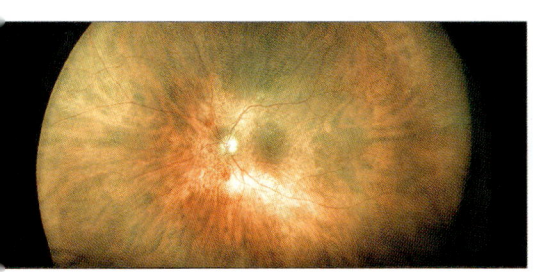

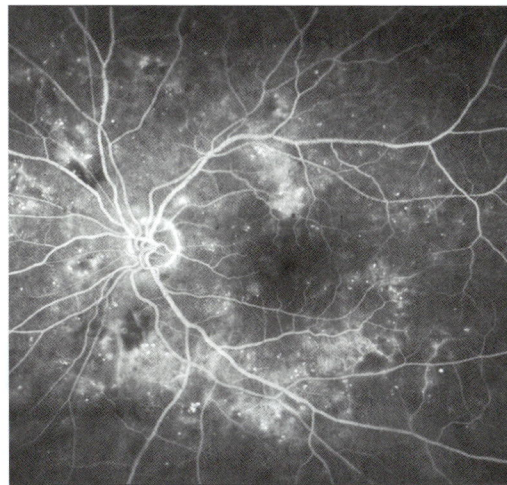

Fig. 8.1. Early background diabetic retinopathy. The wide-angle pseudo-colour image shows only minimal changes. The FA, however, shows extensive leaking microaneurysms and early capillary non-perfusion.

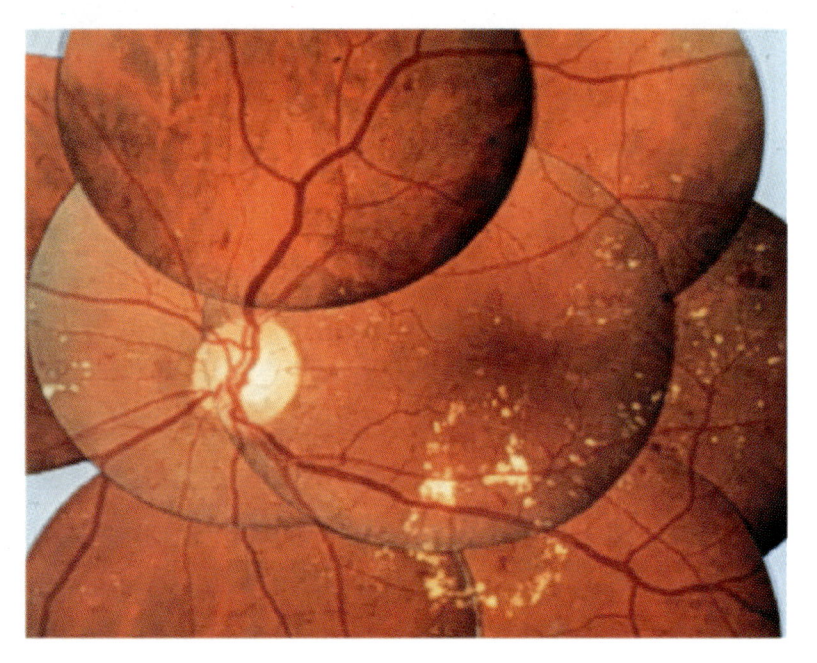

Fig. 8.2. Background diabetic retinopathy showing scattered exudates and haemorrhages near the fovea. Normal vision (6/6). Laser photocoagulation is indicated.

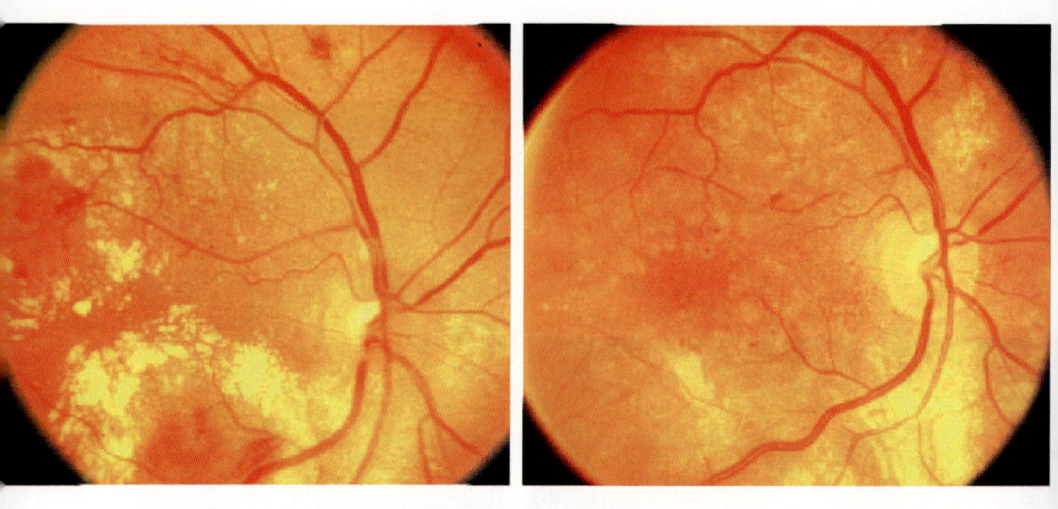

Fig. 8.3. Advanced background diabetic retinopathy before and after laser.

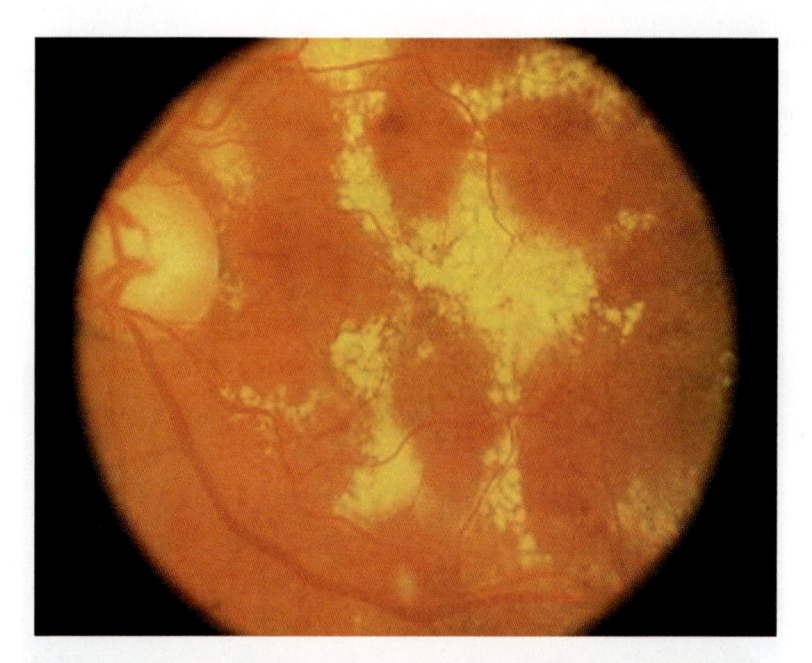

Fig. 8.4. Background diabetic retinopathy with severe maculopathy. Hard exudates at the macula. Vision 6/60. Central vision is permanently lost.

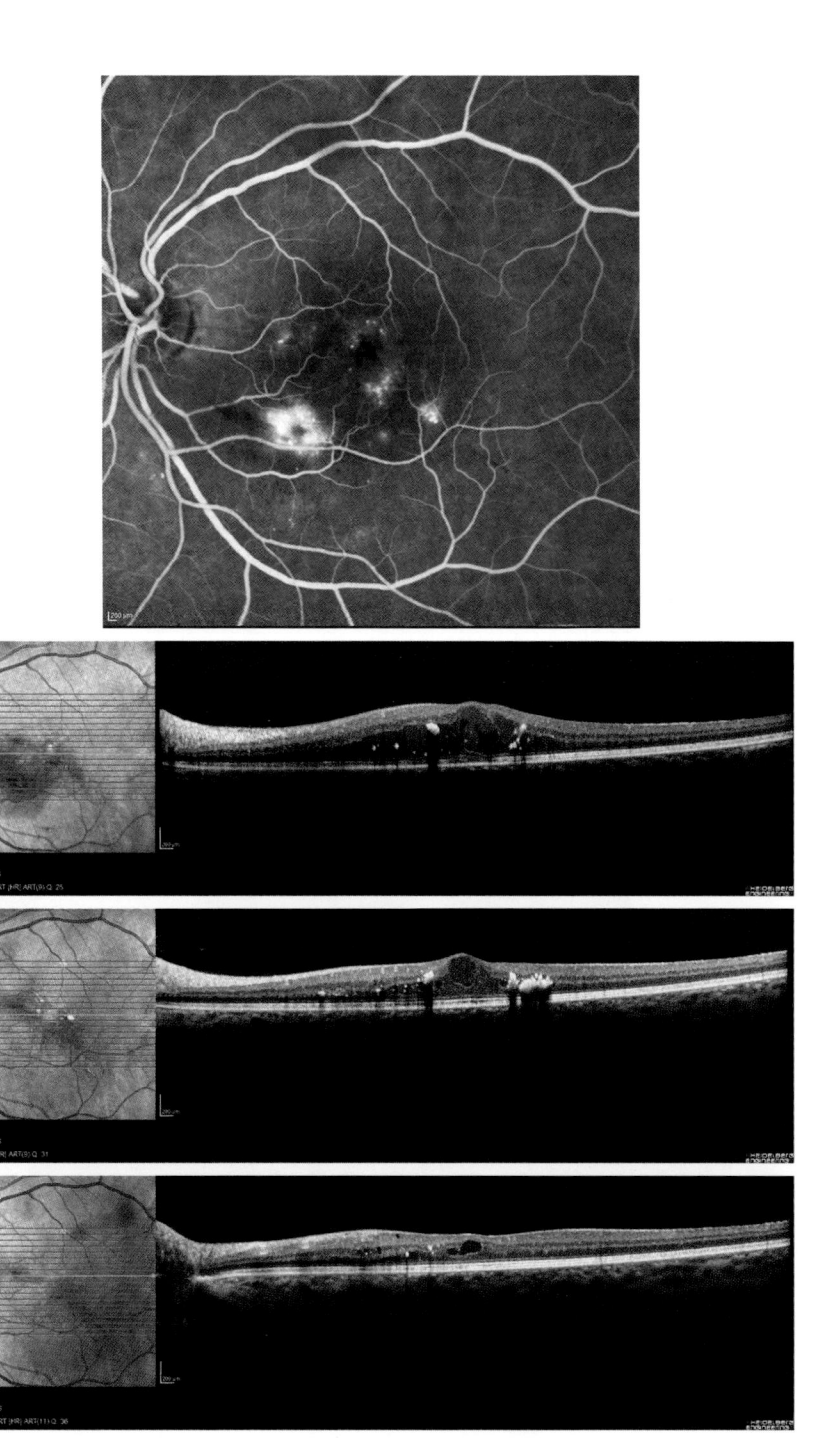

Fig. 8.5. Diabetic macular oedema with progressive decrease in swelling on OCT after 6 injections of bevacizumab over 12 months.

Proliferative Diabetic Retinopathy

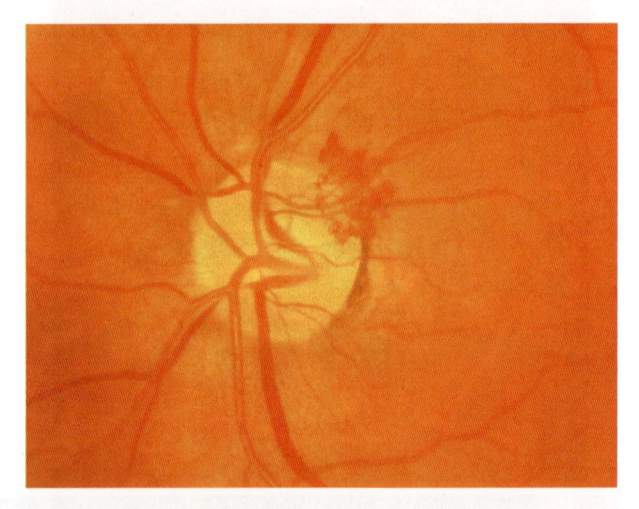

Fig. 8.6. Proliferative diabetic retinopathy with disc neovascularisation. Vision 6/6. Intravitreal anti-VEGF therapy and laser panretinal photocoagulation are indicated.

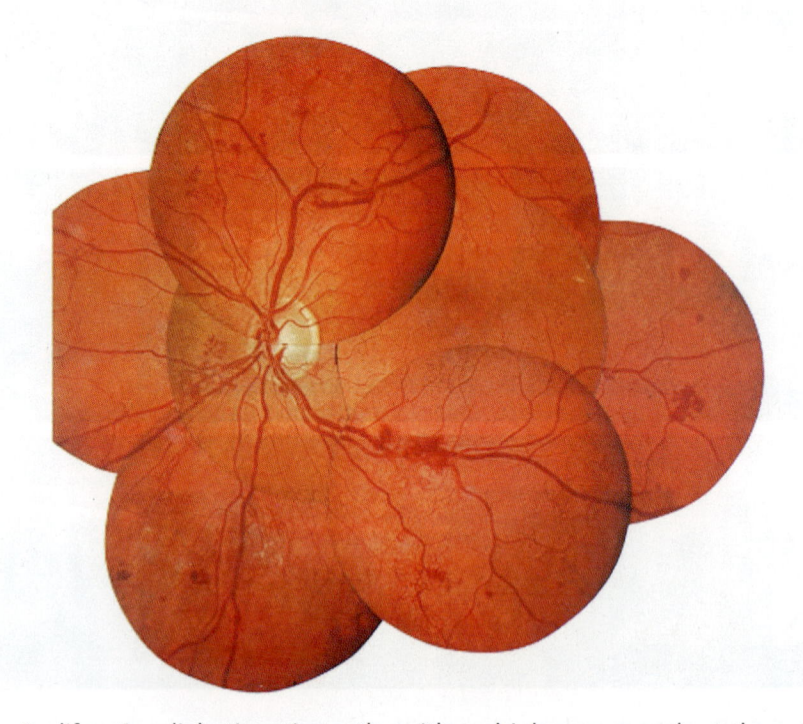

Fig. 8.7. Proliferative diabetic retinopathy with multiple new vessels at the optic disc and retina, with early vitreous haemorrhage. The eye is in danger of becoming blind and requires laser photocoagulation.

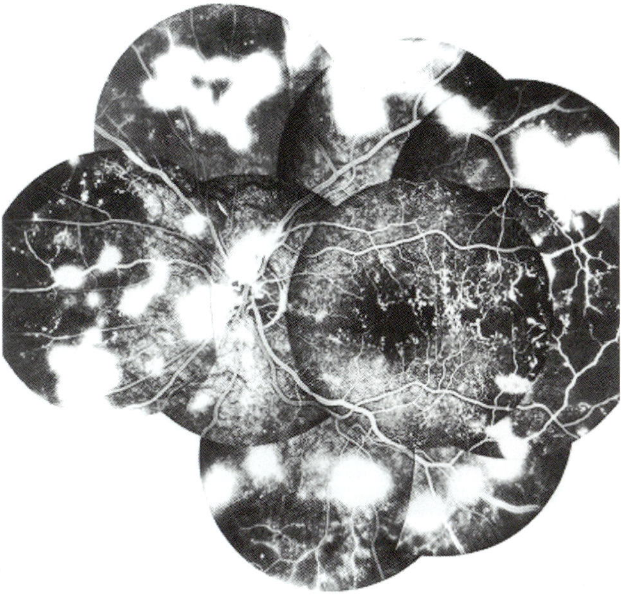

Fig. 8.8. Fluorescein angiography showing extensive dye leakage from new vessels at the optic disc and retinal periphery and areas of capillary non-perfusion. This shows the importance of angiography in evaluation of severity as retinopathy is sometimes not obvious with ophthalmoscopy.

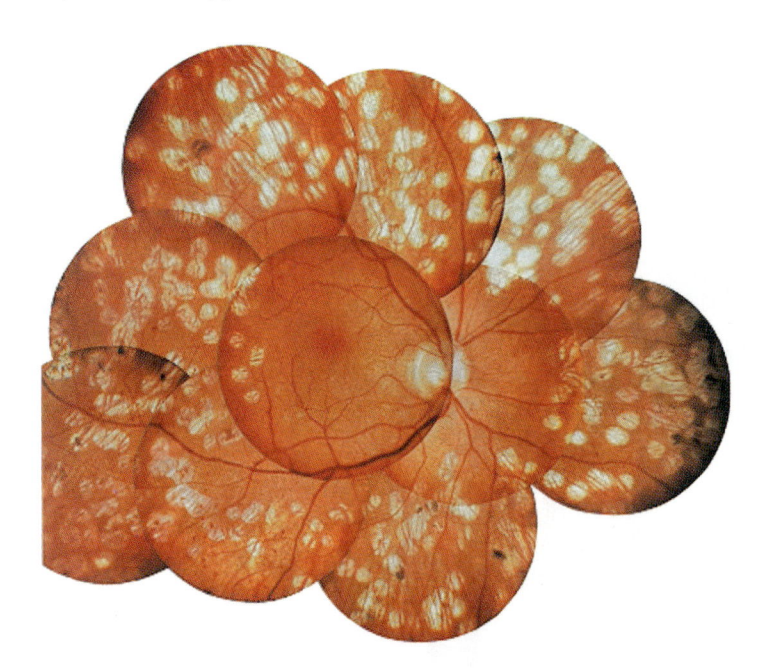

Fig. 8.9. Fully regressed diabetic retinopathy following panretinal photocoagulation.

Fluorescein Angiography in Diabetic Retinopathy

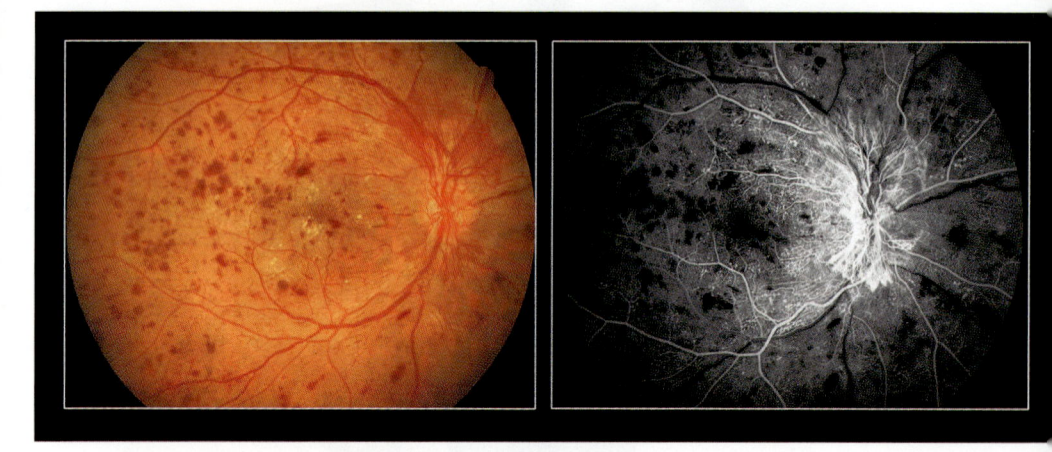

Fig. 8.10. Aggressive diabetic neovascularisation and widespread retinal haemorrhages. This patient requires urgent intravitreal anti-VEGF injections and then panretinal laser photocoagulation.

Anti-VEGF injections combined with photocoagulation and good metabolic control prevents more than 90% of cases of blindness resulting from diabetic retinopathy.

Photocoagulation

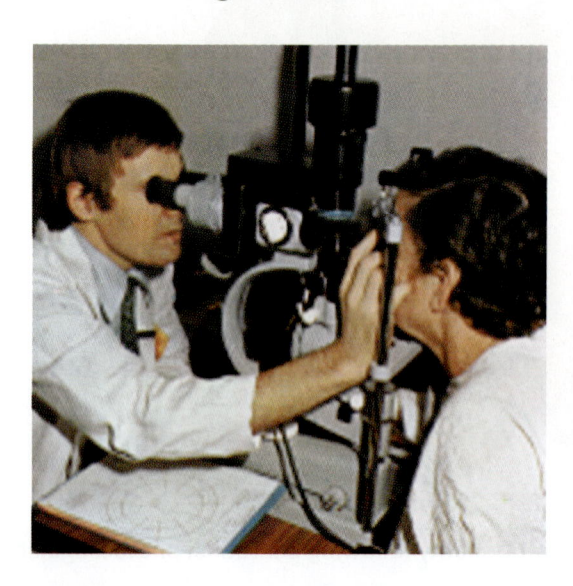

Fig. 8.11. Laser photocoagulation.

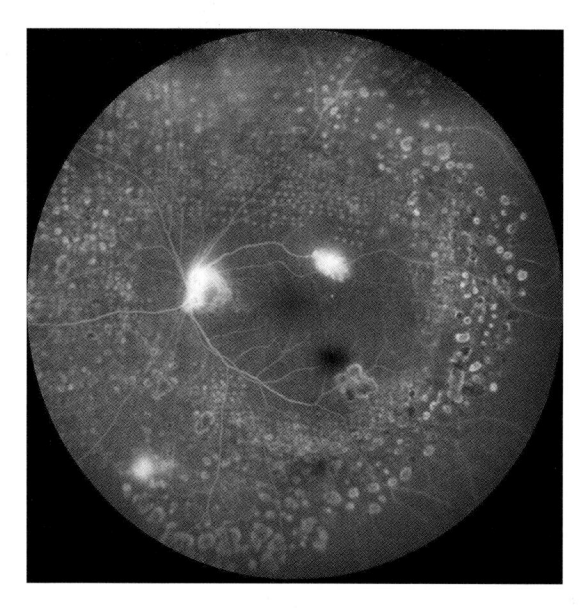

Fig. 8.12. Persisting proliferative diabetic retinopathy with leaks from new vessels on FA despite extensive laser. Further laser or anti-VEGF injections are required.

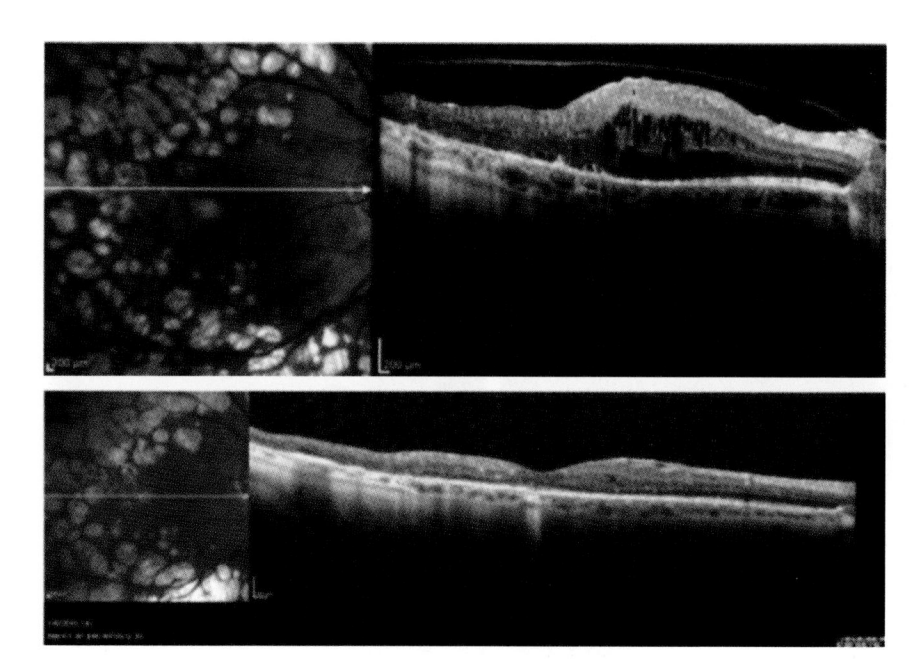

Fig. 8.13. Persistent macular oedema on OCT despite extensive laser PRP. The macula is dry after several aflibercept injections in the vitreous.

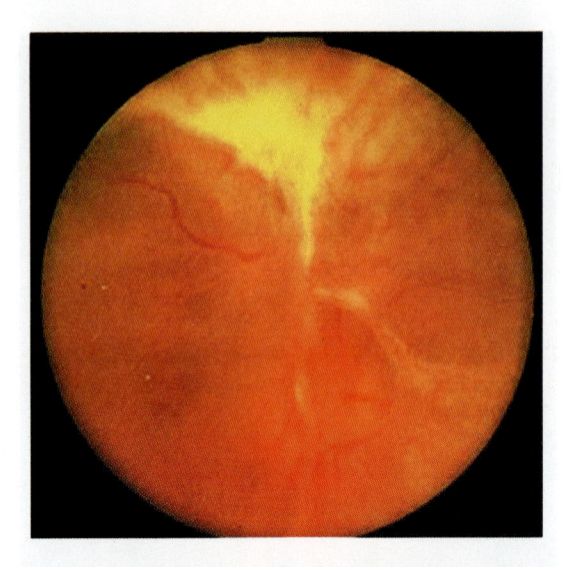

Fig. 8.14. Advanced proliferative diabetic retinopathy with traction retinal detachment resulting from preretinal scar tissue. Vision: hand movement. Too late for laser treatment. Vitrectomy with release of scar tissue traction and then laser and anti-VEGF injection may restore some vision.

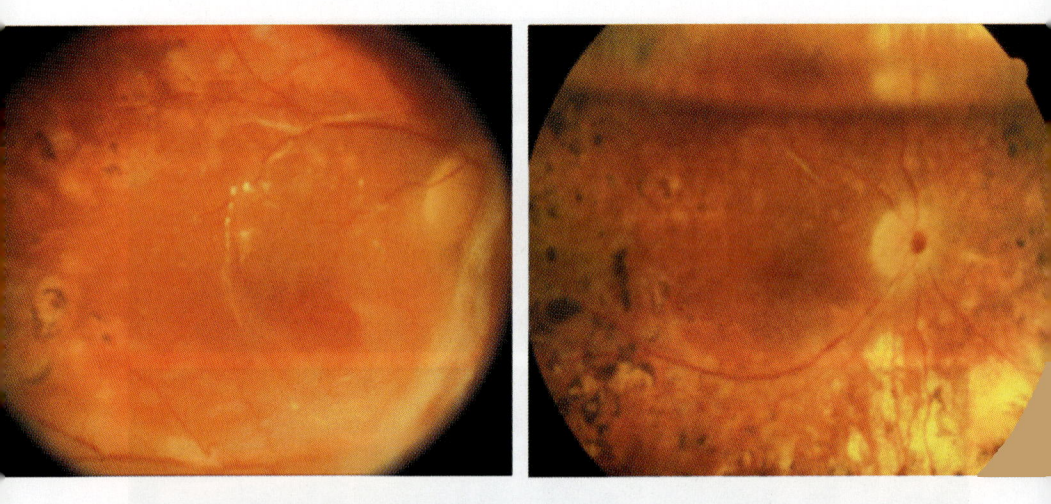

Fig. 8.15. Diabetic traction retinal detachment and appearance after vitrectomy, which cleared out the fibrotic membranes.

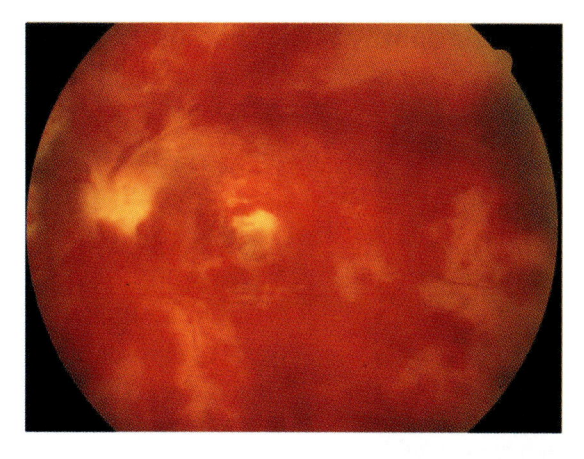

Fig. 8.16. Diabetic vitreous haemorrhage. Unable to laser. Treated with an anti-VEGF injection followed by vitrectomy.

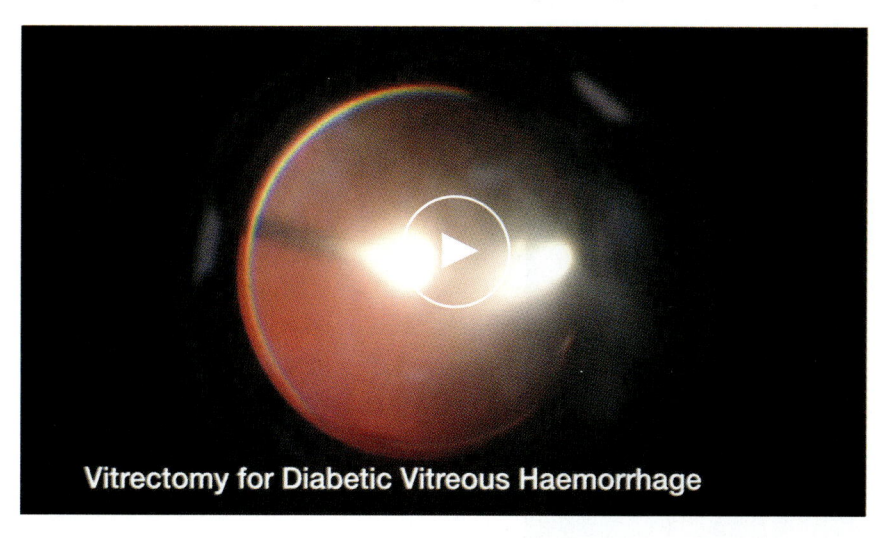

(See video.)

Hypertensive Retinopathy

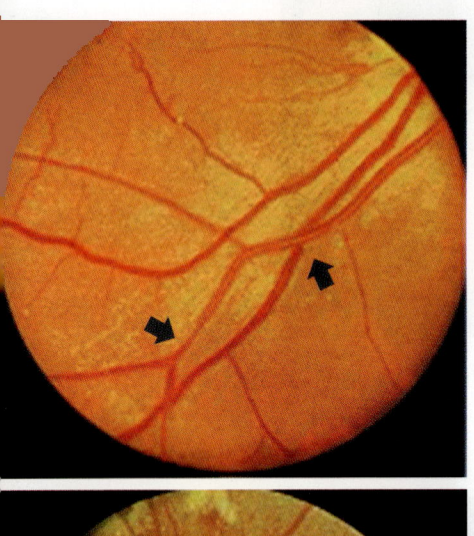

Fig. 8.17. Mild hypertensive retinopathy with focal narrowing of the artery and arteriovenous nipping.

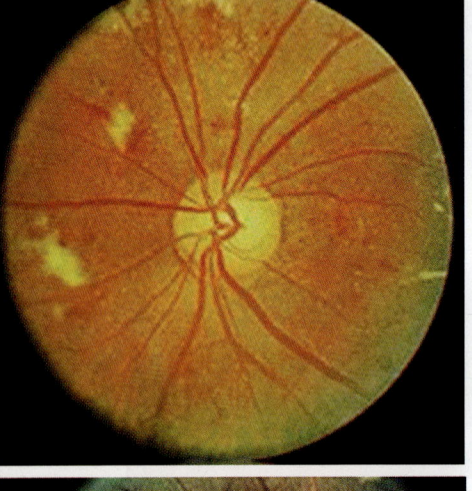

Fig. 8.18. Moderate hypertensive retinopathy with soft exudates, oedema and haemorrhages.

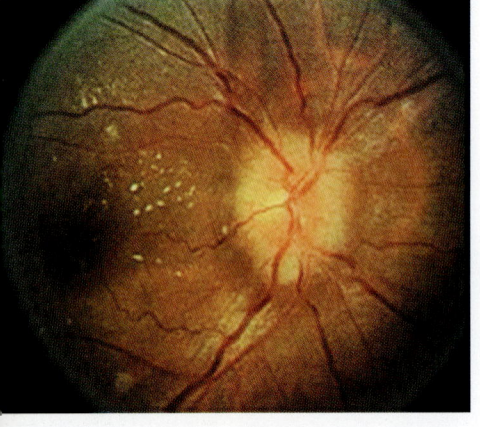

Fig. 8.19. Severe hypertensive retinopathy with papilloedema (malignant hypertension).

Other Vascular Retinopathies

Fig. 8.20. Non-specific retinal haemorrhages with soft exudates seen in severe anaemia.

Fig. 8.21. Fibrovascular proliferation ("sea fan") at the retinal periphery seen in sickle cell retinopathy.

Fig. 8.22. Engorged and tortuous retinal veins and haemorrhages seen in hyperviscosity retinopathy. The appearance is similar to that of central retinal vein occlusion.

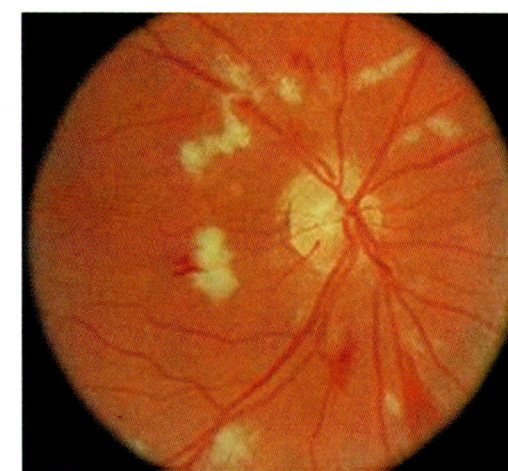

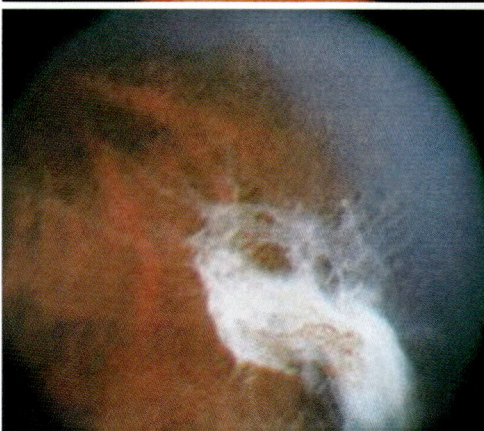

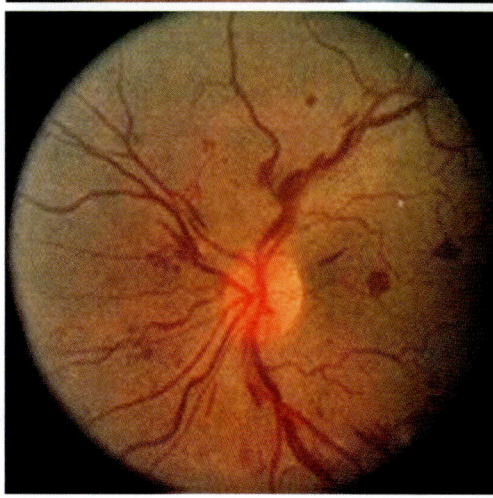

Thyroid Eye Disease

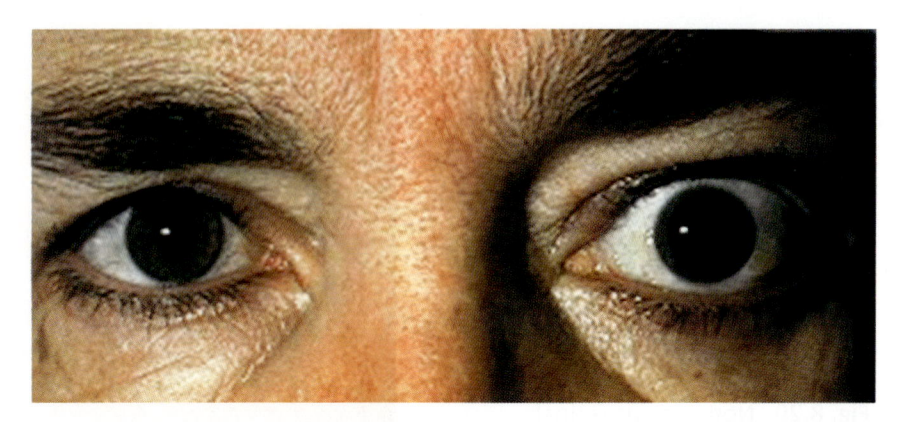

Fig. 8.23. Unilateral left exophthalmos with lid retraction.

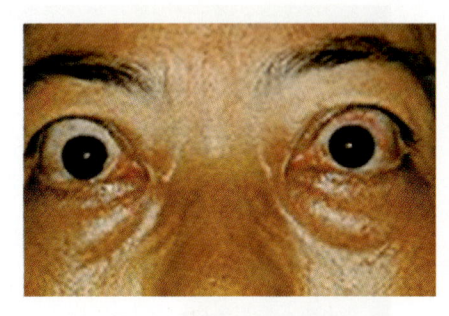

Fig. 8.24. Bilateral exophthalmos with marked lid retraction.

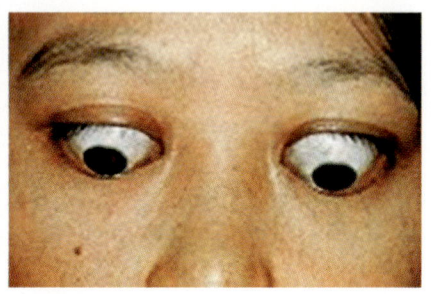

Fig. 8.25. Bilateral lid lag.

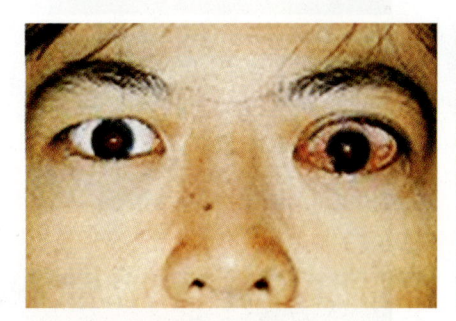

Fig. 8.26. Left exposure keratitis caused by exophthalmos, lid retraction and lagophthalmos (inability to close the eyelid).

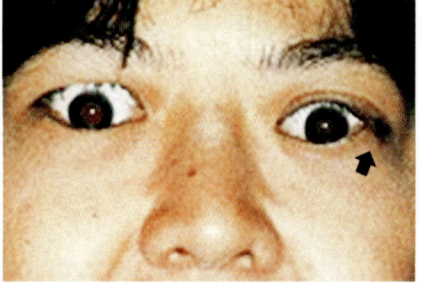

Fig. 8.27. Left lateral tarsorrhaphy to protect the cornea. Same patient as in Fig. 8.26.

Rheumatoid Eye Disease

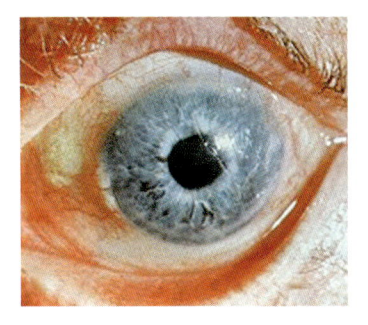

Fig. 8.28. Dry eye with loss of corneal lustre.

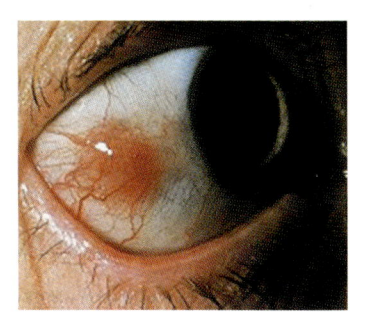

Fig. 8.29. Nodular scleritis.

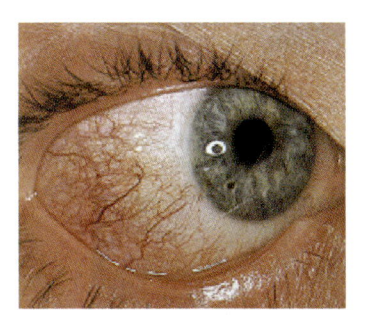

Fig. 8.30. Diffuse scleritis.

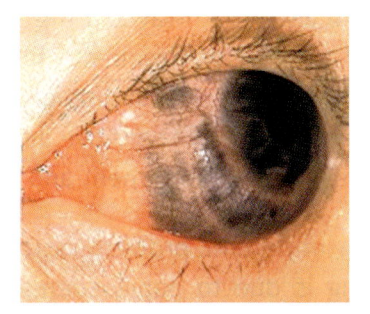

Fig. 8.31. Extensive scleromalacia with dark uveal tissue seen beneath thinned sclera.

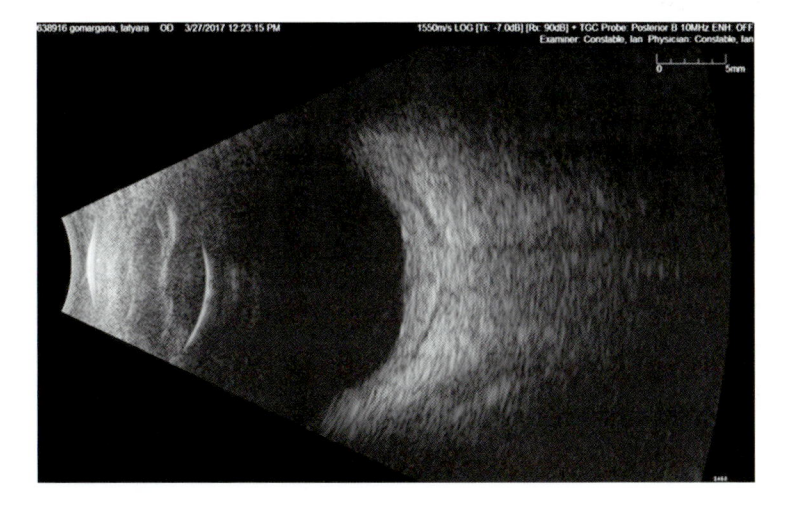

Fig. 8.32. B-scan ultrasound showing thickened posterior scleritis presenting with uniocular pain and a swollen optic disc.

9
NEURO-OPHTHALMOLOGY

INTRODUCTION

The visual pathway and the third, fourth, fifth, sixth and seventh cranial nerves are frequently affected by diseases of the central nervous system. Documentation and analysis of ocular and adnexal function can provide sensitive indicators of neurological diseases and their response to treatment and surgery.

An important problem is to determine whether an optic disc swelling is due to papilloedema, papillitis or ischaemic optic neuropathy. Optic atrophy and diplopia require diagnosis and a full neurological evaluation. A chiasmal lesion causes a bitemporal hemianopic field defect, whereas a post-chiasmal lesion causes a homonymous bilateral field loss.

OPTIC DISC SWELLING

The ophthalmoscopic picture of optic disc swelling consists of blurring of the disc margin and swelling of the optic nerve head, with filling-in of the central physiological cup. The veins are dilated and venous pulsations are absent. There are often small superficial haemorrhages confined to the immediate disc area, as well as oedema of the surrounding retina. With early disc swelling, OCT and fluorescein angiography help to determine its presence.

Papilloedema or Papillitis

The ophthalmoscopic appearance of disc swelling in papilloedema is similar to that in papillitis. Papilloedema is differentiated from papillitis by the presence of other clinical features.

Papilloedema is a passive swelling of the optic disc commonly caused by raised intracranial pressure as a result of the presence of intracranial tumours or malignant hypertension. The condition is usually bilateral. Vision is normal unless the macula is affected by oedema or exudates. Only rarely is the vision diminished because of optic atrophy in severe unrelieved papilloedema. The visual fields and colour vision are also normal, although the blind spot is sometimes enlarged. The pupillary reflex to light is normal.

Papillitis is an inflammation of the optic nerve, frequently of uncertain aetiology. Multiple sclerosis is an important cause. The condition is generally unilateral. Because the optic nerve is inflamed, there is usually marked visual loss. A central scotoma is present and the eye may have defective colour vision, especially with regard to red. The pupil is dilated, with sluggish or no reaction to direct light.

Differential Diagnosis of Papilloedema and Papillitis

	Papilloedema	Papillitis
Visual Acuity	Normal (usually)	Reduced
Pupil	Normal	Poor response to direct light
Visual Field	Normal (enlarged blind spot)	Central scotoma or field defect
Colour Vision	Normal	Defective
	Usually bilateral	Usually unilateral

Ischaemic Optic Neuropathy

Ischaemia to the optic nerve head from arteriosclerosis or giant cell temporal arteritis also causes sudden visual loss with a swollen optic disc in the elderly population. Non-inflammatory anterior ischaemic optic neuropathy often presents with an altitudinal hemianopia, as it may infarct half of the optic nerve head. Risk factors include hypertension and diabetes. It is always important to exclude temporal arteritis using blood erythrocyte sedimentation rate (ESR) and temporal artery biopsy if there is doubt. Systemic steroids will protect the unaffected eye in temporal arteritis. The prognosis for the affected eye is usually poor and optic atrophy usually follows.

Pseudopapilloedema

Pseudopapilloedema is a normal variation in the appearance of the optic disc which is sometimes mistaken for true disc oedema. It should be clearly differentiated from the latter in order to avoid unnecessary investigations and anxiety on the part of the patient.

One common cause of pseudopapilloedema is hypermetropia, where the disc margin is blurred. Other causes include optic disc drusen (yellowish-white deposits in the optic disc) and opaque myelinated nerve fibres. Fluorescein angiography can help to distinguish pseudopapilloedema from true disc oedema (fluorescein leakage at the disc).

RETROBULBAR NEURITIS

Retrobulbar neuritis is an inflammation of the optic nerve with similar symptoms and signs to papillitis except that optic disc swelling is absent. The clinical features include pain on movement of the eyes, sudden blurred vision, defective colour vision, afferent pupil defect and a central scotoma. The cause is usually unknown but some patients have underlying multiple sclerosis or later develop it, confirmed by an MRI scan showing cerebral demyelination plaques. There is no specific treatment but steroids may be used to speed up recovery of the central vision. They do not alter the final vision.

If multiple sclerosis (MS) is confirmed relapses can be reduced with natilizumab or fingolimod therapy.

OPTIC ATROPHY

Because the colour of the optic disc varies in normal individuals, a pale optic disc does not necessarily signify the presence of optic atrophy. Optic atrophy is confirmed where a pale optic disc is associated with defective visual acuity and visual field. OCT may show thinning of the retinal nerve fibre layer around the disc.

There are numerous causes of optic atrophy and they include previous optic neuritis, meningitis, encephalitis, central retinal artery occlusion, chronic ischaemia of the optic nerve, compression of the optic nerve or chiasma, trauma, chronic glaucoma, retinitis pigmentosa, congenital and familial disorders. Numerous systemic factors, such as methyl and ethyl alcohol, heavy metal poisoning, malnutrition, vitamin B deficiency and syphilis, may be causal. The cause is frequently not determined.

Neurological investigation, usually MRI, must be carried out to exclude compression of the optic nerve by intracranial tumours and other treatable causes.

CHIASMAL LESION

A chiasmal lesion causes a characteristic bitemporal hemianopic field defect. A chromophobe adenoma is the most common cause. The presence of optic atrophy and poor visual acuity usually indicate that the condition is already at a very advanced stage. Diagnosis is made by finding the characteristic field defect and confirmed by CAT or MRI scan. It should be differentiated from other causes of a chiasmal lesion, such as a suprasellar cyst (craniopharyngioma) or meningioma.

Post-Chiasmal Lesion

A post-chiasmal lesion causes a homonymous hemianopic field defect. It is usually due to either a cerebrovascular occlusion or a tumour. The optic tract, optic radiation or visual cortex may be affected. If the lesion is further back at the occipital lobe, the homonymous hemianopia tends to be congruous (similar). If the lesion occurs further forward and affects the optic tract, the homonymous hemianopia will tend to be incongruous (dissimilar). At the optic radiation, a homonymous quadrantic field defect may occur because the visual pathway is spread out over a relatively large area.

Computerised Tomography and Nuclear Magnetic Resonance Scans

The MRI scan and (less often) the CT scan are used in neuro-ophthalmic investigations. They permit accurate localisation of the pathology affecting the visual pathway. These investigations are essential in evaluating the extent of intracranial lesions and the serial effects of treatment.

PUPILS

The pupils may be abnormal in size or shape or in their reaction to light and accommodation.

Large Pupil

A large pupil may be caused by mydriatic eye drops, optic neuritis, optic atrophy or oculomotor nerve paralysis. It may also be caused by blunt injury to the eye through damage to the pupillary sphincter (traumatic mydriasis), or by advanced disease of the retina. Less commonly, it is due to Adie's tonic pupil.

Small Pupil

A small pupil can be caused by miotic eye drops such as pilocarpine. Other causes include iritis, an Argyll Robertson pupil due to syphilis, morphine and Horner's syndrome (sympathetic paralysis). In Horner's syndrome, pathology in the sympathetic pathway manifests as an ipsilateral miosis, partial ptosis, apparent enophthalmos and anhidrosis.

Irregular Pupil

A pupil which is irregular may be due to a congenital iris defect, posterior synechiae from iritis, an Argyll Robertson pupil or surgery.

Reaction to Light

A pupil which is not reactive to direct light but which is reactive to consensual light suggests that the eye is severely damaged or blind from disease of the optic nerve or retina (Marcus–Gunn pupil). A pupil which is not reactive to either direct or consensual light indicates a local disease or injury to the sphincter of the iris, or damage to the third cranial nerve, the nerve supply of the pupillary sphincter. Sometimes it is due to the use of a mydriatic.

In an Argyll Robertson pupil, there is no reaction to light but the pupil reacts to accommodation.

EXTRAOCULAR MUSCLES

Paralytic Squints

In severe paralysis of the extraocular muscles, the diagnosis is usually obvious. Lesions of the third nerve lead to ptosis and a relatively immobile eyeball which deviates downwards and outwards. This deviation is due to the paralysis of all the extraocular muscles except for the lateral rectus and superior oblique. The pupil is dilated.

In lesions of the sixth nerve, there will be a convergent squint. In lesions of the fourth nerve, the superior oblique muscle is paralysed. The eye is elevated when it is in an adducted position because of overaction of the inferior oblique muscle. The patient often has a compensatory head posture to avoid double vision.

Numerous conditions may result in paralysis of the extraocular muscles. The cause is often difficult to determine and special investigation may be required. Trauma, diabetes, arteriosclerosis, intracranial aneurysms and tumours are the most common causes.

In slight paralysis, the ocular movements are apparently normal. The patient complains of double vision and the diagnosis can be difficult. The following simple questions may help to confirm the presence of muscle paralysis.

- Is double vision present when both eyes are open? Is double vision present when one eye is closed? Extraocular muscle paralysis causes binocular double vision. If double vision is present when one eye is occluded, it is not due to paralysis of the extraocular muscles.
- Does the separation of images occur side by side or one above the other? In sixth nerve paralysis the separation is side by side, while in third or fourth nerve paralysis the separation is one above the other.
- In which direction of gaze does the maximum separation occur? Maximum separation of images occurs in the direction of action of the affected muscle. For example, there will be maximum separation of images when the patient looks to the left if the left lateral rectus muscle is affected.
- In which eye is the image fainter? The fainter image is seen by the eye with the paralysed muscle. If there is left lateral rectus muscle paralysis, there will be a horizontal separation of images and the fainter image is seen with the left eye.

The cover test for diagnosis of strabismus and special optical tests which dissociate the two eyes are required to investigate patients with diplopia and to chart their progress.

Myasthenia Gravis

Myasthenia gravis causes weakness of the skeletal muscles, especially in young adults. The extraocular muscles are frequently affected. Thus, the patient may present with intermittent and varying double vision and ptosis, which is usually bilateral. The symptoms are classically more pronounced in the evening or with fatigue. They can be precipitated clinically if the patient is asked to keep a sustained upward gaze for a minute or two.

Diagnosis can be confirmed by demonstrating a reversal of symptoms with intravenous Tensilon.

NYSTAGMUS

Nystagmus is an involuntary, oscillatory movement of the eyes.

Jerk nystagmus has a slow and a fast component, and is usually maximum in a particular position of gaze. It is caused by neurological conditions which affect the cerebellum, the vestibular system or their connections. Patients with jerk nystagmus require a full neurological evaluation.

Pendular nystagmus has no slow or fast component. It is caused by poor vision and the patient's inability to fix on targets. As a result, the eyes develop pendular, roving movements.

Both jerk and pendular nystagmus are often congenital.

MIGRAINE

Migraine is a common cause of headaches. Often there is visual disturbance prior to the onset of the unilateral headache. This presents as frequent sparkling or flashing lights followed by a positive field defect. The symptoms are usually unilateral. The headache is often associated with nausea and vomiting. The symptoms are usually relieved by resting quietly in a darkened room. There is frequently a family history of migraine.

Occasionally, migraine-like attacks are due to pathological lesions such as intracranial aneurysms and tumours. Severe, atypical persistent migraine or migraine of late onset requires neurological investigation.

Sometimes the visual symptoms occur in the absence of a headache, particularly in older patients. This is called ophthalmic migraine. It needs to be differentiated from similar transient visual symptoms (amaurosis fugax) caused by carotid stenosis, emboli or mini-strokes.

Disc Swelling

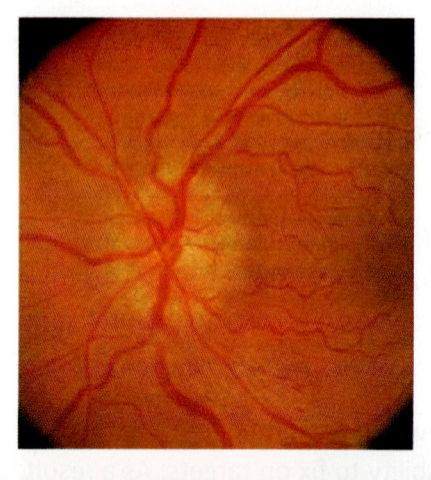

Fig. 9.1. Papillitis due to multiple sclerosis. Afferent pupil defect, central scotoma and decreased visual acuity.

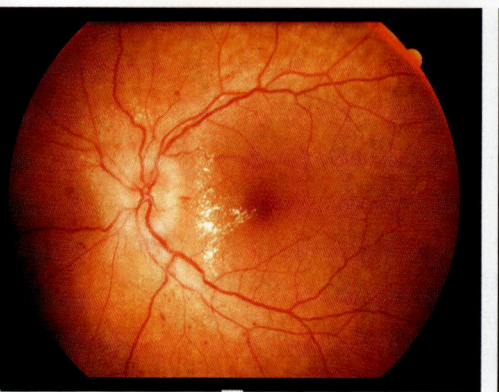

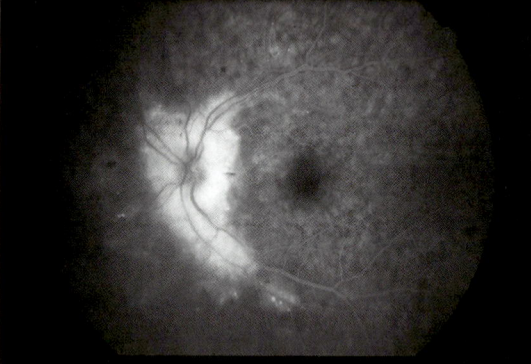

Fig. 9.2. Papillitis with retinal exudates and leakage on FA.

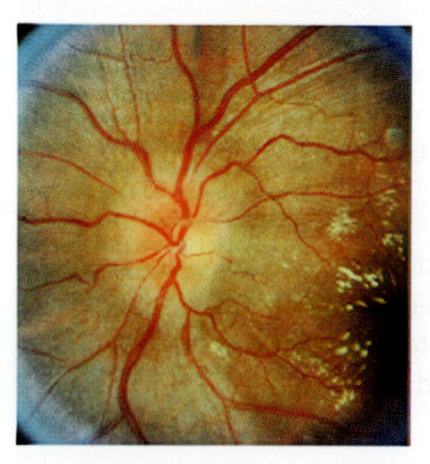

Fig. 9.3. Papilloedema due to malignant hypertension.

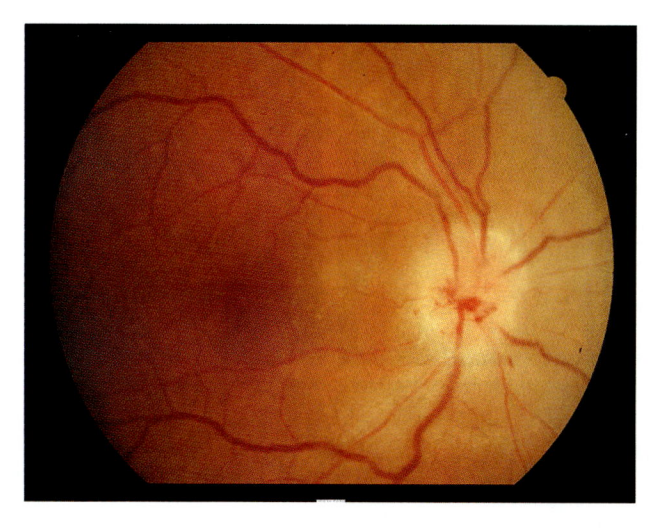

Fig. 9.4. Anterior ischaemic optic neuropathy. Decreased visual acuity, afferent pupil defect and superior or inferior hemi-field defect.

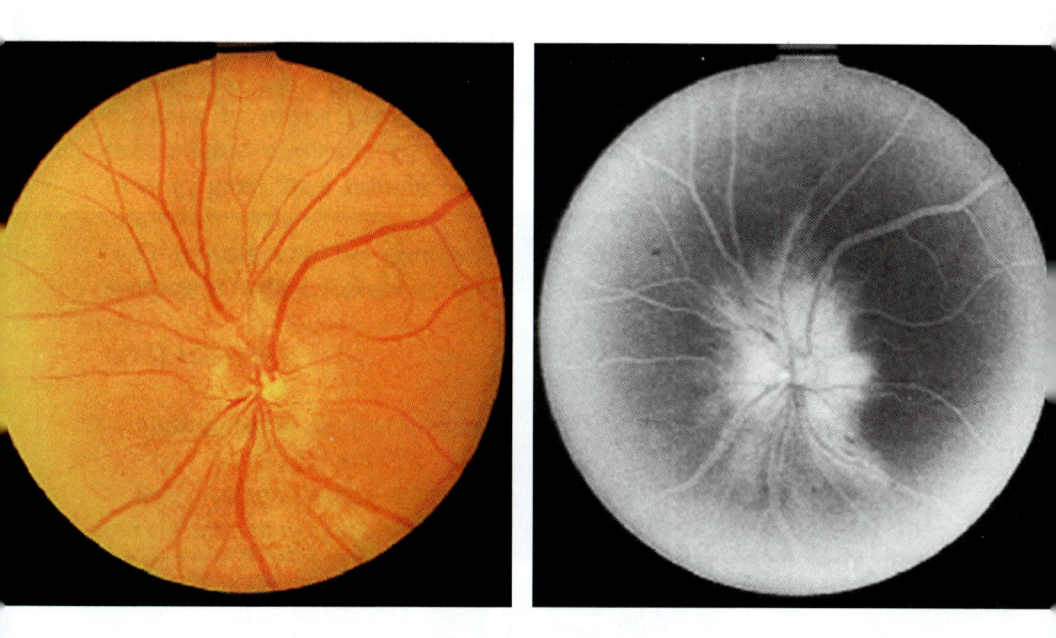

Fig. 9.5. Blurred disc margin suggesting possible papilloedema. Fluorescein angiography confirms leakage of dye from the disc.

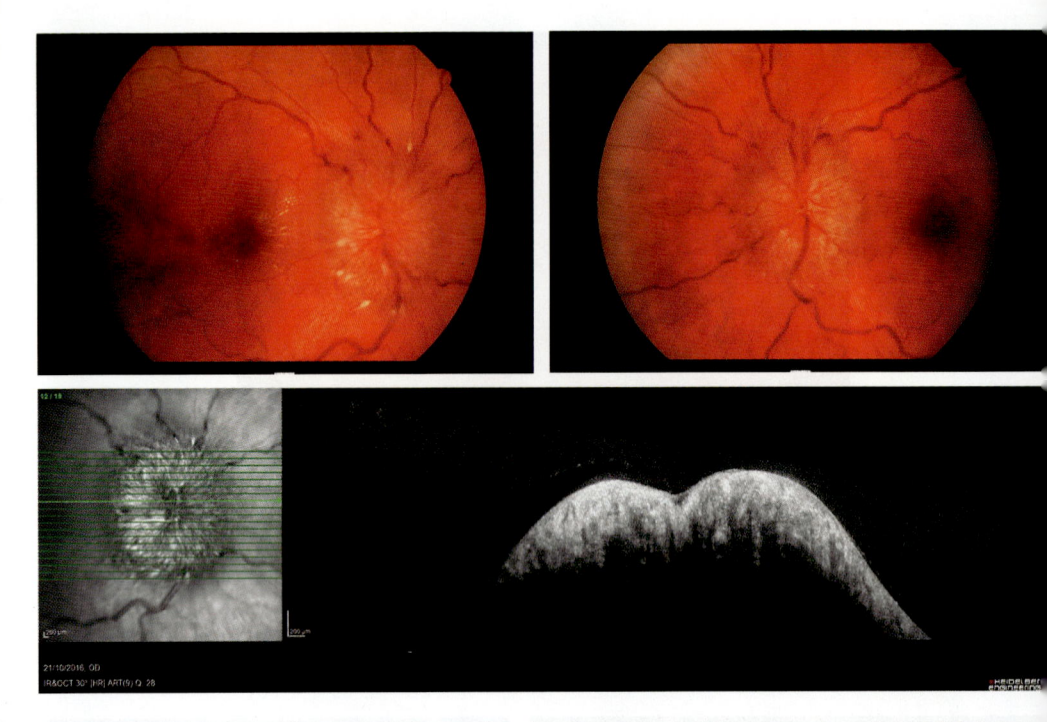

Fig. 9.6. Bilateral papilloedema due to benign intracranial hypertension. OCT highlights swelling. Visual acuity is usually maintained, the pupil is normal and there is a full field with an enlarged blind spot.

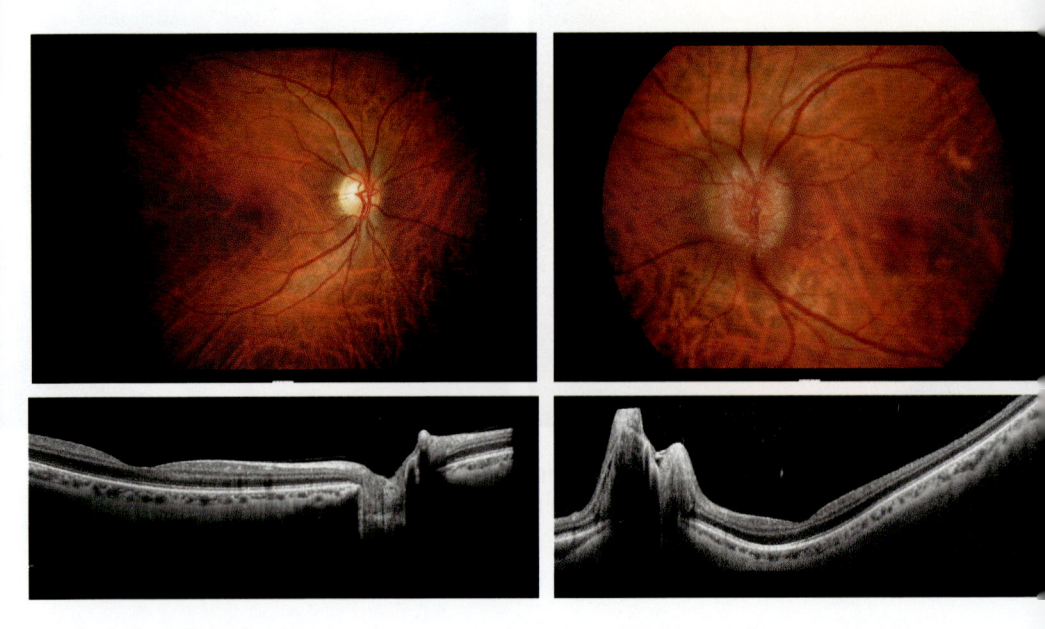

Fig. 9.7. Unilateral disc swelling with OCT comparing the swollen disc to the normal.

Pseudopapilloedema

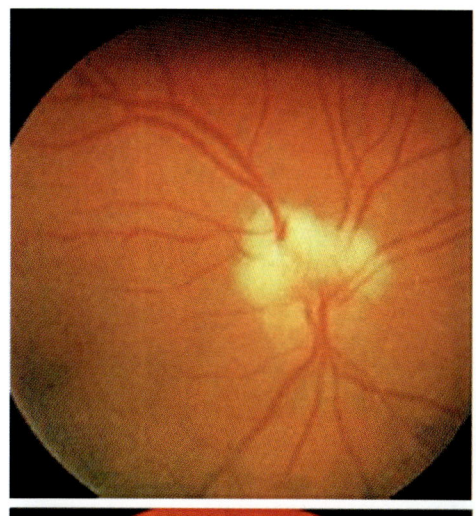

Fig. 9.8. Opaque myelinated nerve fibres.

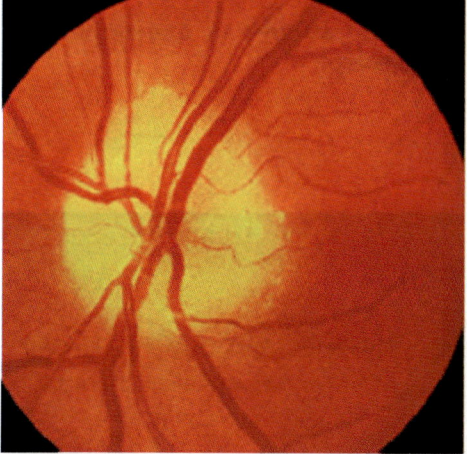

Fig. 9.9. Disc drusen.

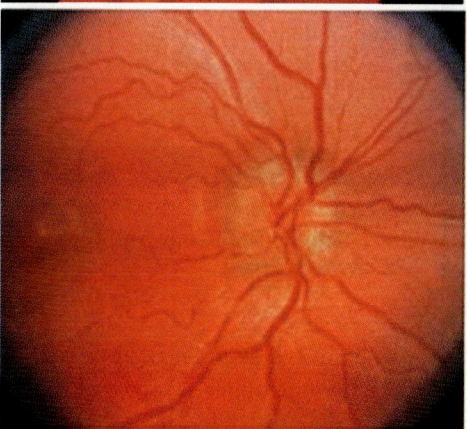

Fig. 9.10. Hypermetropia with a small optic disc and blurred margins.

Optic Atrophy

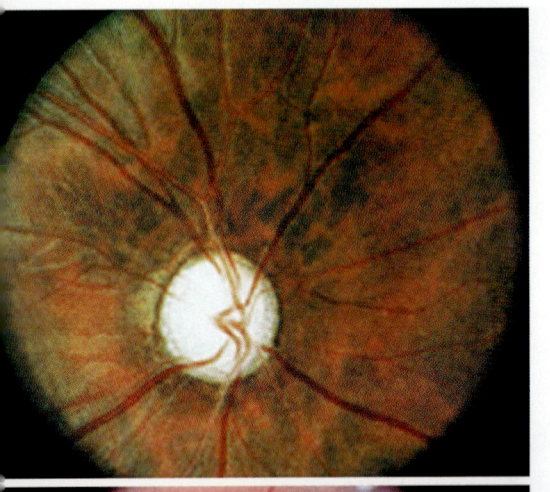

Fig. 9.11. Primary optic atrophy of undetermined aetiology. This requires an MRI scan and exclusion of systemic causes.

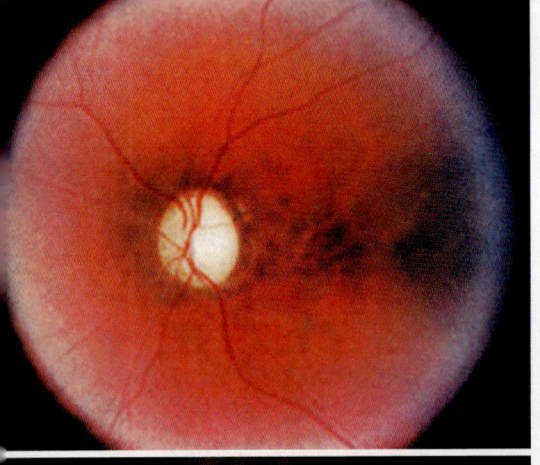

Fig. 9.12. Optic atrophy one year after central retinal artery occlusion. The eye remains blind.

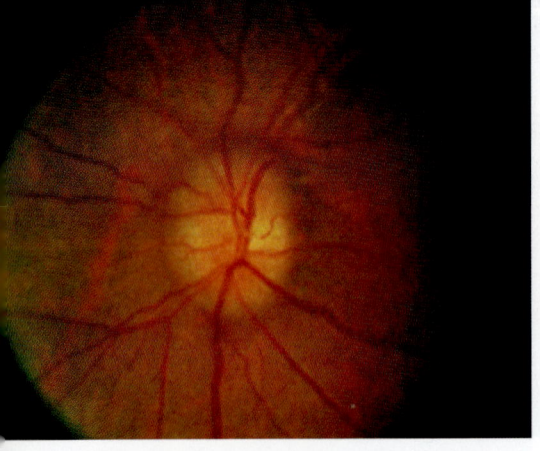

Fig. 9.13. Secondary optic atrophy following papillitis, with a blurred margin and a filled-in optic cup.

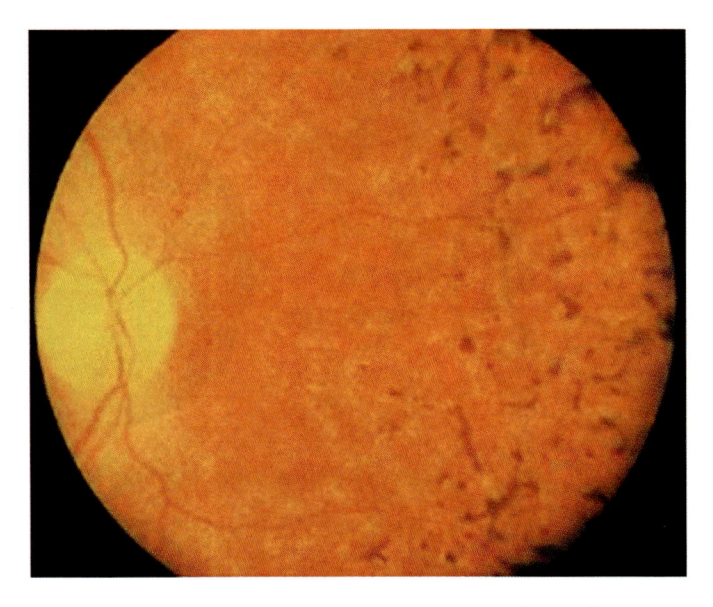

Fig. 9.14. Optic atrophy in retinitis pigmentosa, with a yellow–white optic disc, attenuated retinal vessels and bone spicule retinal pigment.

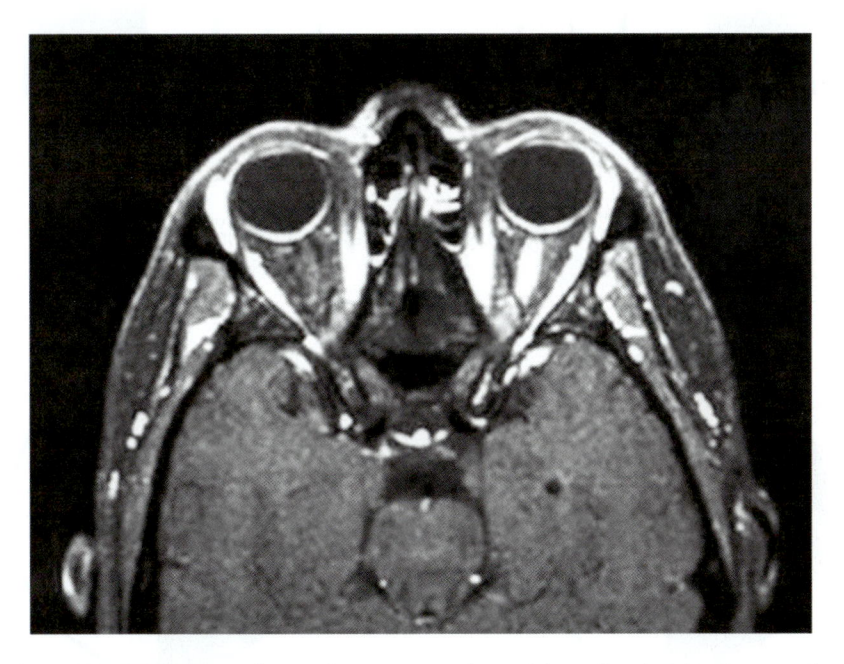

Fig. 9.15. MRI scan of a patient presenting with unilateral optic atrophy, showing an intraorbital optic nerve tumour.

Visual Field Defects

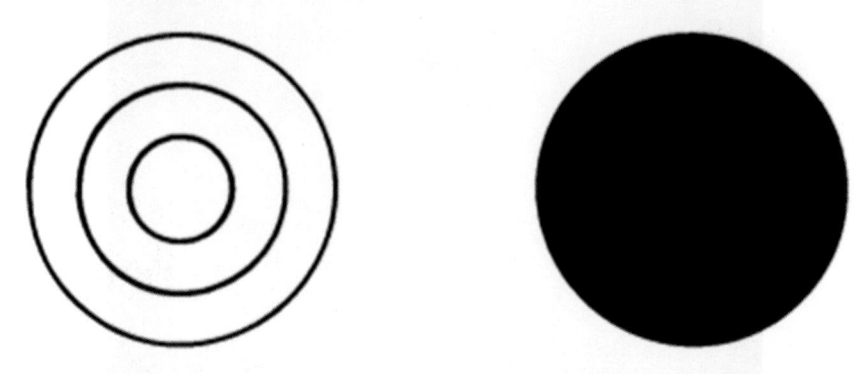

Fig. 9.16. Right optic atrophy with complete field loss.

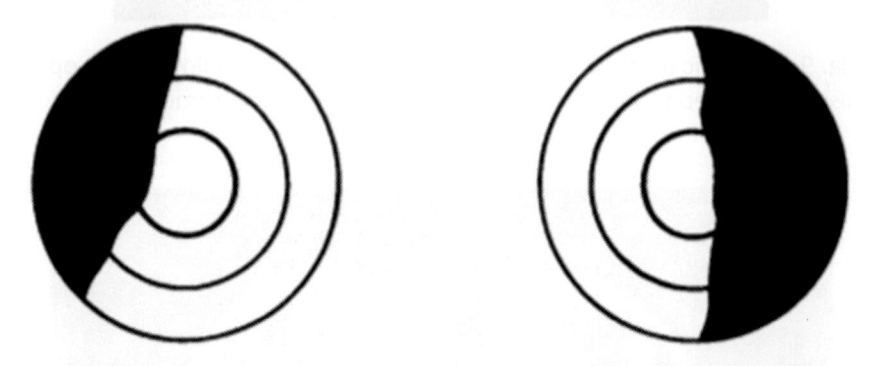

Fig. 9.17. Bitemporal field defect indicating a lesion at the chiasm.

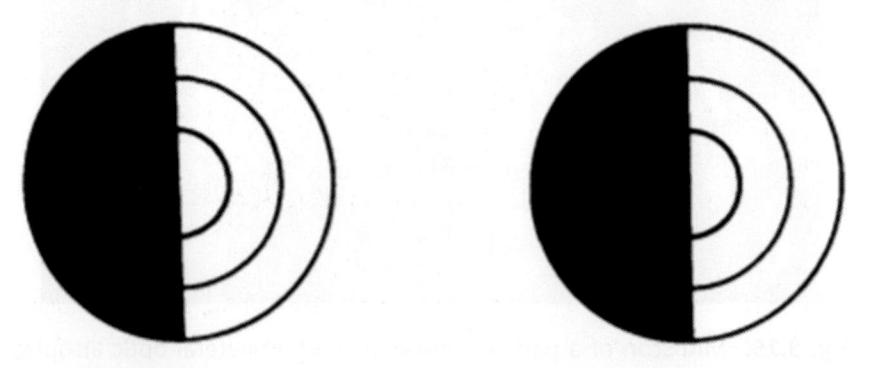

Fig. 9.18. Homonymous (*left*) field defect indicating a post-chiasmal lesion.

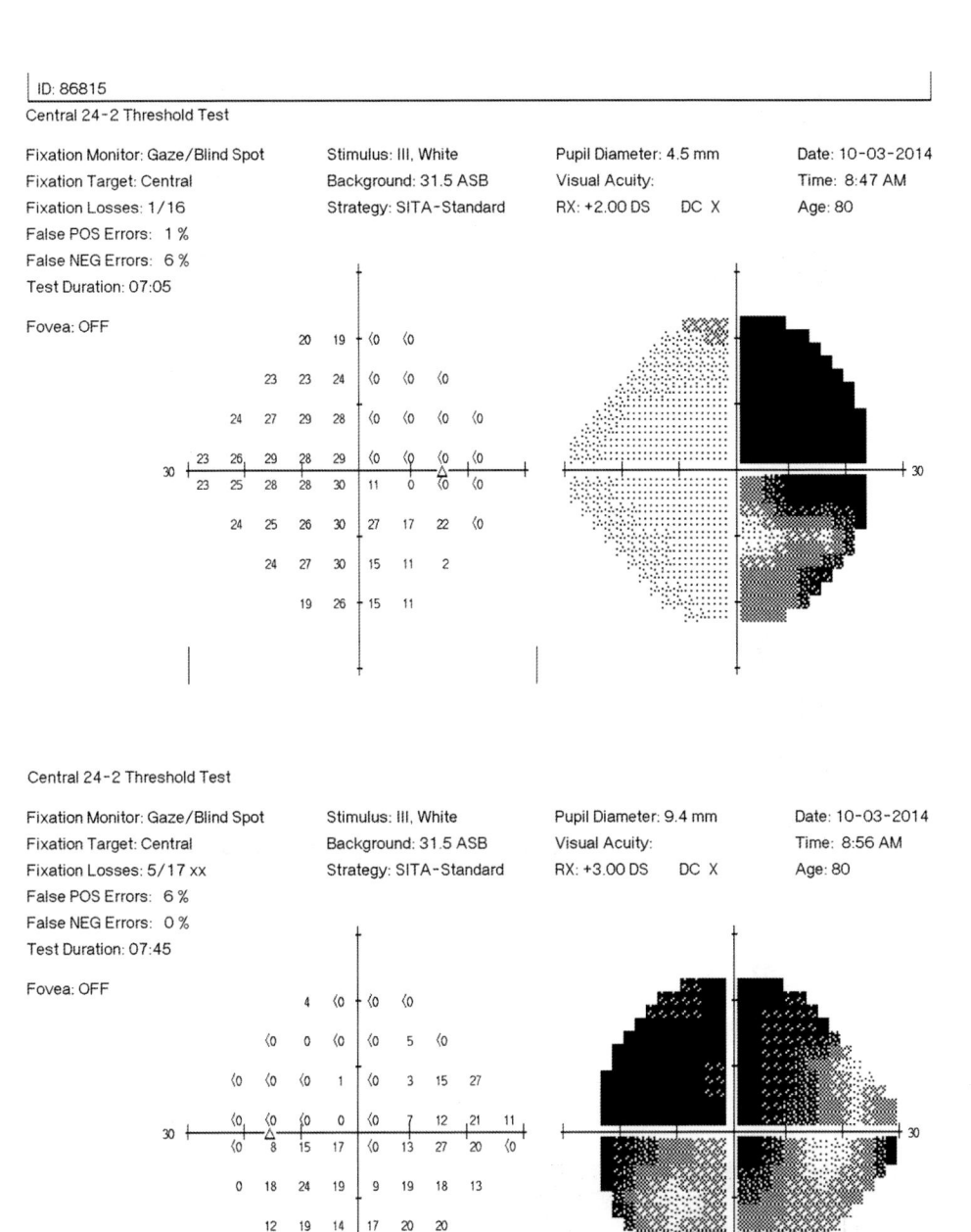

Fig. 9.19. Bitemporal field defect with an extension across the midline and involving central fixation on the left. Pituitary tumour treated by transsphenoidal hypophysectomy.

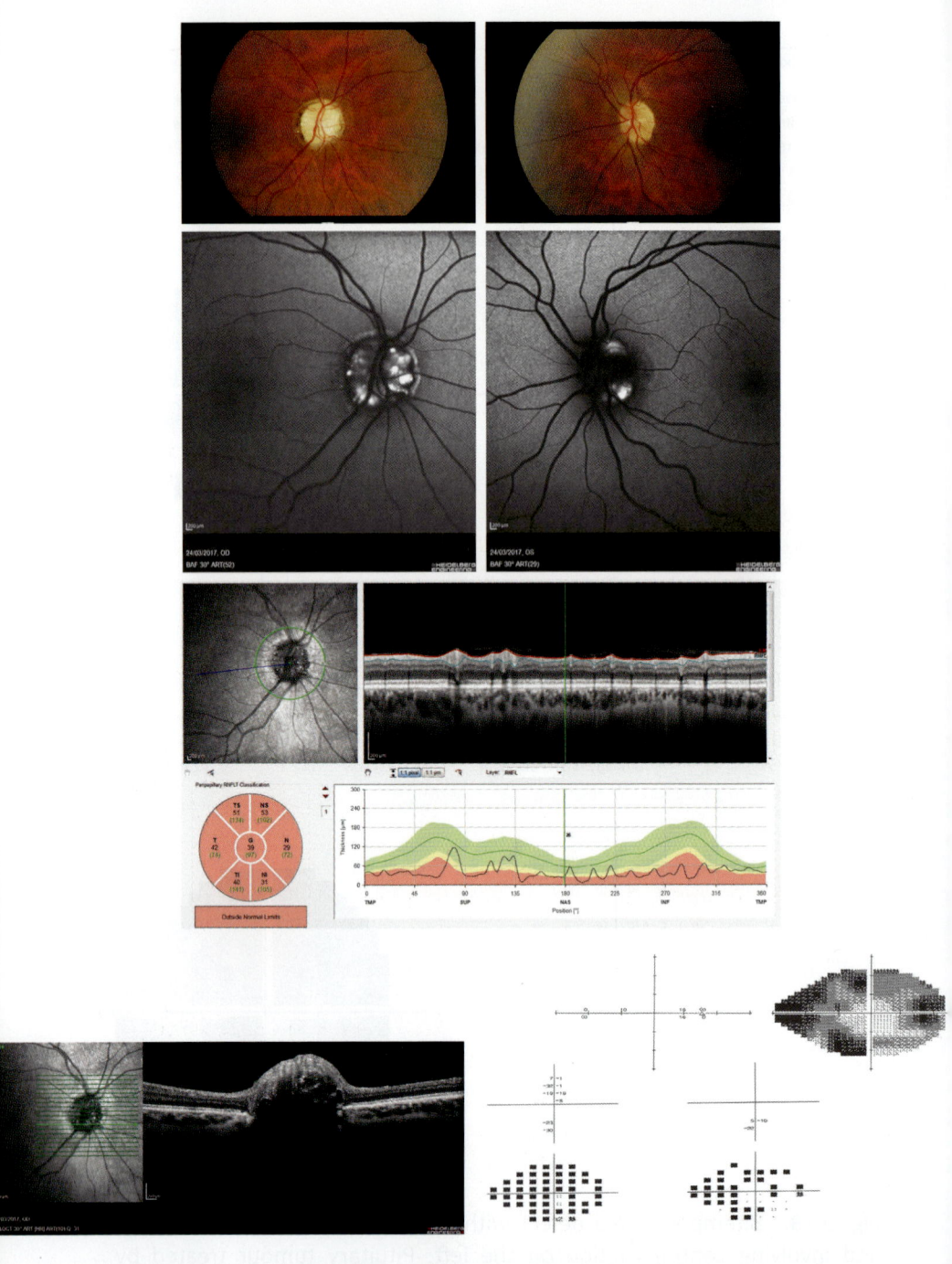

Fig. 9.20. Visual field loss right eye associated with optic nerve drusen which autofluoresce. OCT shows decreased nerve fibre layer thickness and optic disc expansion causing secondary optic atrophy.

Extraocular Muscle Paralysis

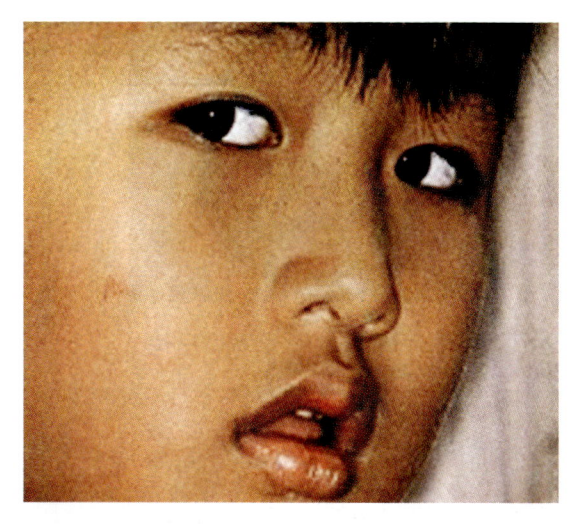

Fig. 9.21. Right superior oblique muscle paralysis leading to head turn and tilt to avoid double vision.

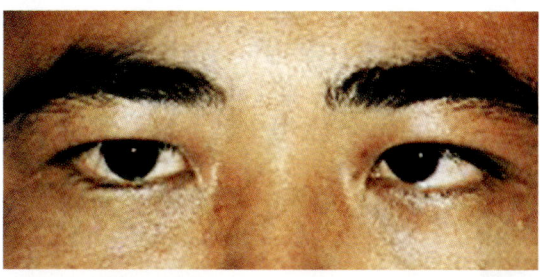

Fig. 9.22. Left lateral rectus paralysis causing a convergent squint.

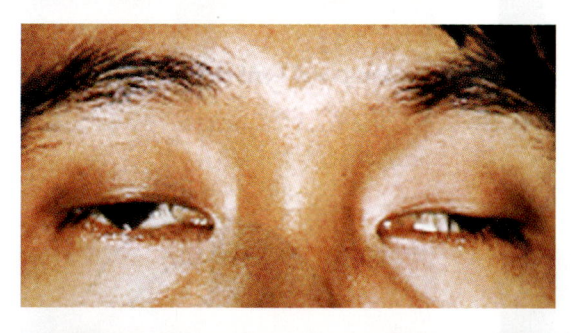

Fig. 9.23. Right third nerve paralysis causing ptosis and a divergent squint.

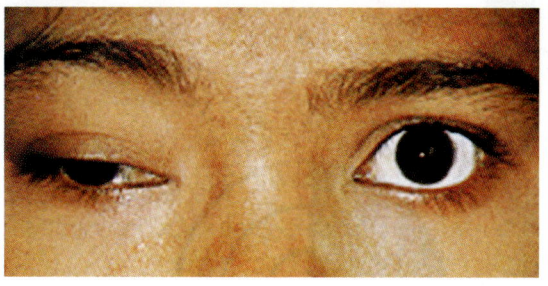

Fig. 9.24. Bilateral ptosis and a divergent squint in myasthenia gravis.

Complete Third Nerve Paralysis

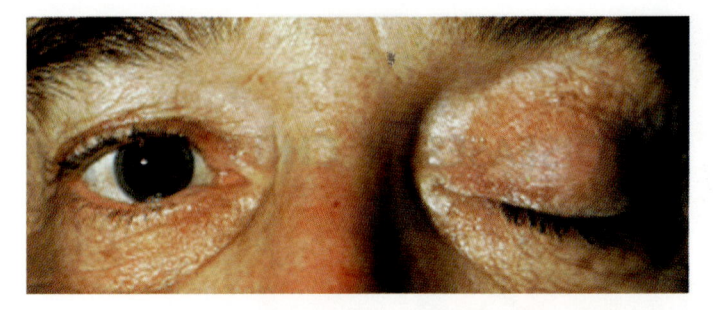

Fig. 9.25. Complete left ptosis (looking straight ahead).

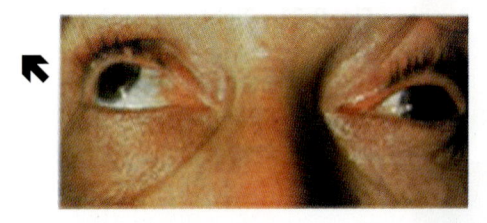

Fig. 9.26. Left inferior oblique paralysis (looking up and right).

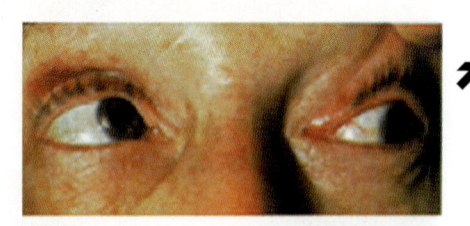

Fig. 9.27. Left medial rectus paralysis (looking left).

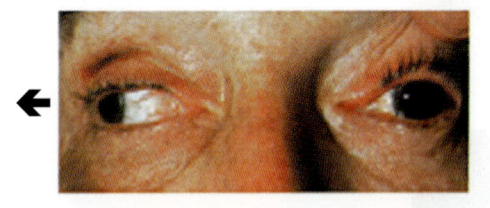

Fig. 9.28. Left superior oblique action is limited (because of inability to adduct: looking down and right).

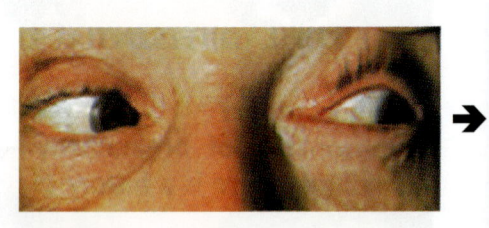

Fig. 9.29. Left superior rectus paralysis (looking up and left).

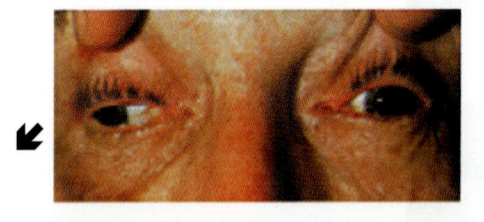

Fig. 9.30. Normal left lateral rectus (looking left).

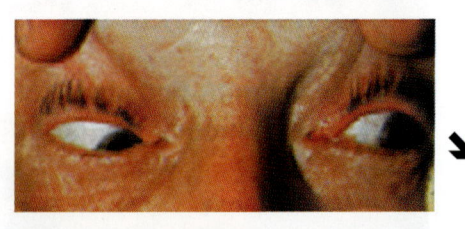

Fig. 9.31. Left inferior rectus paralysis (looking down and left).

Note: The third cranial nerve supplies the levator palpebrae superioris besides the medial, superior and inferior rectus muscles and the inferior oblique.

10
EYE DISEASES IN CHILDREN

INTRODUCTION

A rare but important ocular condition in children is retinoblastoma, a malignant tumour which usually presents as a "white pupil". Early diagnosis may save the life of the child.

Strabismus, or squint, is common in children and should be evaluated and treated early to prevent loss of vision from amblyopia (lazy eye).

Other common ocular conditions in children include conjunctivitis, blocked nasolacrimal duct and congenital cataract.

WHITE PUPIL

White pupil, or leukocoria, is diagnosed in a child when the red reflex is abnormally white. The most important condition to exclude is retinoblastoma. Other causes include:

- Retinopathy of prematurity (retrolental fibroplasia). This affects premature infants with low birth weight following high oxygen concentration during early management.
- Congenital cataract.
- Persistent primary hyperplastic vitreous (persistent fetal vasculature). This is usually unilateral and the involved eye is abnormally small, with a retrolental mass.

- Coats' disease. This is mostly unilateral, affecting boys, and is associated with intraretinal and subretinal exudates secondary to telangiectasia of the retinal vessels.
- Toxocariasis. Chronic endophthalmitis can result in a cyclitic membrane and posterior pole granuloma.
- Severe uveitis.
- Organised old vitreous haemorrhage.

Retinoblastoma

Retinoblastoma is the commonest primary intraocular malignancy in children. It is a developmental tumour of retinal origin. There is a strong genetic component and the patient's family should undergo genetic counselling and screening for possible retinoblastoma. The causal mutation is usually in the rb1 tumour-suppressing gene, which occurs as a hereditary mutation in bilateral cases. Most unilateral cases (2/3) have a random somatic mutation not present in the parents or siblings but can still transmit a risk to their children.

Usually, the condition is detected when an abnormal white reflex appears in the child's pupil. This is most obvious in dim light, when the pupil is partially dilated and usually seen as an abnormally white pupil in photographs. Children with this condition can also present with squint, reduced vision, painful red eye or orbital inflammation. In most cases, the presence of the white reflex indicates that the condition is at an advanced stage.

As retinoblastoma is highly malignant and can spread rapidly, it must be differentiated from other causes of a white pupil. A thorough dilated fundus examination of both eyes is essential. The differential diagnosis can be difficult even for an experienced ophthalmologist. A child with a white pupil should be urgently referred to a paediatric ophthalmologist to establish the cause. Examination under general anaesthesia with full dilatation of the pupils is required to confirm the diagnosis.

Management

Treatment of retinoblastoma involves a multidisciplinary approach, and the treatment choice depends on the stage of the disease. Intravenous chemotherapy is the mainstay of treatment, with usage of agents like carboplatin, etoposide, vincristine and melphalan.

Other treatment options include external beam radiotherapy, transpupillary thermotherapy, cryotherapy, radioactive plaque brachytherapy and enucleation.

An eye with an advanced retinoblastoma usually requires enucleation (removal) as soon as possible, to prevent optic nerve invasion and neural or haematogenous spread.

Retinopathy of Prematurity

Premature babies (born before 32 weeks of gestational age) or weighing 1500 g or less should have their fundus examined by an ophthalmologist in the nursery ward for early signs of retinopathy. Exposure to a high concentration of oxygen in the early neonatal period is a major risk factor. Oxygen causes constriction and obliteration of premature blood vessels in the peripheral retina. This leads to retinal hypoxia, which results in new vessel proliferation, exudation, scarring and retinal detachment. Screening for retinopathy of prematurity (ROP) should commence at 4–5 weeks postnatal age and is repeated every 1–2 weeks, until there is normal retinal vascularisation of the temporal retinal periphery. Treatment involves laser photocoagulation of the avascular retina, cryotherapy or intravitreal injection of anti-VEGF medications. Advanced ROP with retinal detachment may benefit from vitrectomy but vision improves only marginally.

Congenital Cataract

Congenital cataract can be unilateral or bilateral and may be inherited or sporadic. Cataract in children can result from metabolic disorders such as galactosaemia and intrauterine infections during pregnancy, for example toxoplasmosis, rubella, cytomegalovirus and herpes virus. Early recognition and surgery is the key to better visual rehabilitation and prevention of permanent amblyopia.

Persistent Hyperplastic Primary Vitreous

Persistent hyperplastic primary vitreous (PHPV) is usually unilateral, with the involved eye being smaller than the fellow eye. A retrolental mass is seen with elongated ciliary processes attached to it. Secondary cataract and glaucoma can also develop. Early surgery may be beneficial but visual recovery is limited.

Coats' Disease

Coats' disease is mostly unilateral and is more commonly seen in boys, within the first decade. It is associated with intraretinal and subretinal exudates secondary to telangiectasia of the retinal vessels. Massive exudation can lead to retinal detachment. Other complications include cataract, rubeosis iridis and glaucoma. Treatment options are retinal photocoagulation, cryotherapy, anti-VEGF injections and vitreoretinal surgery, depending on the extent of the disease.

STRABISMUS

A strabismus (or squint) is a deviation of an eye, so that its visual axis is no longer parallel to that of its fellow eye.

Squints can be congenital (occurring at birth) or acquired (occurring later in life). They may be latent (suppressed when both eyes are open) or manifest (present all the time). They may also be divided into those associated with paralysis of a muscle (paralytic squint) or where no obvious evidence of paralysis exists (non-paralytic or concomitant squint). In a paralytic squint the degree of deviation of the eyes is not the same in all fields of gaze. In a non-paralytic or concomitant squint the degree of deviation is the same in all directions of gaze.

Paralytic Squint

The ocular manifestations of paralytic squint in children are generally similar to those in adults, except that the young child does not complain of double vision. To avoid double vision, the child suppresses the use of one eye, leading to amblyopia. Sometimes, the child adopts a compensatory head tilt to avoid double vision.

Non-Paralytic Squint

This is the commonest form and can be either horizontal or vertical. Horizontal squints can be either convergent (esotropia), where one of the eyes is turned inwards, or divergent (exotropia), where one of the eyes is turned outwards. In vertical squints, one eye is higher than the other.

A convergent squint (esotropia) is often associated with hypermetropia (long sight). Correction of the hypermetropia with glasses can reduce or control the squint. This type of squint is known as an accommodative convergent squint. It is quite common in Caucasian children. A divergent squint in a child usually develops after the age of three years and is often associated with myopia.

Frequently, a non-paralytic squint is precipitated by illnesses such as measles or chickenpox. An important consideration in young children is that the squint may occasionally be due to poor vision or secondary to ocular diseases, of which retinoblastoma is the most important.

Effects of squint on children

There are three effects of squint on children.

- Amblyopia (lazy eye).
- Failure to develop binocular single vision and stereopsis.
- Cosmetic blemish. This can lead to emotional and socio-economic problems.

Management

The child should be referred to an ophthalmologist as soon as a squint is suspected, for exclusion of ocular pathology like retinoblastoma or congenital cataract and to commence treatment for the prevention of amblyopia.

All children with squint must undergo a thorough dilated fundus exam. Refraction with atropine or other cycloplegics (to reduce accommodation) should be carried out and, where necessary, appropriate glasses prescribed. Glasses for children with accommodative convergent squint may be sufficient to correct the squint and these glasses should be used constantly.

Early diagnosis and treatment may prevent the development of amblyopia or increase the chances of reversing it. Treatment options include occlusion (patching) or atropine instillation (penalisation) of the good eye so that the child is forced to use the amblyopic eye until maximum improvement is obtained. Spectacle correction of any refractive error is essential. Treatment for the prevention of amblyopia is usually supervised by an orthoptist. Patching can be tedious, and needs the co-operation of the child and the parents.

Surgery may be necessary. In a convergent squint, surgery is directed at weakening the medial rectus muscle and strengthening the lateral rectus muscle. The opposite procedure is done in a divergent squint.

In squints which have a vertical element, intervention becomes more complicated as it involves surgery on one of the vertically acting muscles, namely the superior or inferior rectus, or one of the oblique muscles. Although it is common for the eyes to be straightened at one operation, that may occasionally require more than one.

It is important to explain to the parents that even after surgery to straighten the eyes, patching of the good eye and continued supervision are required.

Amblyopia

Amblyopia, otherwise known as lazy eye, is the decrease in best corrected visual acuity, mostly seen in one eye. It can occur because of squint, uncorrected refractive error, sensory deprivation due to ocular pathology or very high refractive error. It is quite common and is present in up to 5% of some populations.

In a squint, whether paralytic or non-paralytic, the child suppresses the use of one eye in order to avoid double vision. Persistent suppression of the eye causes amblyopia.

It is important to treat a child with squint as early as possible, as amblyopia can frequently be prevented or reversed by patching or atropinisation of the good eye to stimulate the squinting eye to function.

Refractive amblyopia is due to anisometropia (difference of refraction in each eye), bilateral high astigmatism, or very high hypermetropia (long sight) or myopia (short sight).

Amblyopia can also be caused by visual deprivation because of ocular pathology such as ptosis, corneal scar, cataract, congenital nystagmus and retinal pathology.

Pseudosquint

Pseudosquint is usually due to marked medial epicanthal eyelid folds which give the appearance of a convergent squint. Diagnosis is confirmed by observing the corneal reflex and by the cover test. As the child grows older, the epicanthal skin folds tend to become less marked. No treatment — only reassurance — is required.

INFECTIOUS CONJUNCTIVITIS

Conjunctivitis occurring in the first 28 days after birth is referred to as ophthalmia neonatorum. In the past, the infection was usually due to gonorrhoea. In recent years, better antenatal care in most countries has made gonorrhoea less common. Other causative organisms include staphylococcus, streptococcus, haemophilus, pneumococcus, coliform organisms, herpes simplex virus and chlamydia (TRIC organism found in the genital tract of females).

In gonococcal infection, there is acute mucopurulent conjunctivitis, which can perforate the cornea and lead to blindness.

If the conjunctivitis is severe, urgent treatment with systemic (IV antibiotics) and local therapy is required. The child may have to be hospitalised with barrier nursing to prevent the spread of the infection. However, many milder cases of conjunctivitis can be treated as outpatients, with hourly applications of antibiotic eye drops until the infection clears. It is important to clean the discharge regularly with sterile (boiled) cotton wool soaked in saline or water.

LACRIMAL SYSTEM (TEARING)

Blockage of the lacrimal drainage system in a child usually occurs at the nasolacrimal duct. Within the first few weeks of life, persistent watering with sticky discharge is seen in the affected eye. Pressure with the finger on the lacrimal sac often produces a reflux of mucopurulent material. This is due to late canalisation of the lacrimal drainage system, which first develops as a solid cord of epithelial cells and normally canalises at about the time of birth.

Treatment is conservative, with daily massage of the lacrimal sac (using the pulp of the index finger) for the first six months. Antibiotics are used only where there is an infection. Most cases will clear by six months. If the condition persists beyond one year, or if the infection is recurrent or severe, the child should be referred to an ophthalmologist for probing and syringing of the nasolacrimal system under general anaesthesia. Surgery to anastomosise the sac to the nasal mucosa (dacryocystorhinostomy) is rarely required in children.

CONGENITAL CATARACT

Congenital cataract with minimal lens change which does not interfere with vision usually requires no surgery. The timing of surgery depends on the density of the cataract. When the cataract is dense, be it unilateral or bilateral, surgery should be performed as early as possible (usually 4–10 weeks of age) to prevent the development of amblyopia secondary to visual deprivation. Dense congenital cataracts should therefore be referred for an ophthalmic opinion as soon as possible. Where the cataract is not dense and where there is a view of the fundus, the decision for surgery can be difficult. It may be advisable to wait until the child is older, when visual acuity can be more accurately determined.

Cataract surgery involves aspiration of lens matter with limited anterior vitrectomy. IOL implantation may be done at the same time or is sometimes deferred. To see clearly after cataract surgery, the child requires spectacles, contact lenses or IOL implantation at a later date. In addition to surgery, an important part of management is to ensure good visual function. The main objective is to prevent amblyopia. Orthoptic support and co-operation from parents are also very important.

CONGENITAL GLAUCOMA

Congenital glaucoma is rare. In infants, raised intraocular pressure causes the cornea to increase in diameter from 11 mm to over 13 mm. Because of the increase in size, this condition is also known as buphthalmos ("ox eye"). It causes tears in Descemet's membrane (Haab striae), leading to corneal oedema, irritation and watering of the eye combined with photophobia. If left unrelieved, the raised intraocular pressure will damage the optic nerve, resulting in glaucomatous cupping and optic atrophy.

Referral to an ophthalmologist of an infant with photophobia and tearing or a large and opaque cornea enables early diagnosis and treatment, and may prevent blindness. Surgical options include gonitomy, trabeculotomy and trabeculectomy. Lifelong follow-up is necessary.

PHAKOMATOSES

Phakomatoses are a group of congenital or hereditary abnormalities which affect the skin, the nervous system and also the eye in varying degrees.

Neurofibromatosis Type 1 (von Recklinghausen's Disease)

This is characterised by pigmented patches on the skin (cafe-au-lait spots) and subcutaneous tumours — plexiform neurofibroma of varying sizes. The brain stem or cerebellum may be affected by tumours. The ocular manifestations include neurofibromas in the eyelids, prominent corneal nerves, Lisch nodules on the iris, hamartomas of the retina and choroid, and optic nerve gliomas.

Tuberous Sclerosis (Bourneville's Disease)

This is a disease in which gliomas of the brain are associated with sebaceous adenoma of the face. These are distributed across the nose and face in a typical butterfly pattern. Occasionally, the retina or optic disc has a yellowish raised nodule which looks like a mulberry.

Sturge–Weber Syndrome

This is a capillary haemangioma or "port-wine stain" affecting the distribution of the fifth nerve on the face. Capillary haemangioma may also affect the cerebral cortex. Sometimes, the eye on the side of the lesion develops congenital glaucoma, which can be difficult to treat. Choroidal angioma may also be present.

Von Hippel–Lindau Disease

This is a condition associated with retinal capillary haemangioma with large feeding retinal vessels and CNS haemangiomas, usually seen in the cerebellum and spinal cord. The haemangioma often causes exudates and haemorrhages in the retina and vitreous, and can lead to retinal detachment. The retinal lesions can be treated with photocoagulation, diathermy or cryotherapy.

Wyburn–Mason Syndrome

This shows dilated and tortuous retinal vessels with arteriovenous communication along with haemangiomas in the midbrain.

DEVELOPMENTAL ABNORMALITIES

There are a large number of developmental ocular abnormalities which may occur in mild or severe forms. Some are associated with antenatal infections, teratogenic drugs and chromosomal abnormalities or hereditary defective genes.

The abnormalities may affect the whole skull and face, giving rise to a number of syndromes, such as craniofacial dysostosis, mandibulofacial dysostosis and meningoencephalocele.

The whole eye may be affected in anophthalmos (absence of one eye, congenital cyst and microphthalmos — small eye).

Coloboma of the iris or choroid is due to incomplete closure of the choroidal fissure during development.

Common congenital abnormalities which affect the lids include congenital ptosis, coloboma of the lid and obstruction of the lacrimal apparatus.

The lens may be abnormal in shape or dislocated, as in Marfan's syndrome and homocystinuria. Persistent hyaloid (embryonic vitreous) artery and hyperplastic primary vitreous which presents itself as a white pupil may also occur.

A number of abnormalities may occur at the optic disc. They include optic disc pits and hypoplasia of the optic nerve, which is an occasional cause of poor vision in childhood.

ANTENATAL INFECTIONS

Antenatal infection, mainly TORCH (toxoplasmosis, rubella, cytomegalovirus and herpes), can lead to ocular complications. Congenital syphilis, rubella or toxoplasmosis can cause profound damage to the eye. The common manifestations of rubella are congenital cataract and nystagmus. Both syphilis and rubella can cause pigmentary changes of the retina. Congenital toxoplasmosis causes a typical localised pigmented chorioretinal scar at the macula, resulting in reduced vision.

Leukocoria

Retinoblastoma

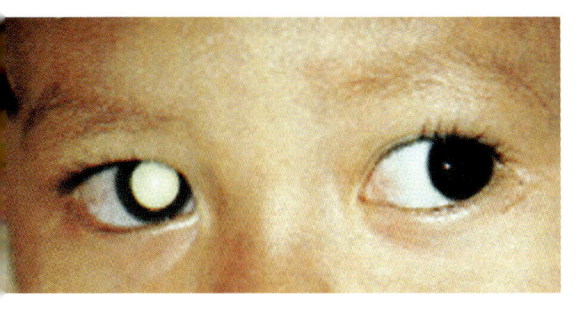

Fig. 10.1. Right leukocoria (white pupil) due to retinoblastoma.

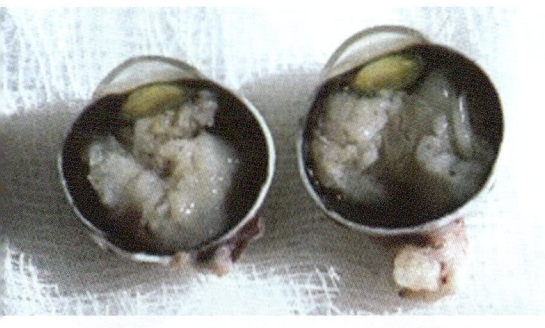

Fig. 10.2. Gross pathology of retinoblastoma.

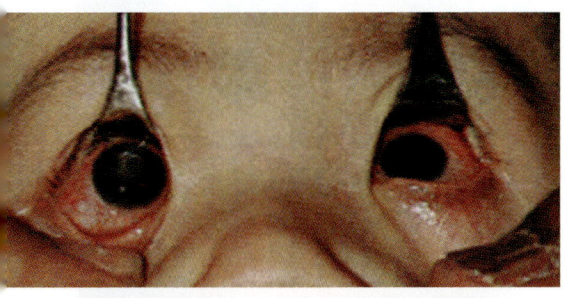

Fig. 10.3. Retrolental fibroplasia. (Note the microcornea of the left eye.)

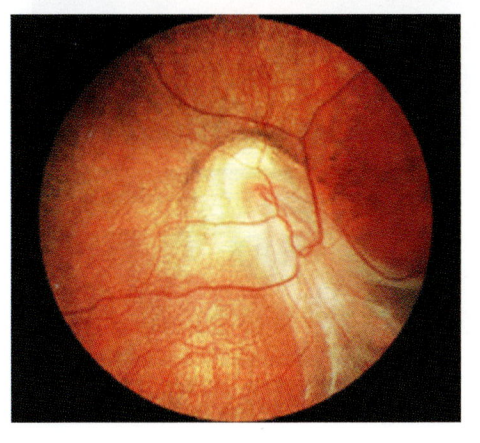

Fig. 10.4. Retinopathy of prematurity with dragging of the optic disc.

Convergent Squint

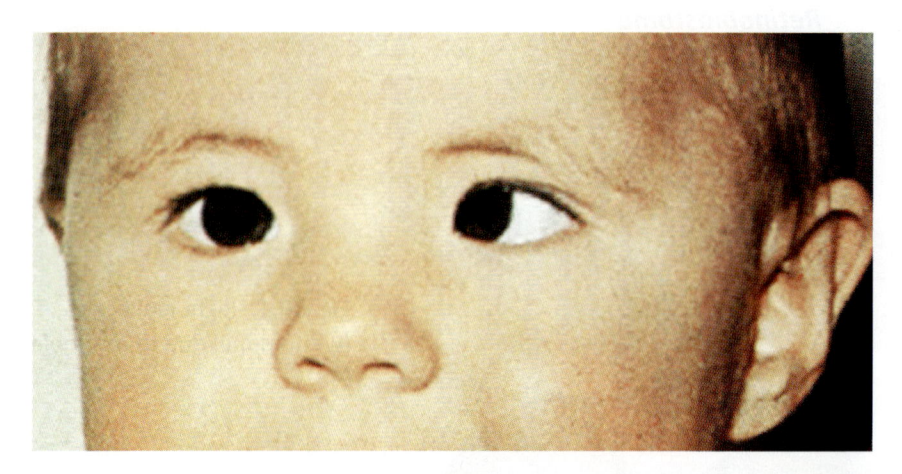

Fig. 10.5. Left congenital convergent squint.

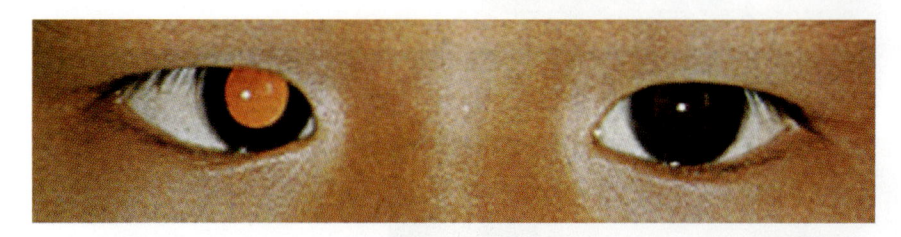

Fig. 10.6. Left convergent squint resulting from retinoblastoma. (Note the loss of the red reflex.)

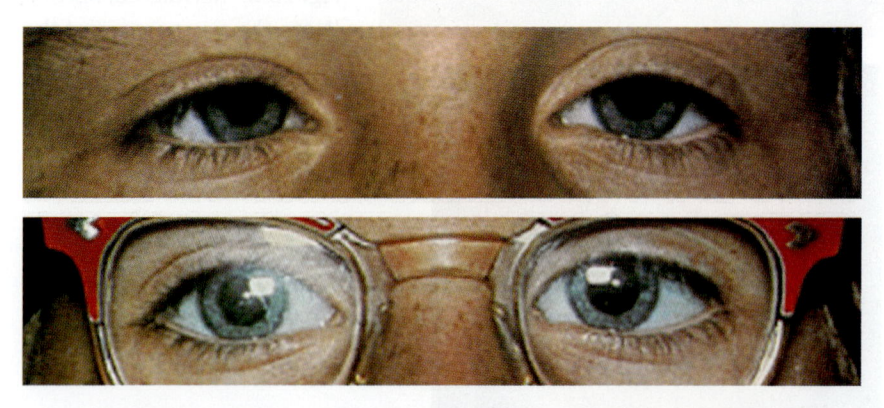

Fig. 10.7. Right accommodative convergent squint straightened with hypermetropic glasses.

Congenital Glaucoma and Congenital Cataract

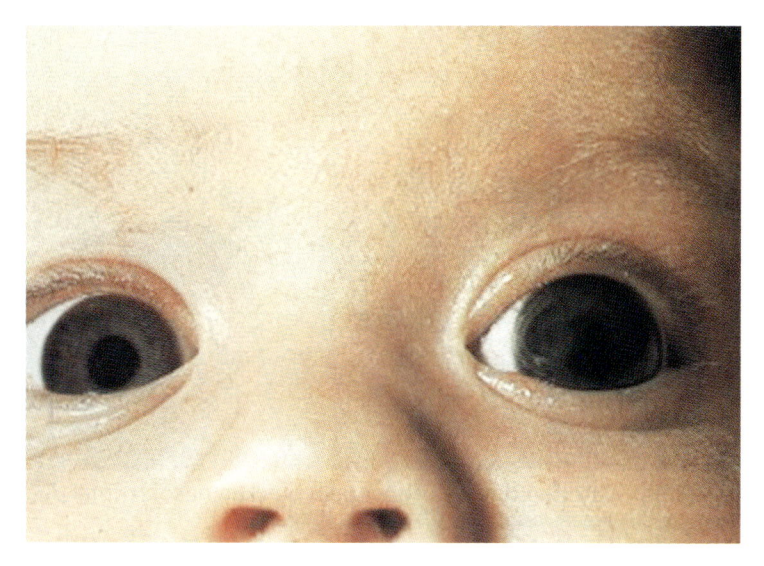

Fig. 10.8. Congenital glaucoma with an enlarged corneal diameter (buphthalmos, or "ox eye"), especially in the left eye.

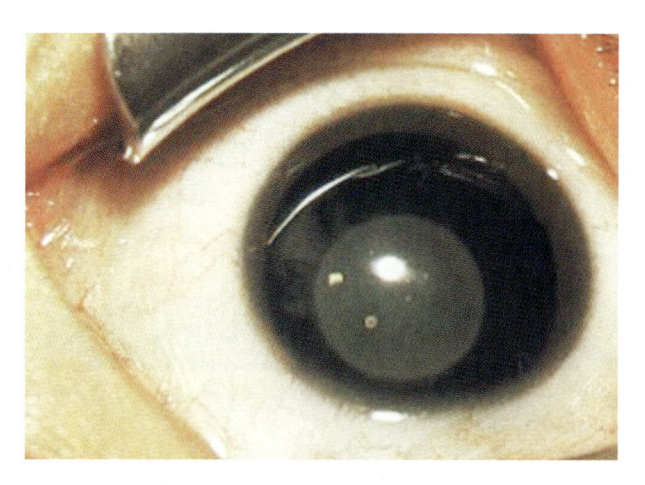

Fig. 10.9. Congenital cataract affecting the nucleus of the lens.

Watering and Conjunctivitis

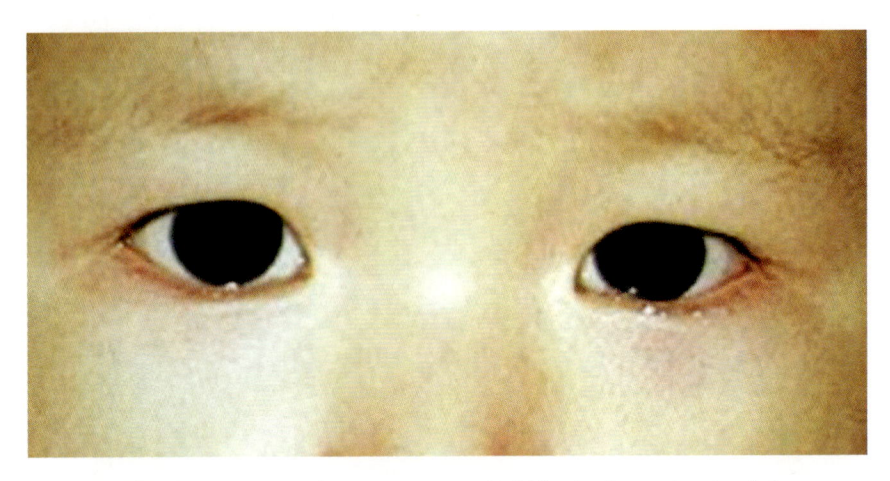

Fig. 10.10. Watering due to a congenital blocked nasolacrimal duct.

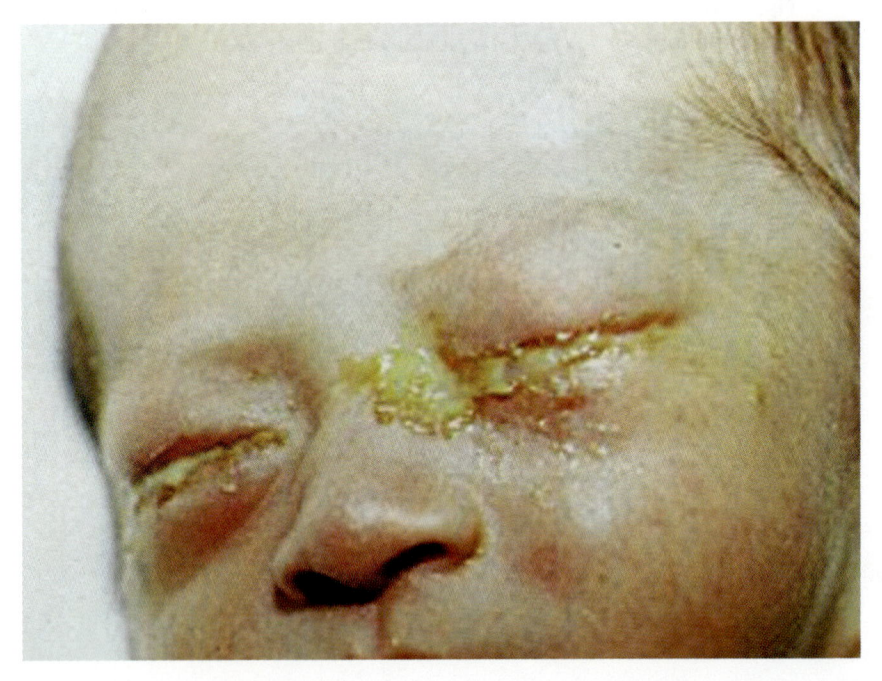

Fig. 10.11. Ophthalmia neonatorum due to gonococcal infection.

Phakomatoses

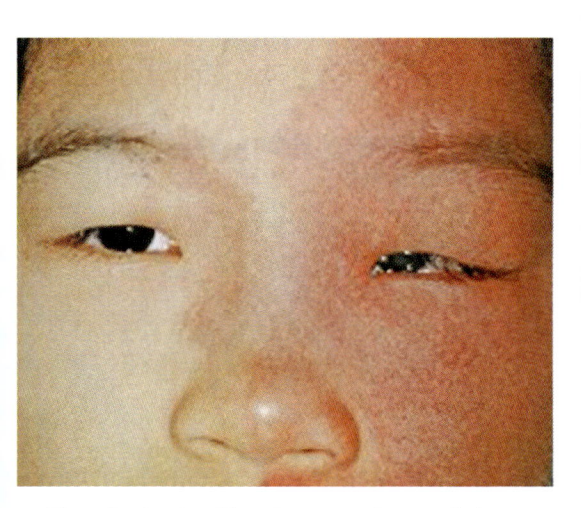

Fig. 10.12. Capillary haemangioma of the left side of the face with unilateral glaucoma in Sturge–Weber syndrome.

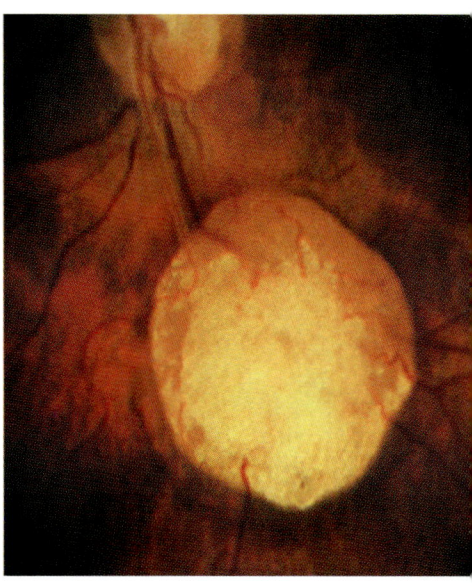

Fig. 10.13. Globular retinal tumour in tuberous sclerosis.

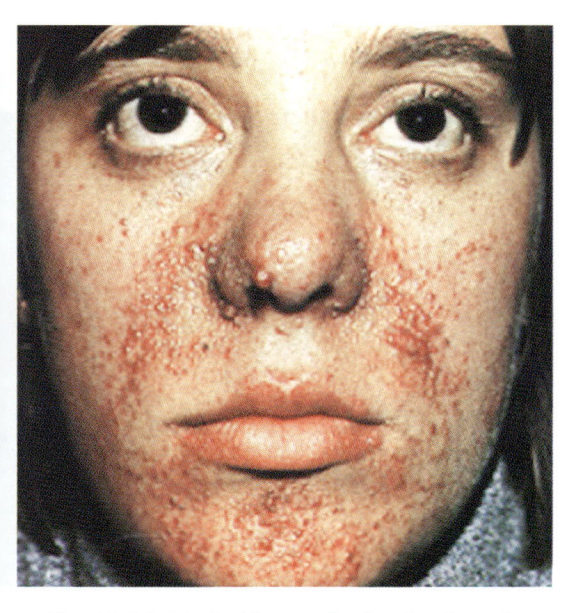

Fig. 10.14. Typical butterfly distribution of sebaceous adenoma in tuberous sclerosis.

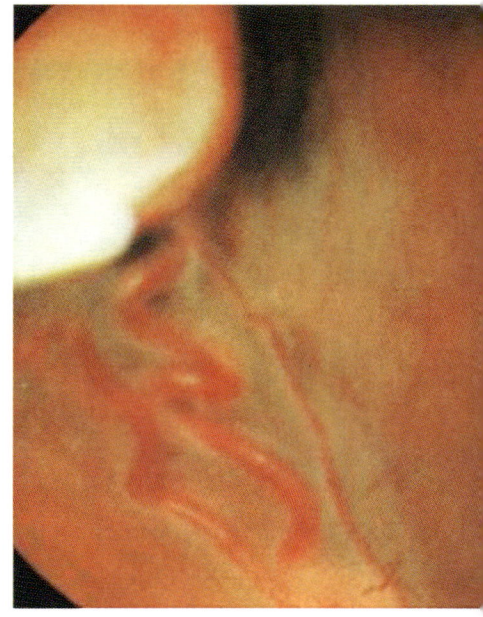

Fig. 10.15. Elevated haemangioma with large feeding retinal vessels in von Hippel–Lindau disease.

Developmental Abnormalities

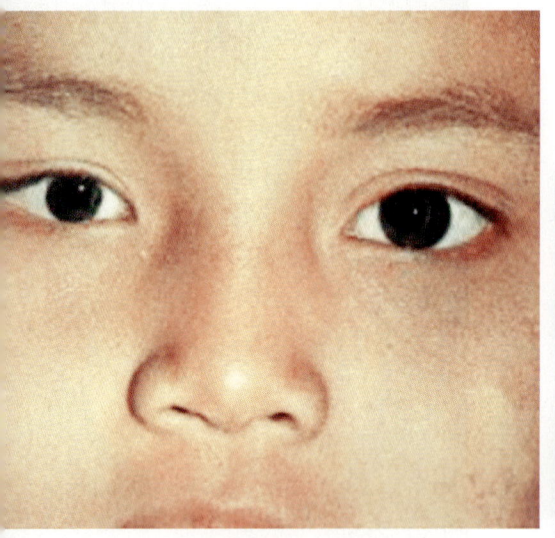

Fig. 10.16. Right microphthalmos.

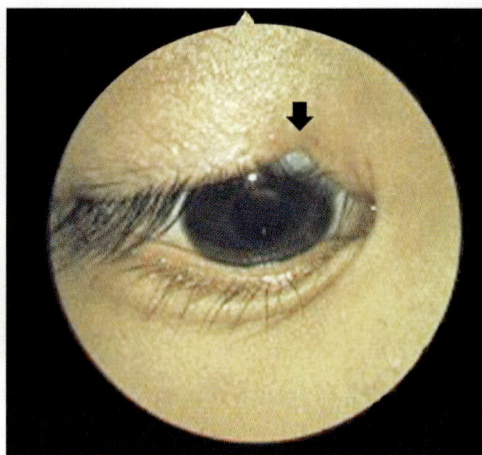

Fig. 10.17. Congenital coloboma of the right upper lid.

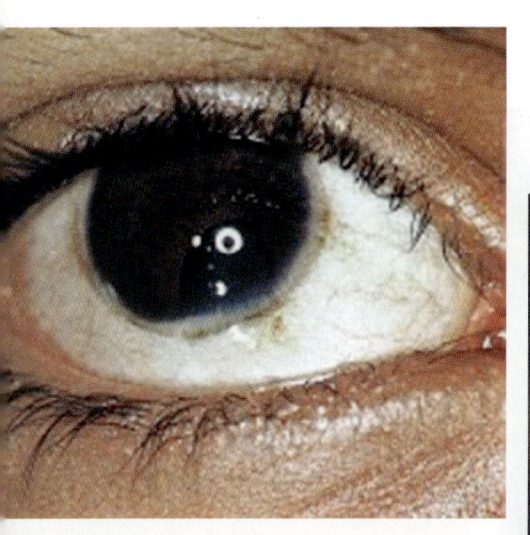

Fig. 10.18. Inferior nasal coloboma of the iris.

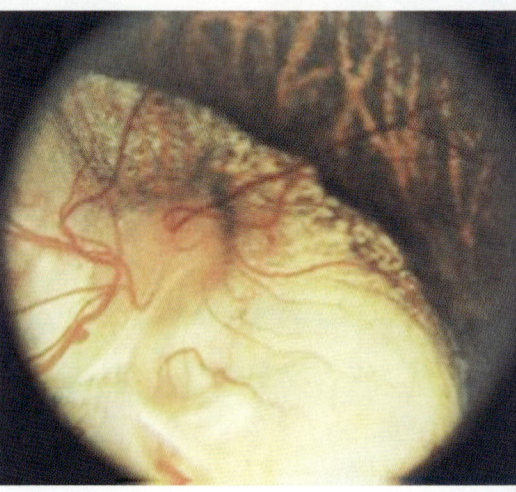

Fig. 10.19. Large choroidal coloboma involving the optic disc and macula.

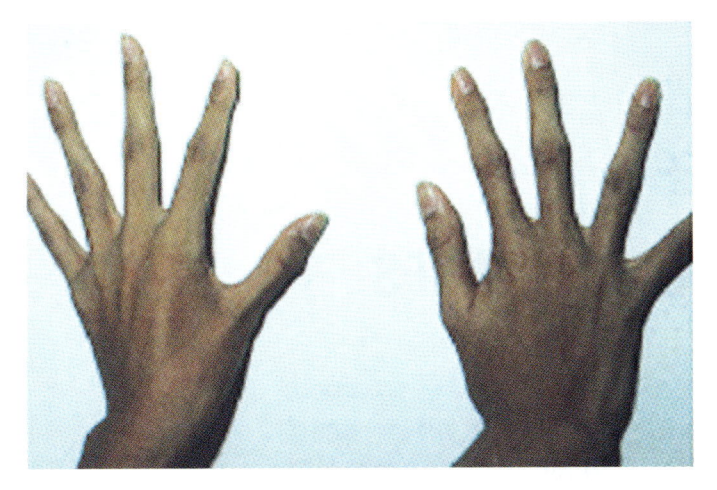

Fig. 10.20. Arachnodactyly in Marfan syndrome.

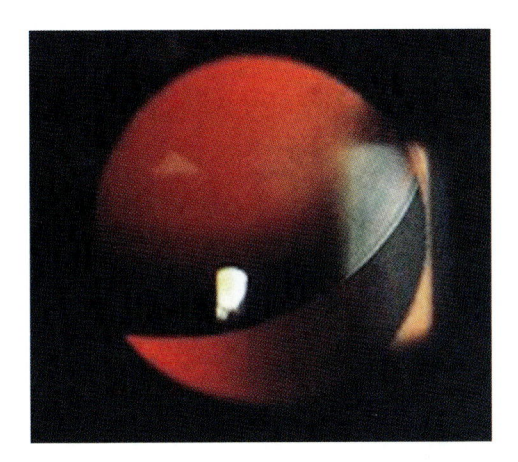

Fig. 10.21. Superior dislocation of the lens in Marfan syndrome.

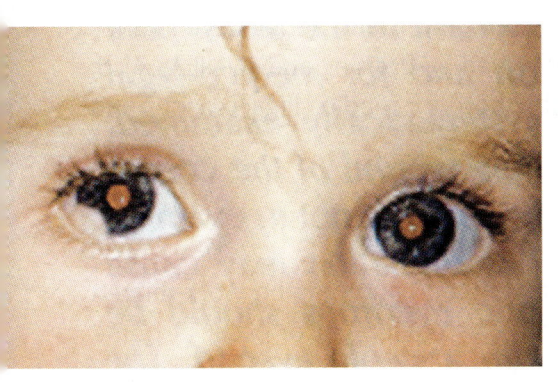

Fig. 10.22. Limbal dermoid.

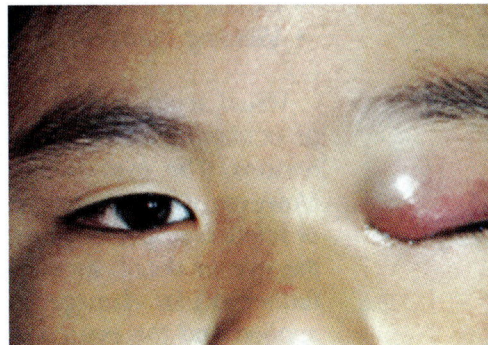

Fig. 10.23. Haemangioma of the left upper eyelid.

11
OCULAR INJURIES

INTRODUCTION

Ocular injuries are common. The severity of these injuries may range from trivial to permanent loss of vision or of the eye itself.

Ocular injuries may be any of the following.

- Chemical injury
- Eyelid trauma
- Superficial injury to the cornea and conjunctiva
- Injury to the globe
- Orbital trauma
- Ocular injury associated with head injury
- Ultraviolet light or welding flash injury

Taking a careful history and making a thorough systematic assessment of the eye and ocular adnexa is important. Serious eye injuries may have subtle signs or be concealed by bruising and swelling. Also, careful documentation is essential both for medico-legal reasons and for prognostication.

PREVENTION

Many ocular injuries are preventable, and may be work-related with lack of use of personal protective equipment or occur at home during play or the pursuit of hobbies.

CHEMICAL INJURY

Chemical injuries are mostly accidental, due to spillage of strong alkalis or acids, and can be potentially blinding, requiring urgent treatment.

It is important to dilute the chemical as soon as possible: it is really quite futile to try to determine whether the chemical is an acid or an alkali — as is frequently recommended in textbooks. The time to act is immediately after the injury has occurred, and it is important that treatment should be started immediately.

The eye should be irrigated with sterile fluid (if available) or else with tap water immediately, and this should be continued for at least 30 min. Conjunctival fornices should be swept with a moistened cotton bud to remove any trapped particles of caustic material. The pH can be checked using litmus paper in the inferior conjunctival fornix if available, after stopping irrigation for at least 5–10 min.

Following first aid measures as described above, one should seek urgent ophthalmological opinion. Patients usually need intensive lubricants, topical steroids, cycloplegics and topical antibiotics.

Alkaline burn injuries are more serious, because the alkali penetrates the eye more deeply than acid. Alkali can destroy internal structures, leading to complications such as cataract, severe iridocyclitis and glaucoma. Acid coagulates collagen and this forms a barrier which may prevent penetration of the chemical into the eye. Therefore, acid causes less severe damage to the internal structures, but it may still result in corneal blindness and a severe dry eye.

Chemical injuries occur in laboratories and in chemical industries. Supervisors, teachers, students and workers should be warned that if any chemical gets into the eye, it should be immediately washed out with any available bland fluid or tap water. Protective glasses or eye shields for those at risk should always be used.

EYELID TRAUMA

The eyelid can be affected by blunt trauma, which usually results in a haematoma or black eye. A sharp injury can result in an eyelid laceration.

In patients with eyelid haematoma, a careful inspection of the globe and recording of visual acuity is necessary in order to rule out globe rupture or penetrating eye injury. Eyelid bruising usually settles spontaneously.

Eyelid lacerations can be superficial or deep and can involve the lid margin. Lid margin laceration needs to repaired very carefully to avoid misalignment and notching of the lid margin.

SUPERFICIAL INJURY TO THE CORNEA AND CONJUNCTIVA

This usually occurs due to injury from "flying" particles or an accidental scratching of the eye. Flying particles generally come from two sources: a working hammer or chisel, or a revolving machine. If the velocity of the foreign particle is great, it will penetrate the eye. Otherwise, it is commonly embedded in the cornea, presenting as a corneal foreign body. This results in severe photophobia, congestion and irritation of the eye. Infection is prevented by the use of antibiotic eye drops. The foreign body is removed after administration of a drop of local anaesthetic with the aid of a loupe or slit lamp and a cotton bud if very superficial.

Foreign bodies within the pupillary area or those more deeply embedded should be referred to an ophthalmologist, as a corneal scar at this site can lead to severe visual loss.

Topical anaesthetic is instilled in the eye and the foreign body removed using a fine gauge hypodermic needle. A sharp instrument such as a hypodermic needle should be used with caution under slit lamp magnification, because of the danger of increased corneal scarring or even inadvertent perforation.

Corneal abrasions usually result from an accidental scratch to the eye. The cornea and conjunctiva should be carefully inspected for the presence of a foreign body. A corneal abrasion in a contact lens wearer is potentially more serious and may require microbiological investigation and fluoroquinolone eye drops. Otherwise antibiotic ointment such as chloramphenicol will usually suffice.

Conjunctival abrasions or lacerations usually heal rapidly on their own. They need to be sutured only if larger than 10 mm or if the underlying extraocular muscle is exposed.

INJURY TO THE GLOBE

Blunt Trauma to the Globe

Blunt trauma can result from a punch, champagne cork, tennis or squash ball, shuttlecock or elastic strap and under a variety of other circumstances at home or work. It can cause injury to the whole range of ocular and orbital tissues.

Conjunctiva: Subconjunctival haemorrhage, conjunctival lacerations
Cornea: Abrasions
Anterior chamber: Hyphaema
Uvea: Traumatic sphincter rupture of the pupil, iridodialysis
Lens: Cataract, lens subluxation and dislocation
Vitreous cavity: Vitreous haemorrhage
Retina and choroid: Commotio retinae, choroidal rupture, retinal detachment, traumatic macular holes, retinal dialysis
Optic nerve: Traumatic optic neuropathy and avulsion.

Globe Rupture

Globe rupture should be suspected if there is deepening of the anterior chamber, limited motility or significant traumatic subconjunctival haemorrhage extending backwards, and if the globe is soft (low intraocular pressure). If there is suspicion, the patient will need urgent B-scan ultrasonography and general anaesthesia for a safer complete examination and primary repair.

Penetrating Eye Injury

A penetrating wound is usually due to a sharp or pointed object which has penetrated the eyeball. Loss of vision may be the result of direct damage to the cornea or the lens, giving rise to a cataract. There may also be intraocular haemorrhage, a retained intraocular foreign body or retinal damage. It is important to obtain a precise history of the nature of the injury. The patient may complain of pain, a watering eye or photophobia. The pupil is sometimes deformed, due to a prolapsed iris.

Treatment is urgent. Antibiotic eye drops are applied locally after the affected area has been cleaned. The eye should be covered with a clear shield to protect it. It is unwise to try to examine the eye in detail, especially if there is a large penetrating wound, as the eye can be further damaged during examination. The patient should be referred immediately to an ophthalmologist. Imaging by CT scan in hospital can exclude a retained intraocular foreign body but surgical repair under general anaesthesia is urgently required.

A retained metallic intraocular foreign body can cause the deposition of iron in the structures inside the eye, mainly the iris, lens and retina, resulting in a condition called siderosis bulbi. The iris becomes hyperchromic (browner in colour) because of the iron deposition, leading to heterochromia, when compared to the fellow eye. Pigmentary retinopathy with atrophy of the retina and RPE can also occur, with profound loss of vision.

SYMPATHETIC OPHTHALMIA

Any patient with a severe injury to the globe must be warned of the risk of sympathetic ophthalmia. This may occur if an autoimmune response to damaged uveal tissue activates an inflammatory response in the undamaged eye. It may occur many years later and be activated by late reconstructive surgery in the damaged eye. Removal of the injured eye with no visual potential within 10–14 days is said to reduce the risk.

ORBITAL TRAUMA

Blowout Fracture

A blunt injury sometimes does not injure the eyeball itself, but may instead fracture one of the thin walls of the orbit, usually the floor. This will cause the contents of the orbit to protrude into the maxillary antrum, giving the eye a sunken appearance (enophthalmos). This usually becomes more obvious at a later stage because of post-traumatic orbital fat atrophy.

Signs of blowout fracture include periorbital ecchymosis, subcutaneous emphysema which is felt on palpating the lower eyelid, anaesthesia in the infraorbital nerve region and double vision. The inferior rectus and inferior oblique muscles may be entrapped and result in both double vision and limited elevation of the eye. Radiological evaluation is necessary. Surgery to free the muscles and repair of the defect in the bony orbital floor is usually required.

OCULAR INJURY ASSOCIATED WITH HEAD INJURY

An ocular injury associated with a head injury is sometimes overlooked, because the lid swelling makes it difficult to examine the eye and also attention is often diverted to other problems.

In patients with severe head injuries, especially if there is bruising around the orbit, it is important to carry out a careful examination of the eyes and orbits. Allowance must be made for this even during emergency neurosurgical care.

ULTRAVIOLET LIGHT OR WELDING FLASH INJURY

Ultraviolet light or welding flash exposure results in severe photophobia, blepharospasm, pain and watering of the eyes. Punctate epithelial erosions are seen on the cornea.

A drop of local anaesthetic can be used to facilitate examination so as to ensure that the symptoms are not due to some other injury. Treatment consists of relieving the symptoms of pain and photophobia with analgesics and patching of the eyes after instillation of an antibiotic ointment. Use of local anaesthetic drops repeatedly for pain relief should be avoided to prevent toxicity to the corneal epithelium. The symptoms of a flash burn usually subside within 24 hr and the patient escapes permanent loss of vision.

Chemical Burn

Fig. 11.1. Acid chemical burn typically affecting the cornea inferiorly.

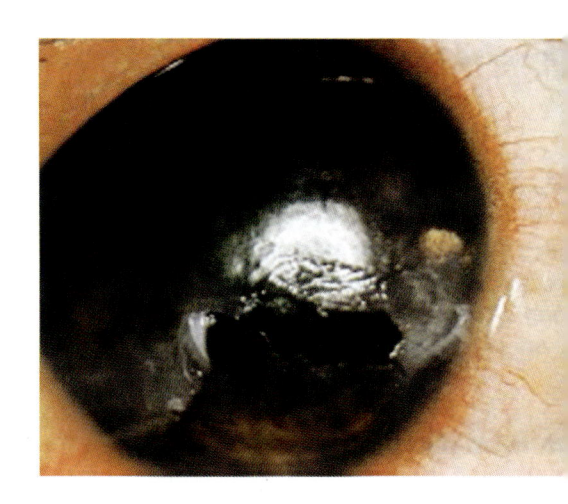

Fig. 11.2. Severe corneal opacity following a lime (alkali) burn.

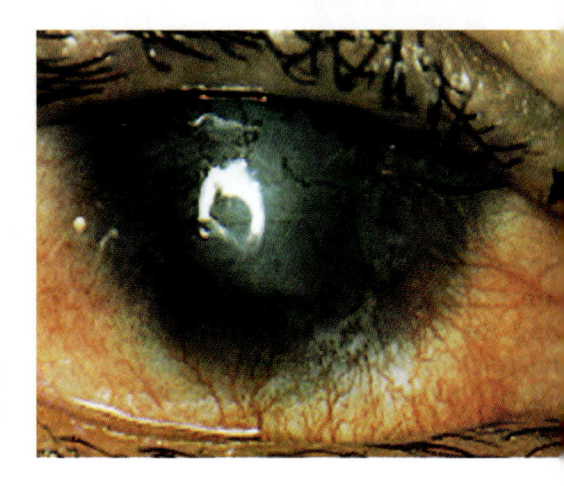

Fig. 11.3. Opaque vascularised cornea after a severe chemical burn.

Foreign Particles

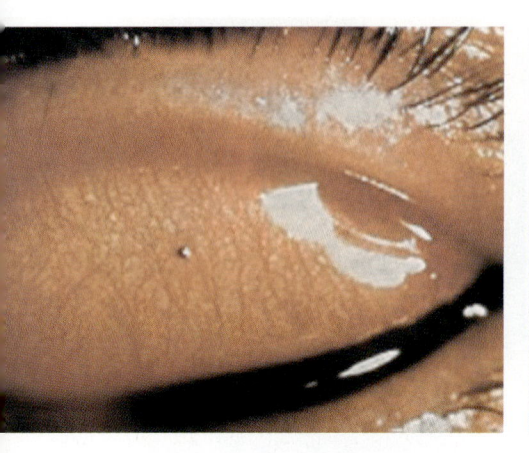

Fig. 11.4. Foreign particle on the upper tarsal conjunctiva (everted upper lid).

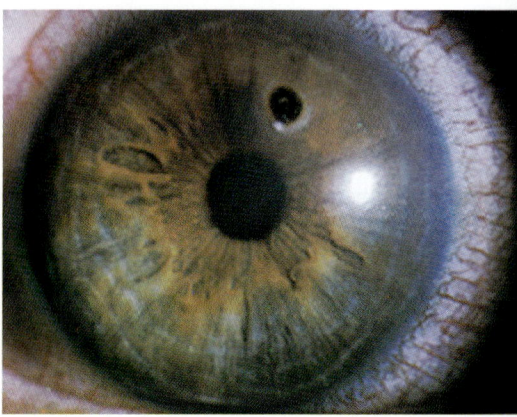

Fig. 11.5. Foreign particle embedded on the cornea.

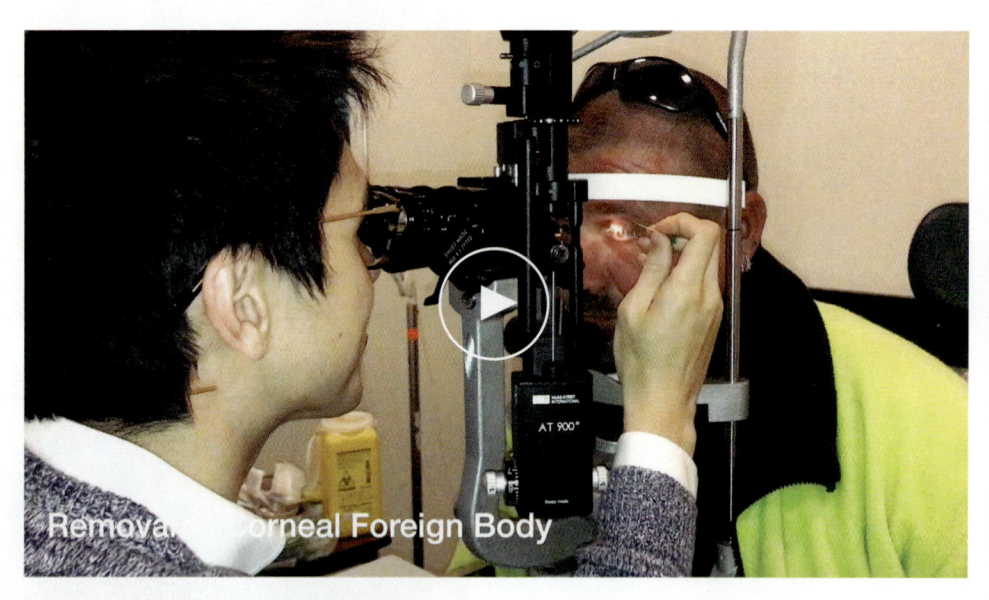

Video of removal of an embedded corneal foreign body.

Intraocular Foreign Particles

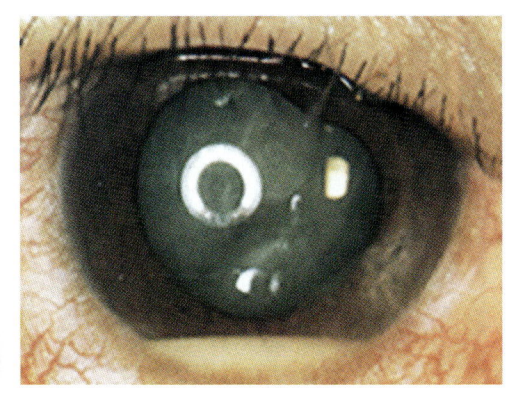

Fig. 11.6. Intraocular foreign body causing cataract and infection with hypopyon (pus in the anterior chamber).

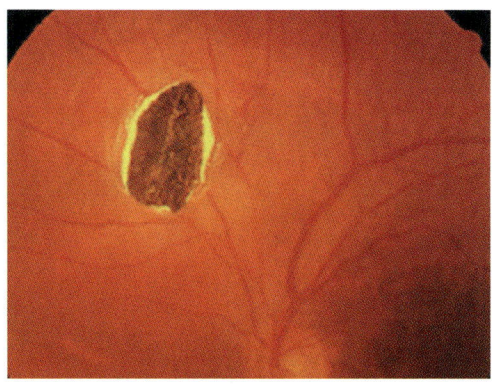

Fig. 11.7. Iron particle in the vitreous.

Fig. 11.8. Siderosis bulbi of the right eye caused by a retained iron particle in the eye. Dilated pupil due to optic atrophy and a discoloured iris.

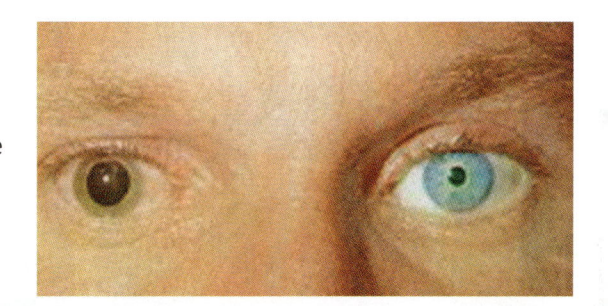

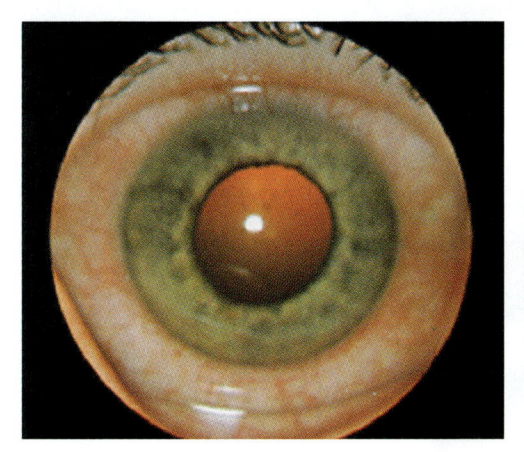

Fig. 11.9. Siderosis bulbi of the right eye. Iris colour changed to brown (same patient as in Fig. 11.8).

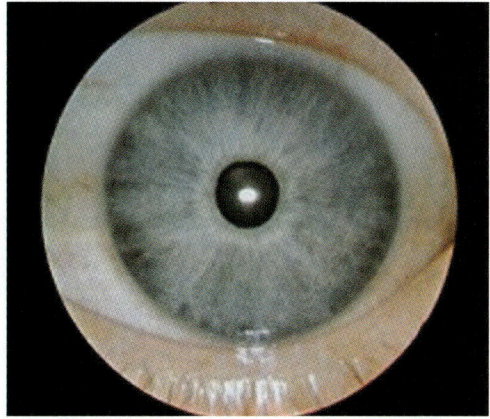

Fig. 11.10. Left eye normal (same patient as in Fig. 9.7).

Injury with Sharp Instruments

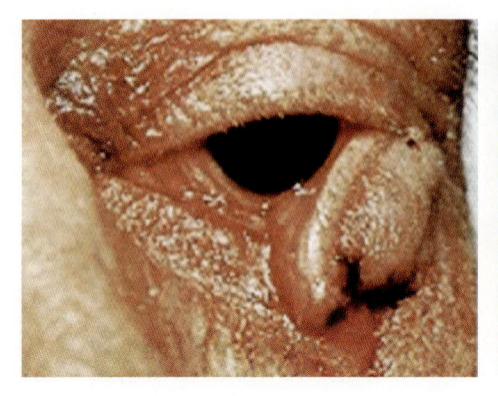

Fig. 11.11. Laceration of the lower lid involving the inferior canaliculus.

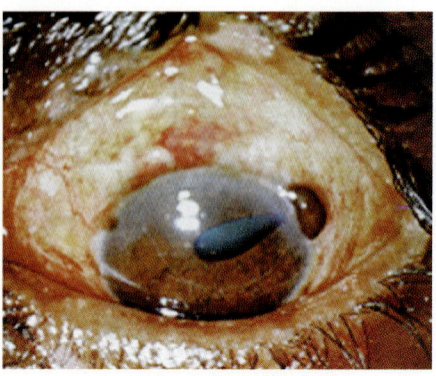

Fig. 11.12. Penetrating corneal laceration with prolapse of the iris. (Note the distorted pupil.)

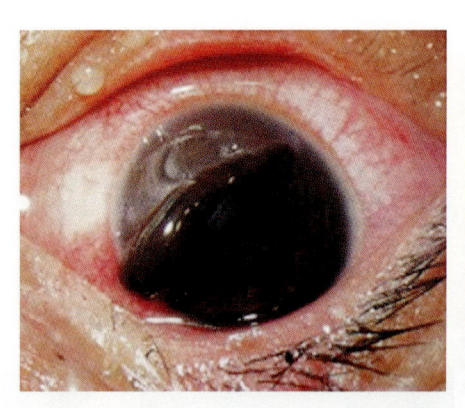

Fig. 11.13. Large corneal laceration with prolapse of blood clot and iris. This requires urgent repair under general anaesthesia.

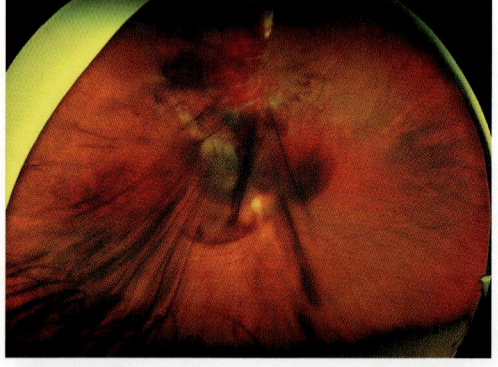

Fig. 11.14. Ruptured globe caused by falling forward onto the edge of a desk. (Note the vitreous and subretinal blood and the scleral laceration above.)

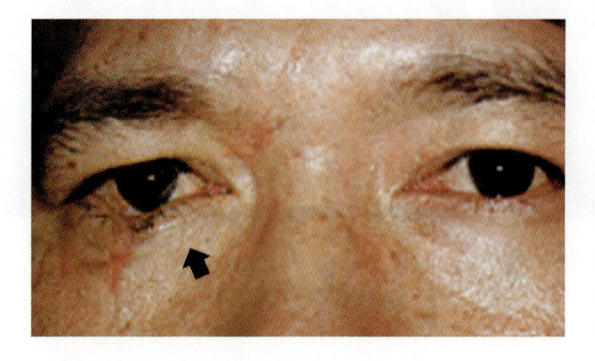

Fig. 11.15. Repaired laceration of both right eyelids, cornea and sclera following a motor vehicle accident.

Blunt Injury Hyphaema

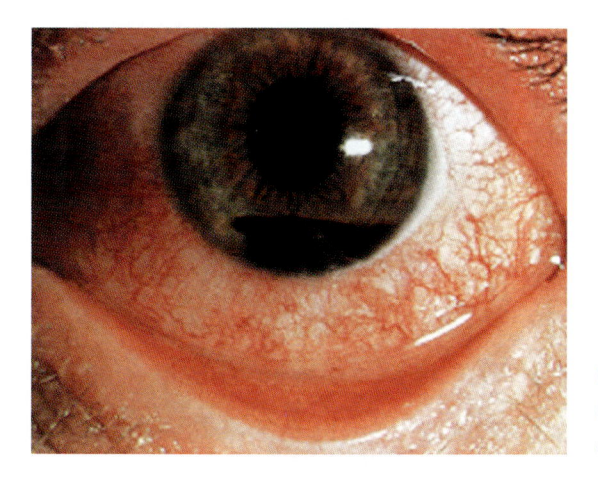

Fig. 11.16. Small hyphaema (blood in the anterior chamber) — characteristic fluid level of blood.

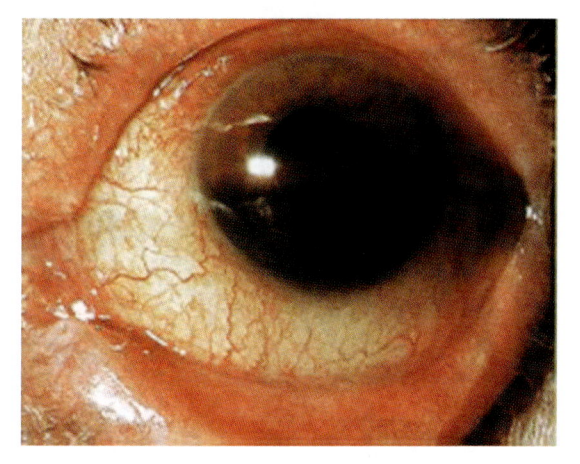

Fig. 11.17. Hyphaema filling more than half of the anterior chamber.

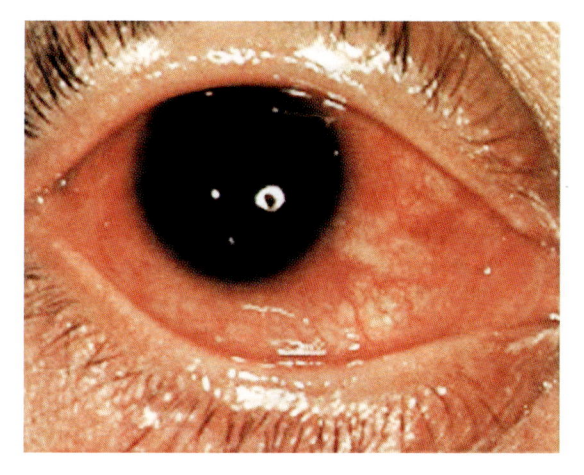

Fig. 11.18. Hyphaema filling the entire anterior chamber, complicated by secondary glaucoma.

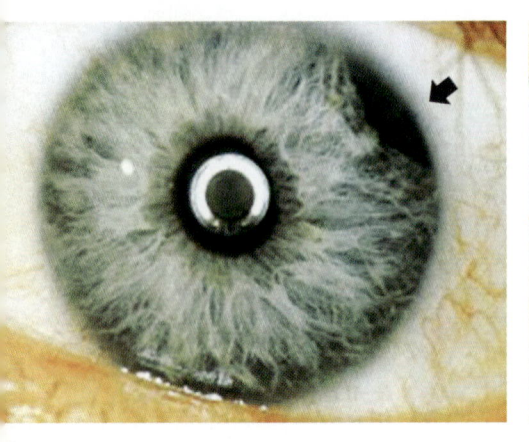

Fig. 11.19. Iridodialysis — iris torn at the root.

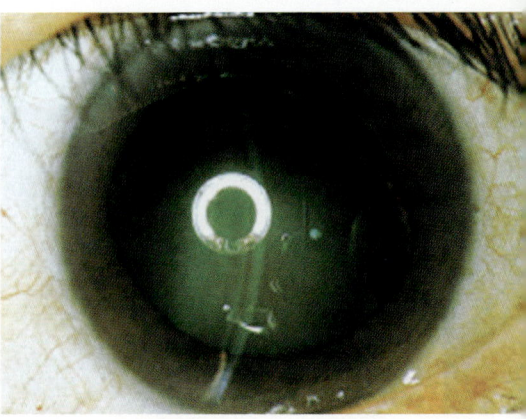

Fig. 11.20. Traumatic dislocation of the lens

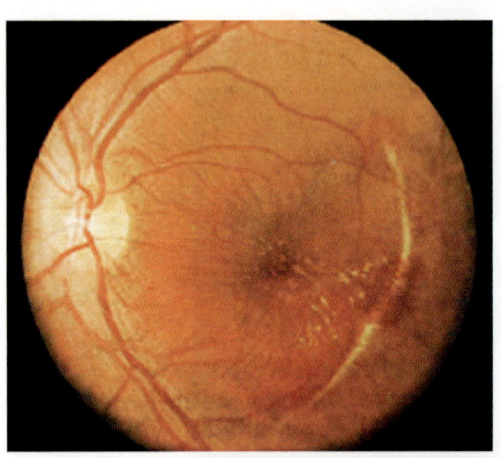

Fig. 11.21. Resolving commotio retinae (traumatic oedema, exudates and haemorrhages at the posterior pole) with a typical curved choroidal rupture temporal to the macula.

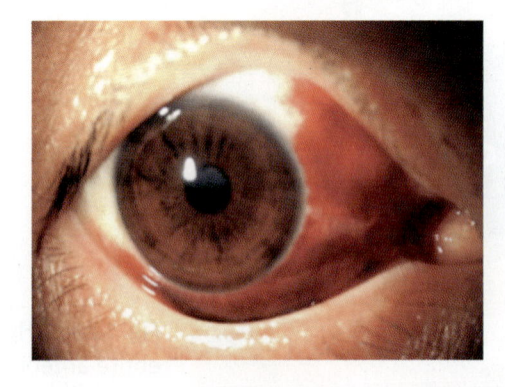

Fig. 11.22. Traumatic subconjunctival haemorrhage.

Fig. 11.23. Right lower lid haematoma and oedema with subconjunctival haemorrhage. (Note the enophthalmos due to a blowout fracture of the inferior floor of the orbit.)

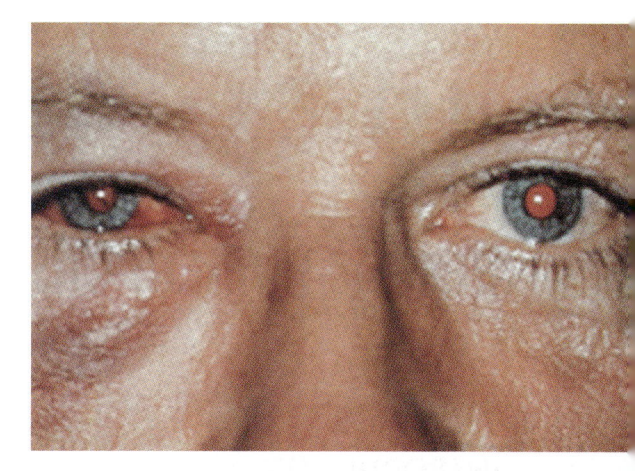

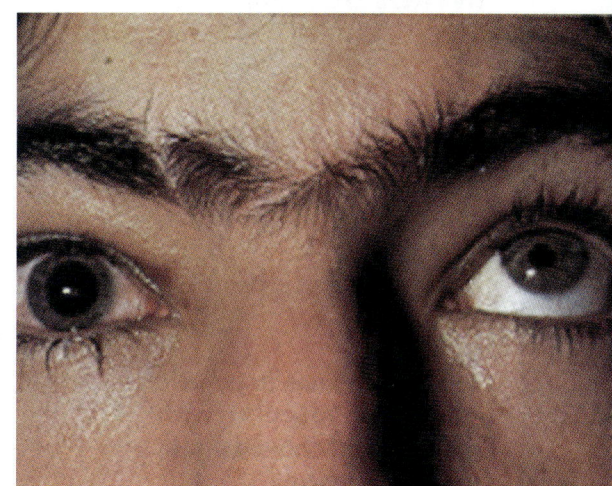

Fig. 11.24. Right blowout fracture with limited elevation of the right eye (right pupil dilated with mydriatics).

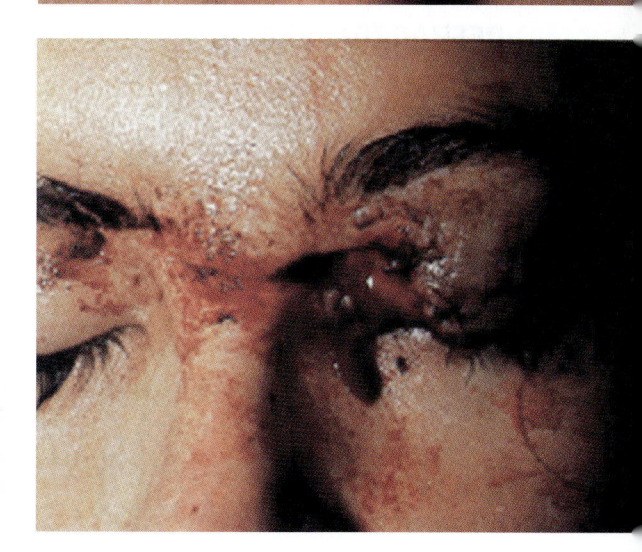

Fig. 11.25. Multiple lacerations of the lids and face by glass fragments in a motor car accident (without seat belt). The cornea was also lacerated.

12
REFRACTIVE ERRORS

INTRODUCTION

The commonest cause of blurred vision is refractive error. This is a physiological condition where the refracting system of the eye fails to focus objects sharply on the retina. It is usually corrected with glasses. A useful rapid test to distinguish between refractive error and disease of the eye is the use of a pinhole.

In modern societies, contact lenses are often preferred to glasses mainly for myopia and for cosmetic reasons. When contact lenses are used, it is important for the wearer to take the necessary precautions to prevent complications from infection and excessive wear, as serious ocular damage may occasionally develop.

REFRACTIVE ERROR

Myopia

Myopia (short-sightedness) is an optical condition where distant objects are focused in front of the retina so that vision for distance is blurred but near vision is normal. It is measured by the power in dioptres of the concave lens needed to focus light onto the retina.

Myopia is common in Asians, especially the Chinese. Studies have shown that up to 80% of the Chinese student population may be myopic, as compared with 25% in Caucasians. In addition, there are indications that myopia is becoming more common and more severe with time. It exerts a socio-economic burden on society.

A strong genetic component probably exists in myopia but there is also evidence that it is related to changing environmental factors, especially in Asia. These include increasingly prolonged close work or play and absence of extended outdoor activites at a young age.

There are two types of myopia. The commonest form of myopia is known as simple or physiological myopia. It is usually slow or non-progressive and not associated with any degenerative changes of the retina.

It is important to distinguish simple myopia from the other form, pathological myopia. The latter is more serious but is found in only a small percentage of patients. Pathological myopia is usually seen in people with more than 6 dioptres of myopia associated with progressive degenerative changes of the retina, affecting in particular, the macula. This degeneration, known as myopic maculopathy, sometimes leads to blindness. In addition, patients with pathological myopia have a higher risk of developing glaucoma, cataract, retinal tears or retinal detachment.

Glasses are the usual way of correcting myopia, and they are usually prescribed by an optometrist. Contact lenses are also a popular and efficient means of correcting myopia. Laser refractive surgery is increasing in popularity as a permanent means of correction for myopia of up to 8 dioptres. Higher degrees of myopia can be corrected by invasive surgery with an intraocular contact lens or clear lens extraction and replacement with a suitable IOL, as in cataract surgery.

Extensive community-based trials have focused on preventing or slowing down the progression of myopia. They have included the use of bifocal glasses, contact lenses and eye drops (atropine).

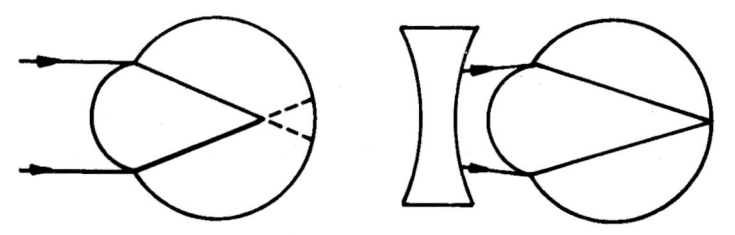

Fig. 12.1. Simple myopia corrected with a concave lens.

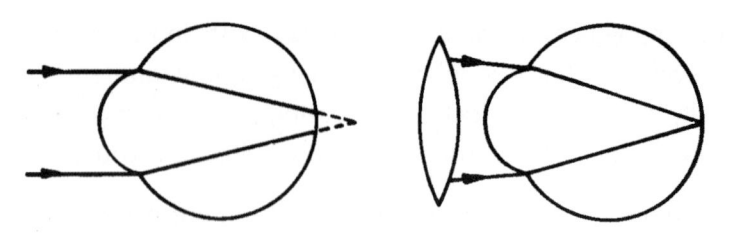

Fig. 12.2. Hypermetropia corrected with a convex lens.

Hypermetropia

Hypermetropia (long-sightedness) is a condition where a distant object is focused behind the retina. In the young, hypermetropia is compensated by because of the strong accommodative power of the lens. With age, however, the power of accommodation decreases and the patient is unable to focus on near objects, and later also on distant objects. Because of this, the patient requires the use of reading glasses earlier in life than normal. With time, glasses are required for distant vision as well.

Astigmatism

Astigmatism is a condition where the image cannot be focused sharply on a point because either the cornea or the lens is not spherical and has greater power in one meridian. Marked astigmatism causes poor vision, both distant and near. It is corrected with a cylindrical lens. A cylinder is shaped like a food can with no power in one axis and maximum power at right angles to that axis. Sometimes the astigmatism is irregular. This is caused by corneal scarring or keratoconus (conical cornea). Irregular astigmatism is usually difficult to correct with glasses and requires contact lenses.

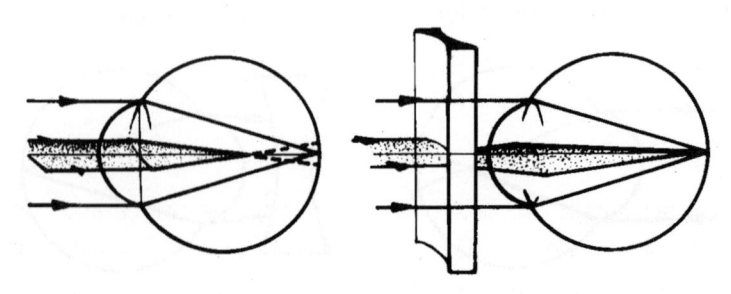

Fig. 12.3. Astigmatism corrected with a cylindrical lens.

Presbyopia

Presbyopia (old-age sightedness) is a condition of weak accommodation brought about by age. A young child has considerable ability to accommodate. This diminishes with age, owing to progressive enlargement and stiffening of the lens. In middle age, near vision becomes progressively worse. Glasses for near vision are required even though the distant vision is perfect. For people who require correction for both distant and near vision in a single pair of glasses, bifocals or multifocal progressive power lenses are prescribed.

Another alternative refractive solution for presbyopia is to correct one eye for distance (emmetropia) and make the other eye myopic for near vision (monovision). This can be achieved with both contact lenses and intraocular implants.

EYE STRAIN

Uncorrected refractive errors or wrongly prescribed glasses may lead to symptoms which include red eyes, blurring, watering, tired eyes and headaches which may be ocular, frontal or diffuse. There is often a close relationship between eye strain and the use of the eyes for reading, driving, or an occupation which requires close visual concentration. Patients show great individual variations in tolerance of refractive errors. Some are sensitive to minor changes in their glasses, while others are not bothered by gross refractive errors.

The symptoms of eye strain may also be due to muscle imbalance, poor convergence, the patient's psychological state, or a variety of drugs, macular diseases and, occasionally, systemic diseases.

In presbyopic patients, the symptoms are relieved by the use of reading glasses and stronger light when they are reading.

CONTACT LENSES

Contact lenses are widely used, for both refractive and cosmetic reasons. There are a variety of contact lenses — hard, soft and oxygen-permeable. Hard contact lenses have been available for more than 60 years. However, they are not as comfortable to wear and require careful fitting. For this reason, soft lenses have become more popular, being easy-to-fit, well-tolerated and disposable.

Optically, contact lenses function in the same way as glasses. They help to focus the image sharply on the retina.

There are many reasons why contact lenses are used. They result in better vision than glasses, with less optical distortion in higher refractive errors. They are sometimes the only practical method of vision correction for keratoconus and irregular astigmatism. Contact lenses are very popular also for cosmetic considerations. Many young myopic patients are willing to tolerate discomfort and the inconvenience of meticulous daily management for their resultant appearance.

Contact lenses are also used by sportsmen who find that glasses fog with perspiration, as well as stage or television personalities who find it less attractive to wear glasses. Contact lenses may be contraindicated in dusty or industrial conditions. They are not easily tolerated in the presence of dry eyes.

Soft contact lenses are sometimes used therapeutically to bandage a corneal ulcer which fails to heal or to prevent discomfort from chronic corneal epithelial disturbance. Bifocal contact lenses are also occasionally used to correct both distance and near vision.

Complications of Contact Lens Wear

A common complication, especially with hard lenses, is overwear. The prolonged relative lack of oxygen supplied via the tear film from the atmosphere leads to corneal oedema. The patient gives a history of having used the lenses longer than usual and complains of pain, watering, photophobia and eyelid spasm (blepharospasm). Because of the complications, any contact lens wearer who complains of persistent pain or discomfort should have the cornea assessed by an optometrist or ophthalmologist.

Prolonged contact lens wear can induce peripheral corneal vascularisation which may resolve with cessation of use, by changing to smaller diameter lenses or a type of lens giving improved oxygen permeability.

The main problem with soft contact lenses, however, is the risk of corneal infection, which may lead to corneal ulcers or blindness. The source of infection may be contaminated fingers handling them or the lens storage medium.

Another occasional problem with soft lenses is the development of giant papillary conjunctivitis due to a hypersensitivity reaction through contact of the lens material with the subtarsal conjunctiva. The patient complains of redness, itching, irritation and mucoid discharge. Eversion of the upper lid will reveal characteristic giant papillae. If the condition is severe, the patient should stop wearing the contact lenses.

REFRACTIVE SURGERY AND THE EXCIMER LASER

Correction of refractive errors by laser reshaping of the cornea or by intraocular lens surgery also has an established place in the management of refractive errors.

Initially, radial keratotomy, which involved partial-thickness radial incisions into the peripheral cornea to change the curvature, was developed to reduce simple myopia. It was superseded by photorefractive keratectomy using the excimer laser, which was found to have less complications and to be more predictable. Photorefractive keratectomy involves the use of ultraviolet light to remove a few microns of superficial corneal tissue. This reduces the refractive power by reshaping the anterior surface of the cornea and so reduces myopia. However, photorefractive keratectomy is painful and can cause surface scarring.

LASIK (laser-assisted intrastromal keratomileusis) is the preferred method for corneal refractive surgery. In this technique, a flap of cornea is created with a photo-disruptive high-frequency laser and then the excimer laser is applied to the corneal stromal bed to remove the required tissue, as in photorefractive keratectomy. The flap is replaced at the end of the procedure. LASIK has been found to achieve excellent results for myopia of up to about −8 dioptres. Higher power corrections require removal of more corneal tissue and tend to give less accurate results and more post-operative glare.

Insertion of an intraocular lens in front of the normal crystalline lens may be performed effectively in high myopia. Clear lens extraction and replacement can also be done. Both have the risks of intraocular surgery.

APHAKIA

Aphakia is an optical condition of the eye without its lens (following cataract extraction). A strong convex (plus) lens has to be used to replace the power of the removed lens so that images can be focused on the retina. Thick cataract glasses cause adjustment difficulty because of optical distortion and the increased image size. Contact lenses decrease the adjustment problems but are difficult to manage with older people. As a result implanted intraocular lenses are almost universally the chosen method for correction of aphakia. Small-incision cataract surgery with phacoemulsification gives a fairly predictable post-operative astigmatism. Pre-operative measurement of the corneal curvature and axial length allows calculation of the corrective lens needed. Toric (astigmatic) lenses may be used, which will correct both the spherical and astigmatic components and result in excellent vision without distance glasses. Near glasses are still needed unless a multifocal intraocular lens is inserted or one eye is overcorrected to induce unilateral myopia for near vision.

Myopia

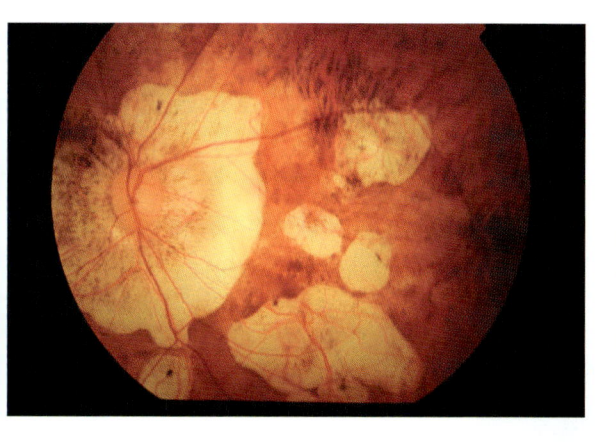

Fig. 12.4. High myopia with degeneration of the macular area. The large myopic eye may stretch posteriorly, causing a staphyloma and degeneration of retinal and choroidal tissue.

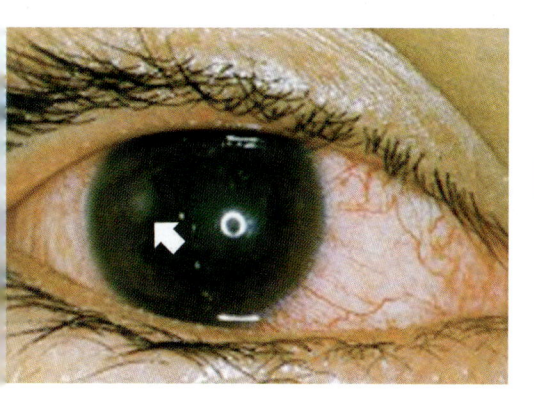

Fig. 12.5. Small corneal ulcer caused by a staphylococcal infection from the use of soft contact lenses.

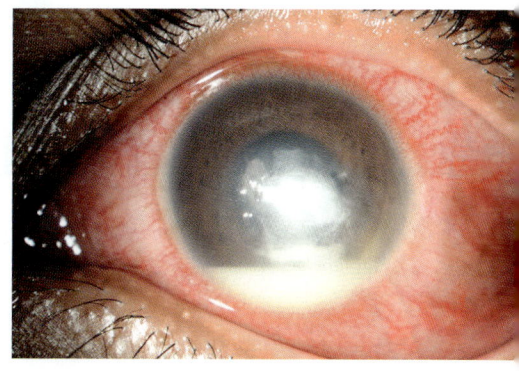

Fig. 12.6. Bacterial corneal ulcer and hypopyon associated with a contaminated contact lens solution.

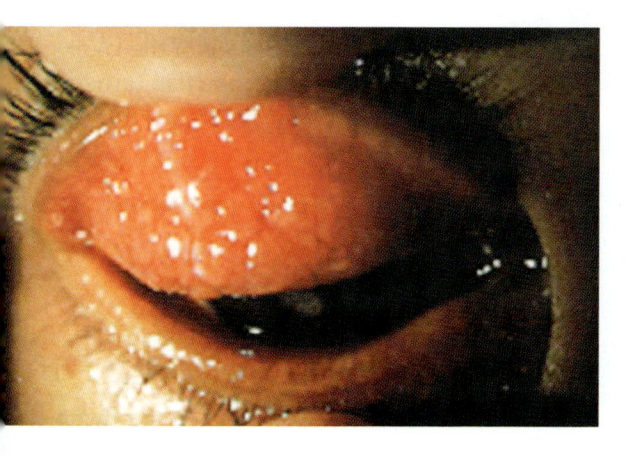

Fig. 12.7. Severe giant papillary conjunctivitis associated with contact lens wear.

Refractive Surgery

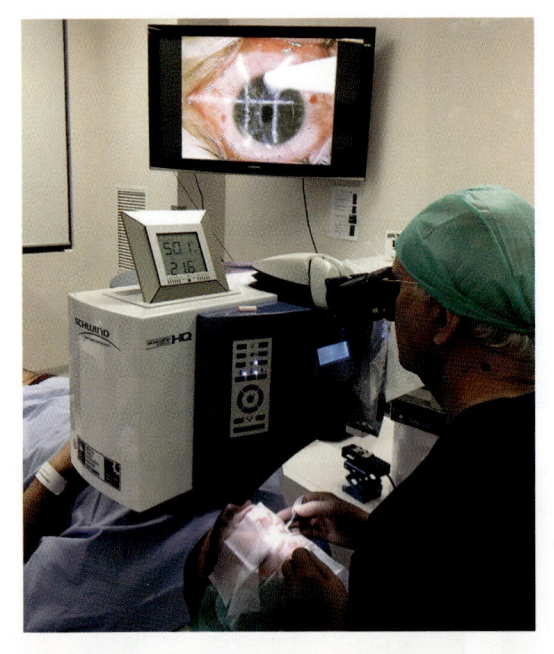

Fig. 12.8. Excimer laser in progress.

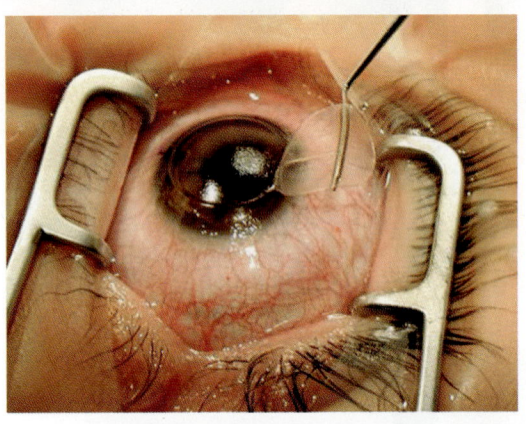

Fig. 12.9. Close-up of the LASIK procedure with the flap turned back.

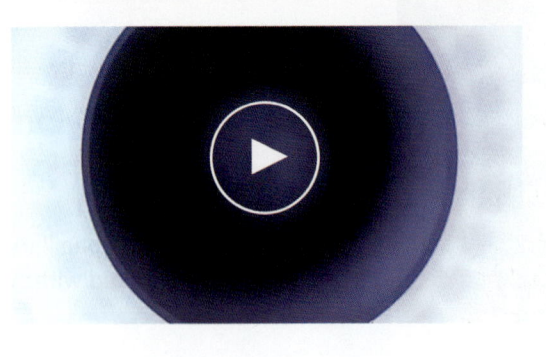

Video of LASIK surgery for myopia.

13
OPHTHALMIC MEDICATIONS

INTRODUCTION

Ophthalmic medications can be given topically in the form of eye drops or ointments, and are effective for conditions affecting the anterior part of the eye. In general, eye drops are preferred as they do not blur vision and can deliver the drugs in a higher concentration. Conditions affecting the back of the eye usually require subconjunctival, retrobulbar or intravitreal injections and systemic therapy. Intravitreal injections are highly effective as they bypass the blood–vitreous barrier and are widely used for retinal conditions including age-related macular degeneration, diabetic retinopathy and retinal vein occlusions.

TOPICAL THERAPEUTIC DRUGS

These drugs are usually dispensed as eye drops, but may be used as eye ointments.

Antibacterial

The commonly used antibiotic eye drops are those which are seldom used systemically and have a broad spectrum of action. They are chloramphenicol, neomycin, soframycin, gentamycin and polymyxin. Tetracycline or sulphur derivatives are particularly useful in the treatment of trachoma. Fortified preparations are available for treatment of severe corneal infections, including fortified cephazolin, gentamycin and vancomycin. Newer drugs such as fluoroquinolones have increased efficacy and a broader antibacterial spectrum, and are considered the first line of treatment for contact lens keratitis. Some of the commonly used fluoroquinolones are ciprofloxacin, ofloxacin, levofloxacin, moxifloxacin and gatifloxacin. Prolonged usage of fluoroquinolones can result in corneal deposits.

Antiviral

Idoxuridine, adenine arabinoside, acycloguanosine and trifluorothymidine eye drops or ointments are used for herpes simplex infection of the eye. However, their availability can be limited in certain countries. The first line of treatment is aciclovir 3%, which is in ointment form. Aciclovir ointment is used five times a day for herpetic corneal infections. Prolonged usage of aciclovir can cause severe punctate epithelial erosion. More recently, ganciclovir in ointment form has been developed for the use of herpetic corneal infections, with a reduced side effect profile.

Glaucoma Therapy

There are a variety of eye drops for the treatment of glaucoma. They include pilocarpine, beta adrenergic blockers, adrenaline, prostaglandin agonists and topical carbonic anhydrase inhibitors.

Prostaglandin analogues

These are prescribed as the first line of treatment for glaucoma. The commonly used prostaglandin analogues are latanoprost, travoprost, bimatoprost and tafluprost. They lower intraocular pressure by increasing uveoscleral outflow of aqueous humour. The usual dosing regime is once daily. The potential side effects include longer eyelashes, darkening of the iris, redness of the conjunctiva, periorbital pigmentation and periorbital fat atrophy.

Beta blockers

This class of drugs was the first line of treatment before the advent of prostaglandin analogues. The commonly used beta blockers are timolol, betaxolol and metipranolol. They lower intraocular pressure by reducing aqueous production. They are usually used twice daily. However, there are long-acting gel preparations which allow once-daily dosage. The common side effects are bradycardia, shortness of breath, worsening of asthma, lethargy and (rarely) impotence. They should be used with caution in patients with type 1 diabetes, as they can mask the reactive symptoms of hypoglycaemia. They are also available in fixed dosing combinations with prostaglandin analogues, like a latanoprost–timolol combination (Xalacom®), a travoprost–timolol combination (Duotrav®) or a bimatoprost–timolol combination (Ganfort®), and can then be used once daily.

Carbonic anhydrase inhibitors

These drugs can be used on their own or in a fixed combination with beta blockers. They reduce IOP by decreasing aqueous production and are taken twice daily. The commonly used carbonic anhydrase inhibitors are brinzolamide and dorzolamide. The common side effects are redness, soreness and grittiness of the conjunctiva.

Alpha adrenergic agonists

The drugs in this class are brimonidine and apraclonidine. They reduce IOP by decreasing aqueous humour production and increasing outflow of aqueous, and are used twice daily. Brimonidine is available in a fixed combination with timolol. Apraclonidine is short-acting and is commonly used after laser procedures like capsulotomy, iridotomy and selective laser trabeculoplasty to prevent an IOP spike. The adverse reactions of this class of drugs are hyperaemia of the conjunctiva, a gritty sensation and allergic blepharoconjunctivitis.

Pilocarpine

This is a miotic which stimulates the parasympathetic system. It is commonly used in narrow-angle glaucoma, where it enables widening of the anterior chamber angle by causing miosis. The common side effects include headache, miosis exaggerating the effect of central lens opacities, iris cysts and retinal detachment.

Decongestants and Antihistamine Eye Drops

There are numerous combinations of decongestants and antihistamine eye drops used for non-specific conjunctivitis and mild allergies and also as a placebo for tired or irritable eyes. The commonly used ones are phenylephrine for temporary vasoconstriction, and anti-allergy drops such as naphazoline or ketotifen.

Dry Eye Therapy

Tear substitutes are used to treat dry eye. The treatment depends on the underlying causative pathology. They are available in both preserved and non-preserved form. Normal saline eye drops can be used as an ocular lubricant in dry eyes but are not retained in the conjunctival sac. Preserved tear substitutes are usually the first line of treatment. They are available in drop and gel form. They replace the aqueous component of the tear film, and the frequency needs to be tailored based on the symptoms and severity of the disease. The common preparations include:

- Cellulose derivatives. Carboxymethyl cellulose (CMC) — Refresh Tears®, etc. — and hydroxypropyl methyl cellulose (HPMC) — Tears Naturale® etc. — are effective in mild dry eye.
- Gylcerin-containing products. These are usually combined with CMC (Visine®, Optive®) or HPMC (Tears Naturale Forte®).
- Polyethylene glycol and propylene glycol. The glycol derivatives help balance the viscosity and elasticity of tears, allowing a longer retention time with minimal blur (Systane Ultra®).
- Hyaluronic acid derivatives. Sodium hyaluronate drops are useful for improving subjective symptoms and are frequently chosen.
- Polyvinyl alcohol derivatives. These lubricate the ocular surface and also address hyper-osmolarity issues.
- Cyclosporine 0.05%. Cyclosporine eye drops are very effective in treating inflammatory dry eye. They are used twice a day. The common side effects include stinging and a burning sensation.

Mydriatics and Cycloplegics

Mydriatic and cycloplegic eye drops are used routinely for eye examination and in uveitis to dilate the pupil and to paralyse the muscles of accommodation in order to relieve pain and to prevent adhesion of the iris to the lens (posterior synechiae). They are also used in the treatment of amblyopia and sometimes after surgery. The common eye drops used for longer action in therapy are atropine and homatropine.

Steroids

Steroids are used for treating inflammation from many conditions, such as iridocyclitis and surgical trauma. The most commonly used topical steroids in ascending order of potency include fluorometholone, loteprednol etabonate, betamethasone, dexamethasone and prednisolone. Steroids need to be tapered slowly so as to prevent rebound inflammation. Because of their many complications, some of which can lead to severe visual loss, there should be specific indications for their use.

Prolonged usage of steroids without monitoring can give rise to complications such as glaucoma, cataract and aggravation of corneal infection, especially from herpes simplex and fungus.

TOPICAL DIAGNOSTIC DRUGS

Short-acting mydriatic eye drops are used to dilate the pupil to examine the lens and for ophthalmoscopy of the retinal and retinoscopy to measure the refractive error. They include tropicamide, cyclopentolate and phenylephrine. Side-effects include a topical allergic reaction, a rise in intraocular pressure in a patient at risk of narrow-angle glaucoma, glare and blurred vision until they wear off. Patients should be warned not to drive with dilated pupils. Phenylephrine may cause a significant rise in blood pressure.

Local anaesthetic eye drops are used for ocular examinations to overcome blepharospasm and for tonometry. They include proparacaine, tetracaine and idicaine. Besides their diagnostic uses, they are employed in the removal of corneal or conjunctival foreign bodies and for cataract surgery.

Fluorescein is used in strip form or as a single dose minims in the assessment of corneal injury and suspected ulceration. It is also used as an intravenous preparation for fluorescein angiography.

INTRAVITREAL THERAPY

Intravitreal injections are now the mainstay of treatment for wet, age-related macular degeneration, diabetic retinopathy and retinal vein occlusion. This form of treatment is also used for severe or persistent intraocular inflammation (uveitis), infections like viral retinitis and endophthalmitis.

The commonly used intravitreal medications for wet AMD, diabetic retinopathy and retinal vein occlusion are:

- Bevacizumab (Avastin®) — 1.25 mg in 0.05 mL. This is a humanised whole antibody which targets vascular endothelial growth factor A (VEGF).
- Ranibizumab (Lucentis®) — 0.5 mg in 0.05 mL. This is a monoclonal antibody fragment which targets and inhibits angiogenesis by inhibiting VEGF-A.
- Aflibercept (Eylea®) — 2 mg in 0.05 mL. This is a recombinant fusion protein that binds VEGF-A and placental growth factor (PIGF), thus inhibiting angiogenesis.

This class of drugs carry a possible risk of thrombotic stroke or myocardial infarction but after millions of injections world-wide the evidence is inconclusive.

Steroids can also be used intravitreally in the form of triamcinolone injections, which are usually given in the dosage of 4 mg in 0.1 mL. However, there is a risk of cataract formation and elevation of IOP. Sustained release implants (Ozurdex® and fluocinolone acetonide) have also been developed. They are biodegradable and elute the drug over 3–6 months. Steroid injections are commonly used for treatment of diabetic macular oedema, cystoid macular oedema and persistent intraocular inflammation.

MISUSE OF EYE DROPS

If misused, eye drops can lead to a number of complications.

Steroid Eye Drops

The most important and common problem is the indiscriminate use of steroid eye drops. These may cause dangerous complications with prolonged use. The complications include:

- Glaucoma
- Cataract
- Herpes simplex and fungal infection

Contaminated Eye Drops

Eye drops which have been opened and left unused for many months can be contaminated. It is important that unused eye drops are discarded. Many countries warn consumers to discard eye drops one month after they are opened. Drops formulated without preservative should be used only once.

Systemic Effects

Local eye drops, especially atropine and related anticholinergics, may lead to systemic effects, particularly in children and infants. Pilocarpine eye drops, if used intensively in acute glaucoma, can also have systemic effects. 10% phenylephrine drops may cause serious cardiovascular effects, including tachycardia and sudden increase in blood pressure, and should be replaced with 2.5%. Timolol may aggravate asthma.

Local Anaesthetic Eye Drops

Local anaesthetic eye drops should never be prescribed for ocular pain, as they can de-epithelialise the cornea and mask serious eye complications by relieving the pain. When local anaesthetic drops are used for diagnostic purposes, it is important that the patient is told not to rub the eye immediately after application in order to avoid corneal abrasion.

Antibiotic Eye Drops

The prolonged use of antibiotic eye drops locally may sometimes cause chronic conjunctivitis or mask opportunistic infection with fungus or protozoa. They may also contribute to the development of resistant strains of bacteria.

Diagnostic Eye Drops

Main Uses	(Chemical) Names	Remarks
Ophthalmoscopy	*Dilators*: • Tropicamide 0.5%–1% • Cyclopentolate 1%–2% • Phenylephrine 2.5%	Short-acting (6 hr).
Examination (blepharospasm and tonometry)	*Local anaesthetics*: • Proparacaine • Tetracaine	Not to be used for pain relief.
Staining cornea	Fluorescein	Use strips or single-dose capsules. Drops may be contaminated.

14
GLOBAL BLINDNESS AND ITS PREVENTION

INTRODUCTION

Blindness and visual impairment are major public health problems. Visual impairment leads to poor quality of life, depression, social isolation, falls or medication errors and imposes a heavy socio-economic burden on the patient, the family and society. It is therefore important that general physicians and healthcare workers play essential roles in preventing vision loss.

Most blinding eye disorders are initially asymptomatic and often go under-diagnosed or undetected for long periods of time. Therefore, screening, early detection and timely referral to eye care professionals (ophthalmologists or optometrists) and intervention are important in the prevention of vision loss and blindness.

Globally, the major causes of blindness and visual impairment are the following.

- Cataract
- Age-related macular degeneration (AMD)
- Glaucoma
- Diabetic retinopathy (DR)
- Uncorrected or under-corrected refractive error (myopia, hyperopia and astigmatism)
- Corneal diseases
- Infectious diseases

Spectacles and cataract surgery will successfully restore sight for uncorrected refractive error and cataract, respectively. Visual impairments as a result of AMD, glaucoma and diabetic retinopathy can be prevented if they are identified early enough, with appropriate treatment.

DEFINITION OF VISUAL IMPAIRMENT AND BLINDNESS

For distance vision, visual impairment is defined as presenting a visual acuity worse than 6/18 but better than or equal to 6/120 in the better eye. Blindness is defined as a visual acuity worse than 6/120, or a corresponding visual field loss to less than 10% in the better eye. Thus, low vision includes both visual impairment and blindness.

Near visual impairment (functional presbyopia) is defined as presenting near vision worse than N6 or N8 at 40 cm when the best-corrected distance visual acuity was better than 6/12.

EPIDEMIOLOGY OF BLINDNESS AND VISUAL IMPAIRMENT

Globally, of the 7 billion people in 2015, an estimated 36 million were blind and 250 million had visual impairment.

Functional presbyopia affects an estimated 1 billion people aged 35 years or older.

The major causes of moderate-to-severe visual impairment are uncorrected or under-corrected refractive error (50%) and cataract (25%), followed by AMD (4%), glaucoma (2%) and diabetic retinopathy (1%). Other causes are corneal opacities, trachoma and onchocerciasis.

The heaviest burden of eye diseases is on patients aged 80 years or older, but common age-related eye diseases start when the patients are aged 60 years or older.

In the least-developed countries, such as several in Africa, the causes of avoidable blindness are still cataract (50%) and glaucoma (15%), but corneal opacities (10%), trachoma (7%), childhood blindness (5%) and onchocerciasis (5%) have become more important.

Over 80% of all vision impairments can be prevented or cured.

About 80% of people who are blind or have visual impairment are aged 50 or above. With ageing populations, many more people will be at risk of visual impairment.

Concurrently, children below age 15 are also at risk. An estimated 20 million children are vision-impaired. Of these, 12 million have a vision impairment due to refractive error.

CATARACT

Cataract is the main cause of treatable blindness in developing countries, affecting more than 20 million people worldwide. The prevalence of cataract increases steadily with age, from 7% of people aged 50–59 to 43% of those aged 70–79. By the age of 80, 70% have cataract.

In addition to age, cigarette smoking has been consistently associated with increased risk of cataract, especially nuclear cataract. Other possible risk factors include long-term exposure to sunlight, diabetes, heavy alcohol consumption and poor nutrition.

There is still no clinically established method to prevent or slow the progression of cataract. Researchers have recommended using ultraviolet-coated sunglasses to reduce exposure to sunlight, decreasing or discontinuing smoking or alcohol intake, and close control of the blood sugar level if the patient has diabetes.

Cataract surgery successfully restores sight in more than 95% of patients, and is considered among the most cost-effective interventions in healthcare leading to improvement in vision, functional status, driving ability and satisfaction with vision in most patients.

AGE-RELATED MACULAR DEGENERATION

AMD is another major cause of blindness in older adults, and is estimated to affect 100 million people. The prevalence of early and late AMD has been estimated to be 8% and 0.4%, respectively, in adults aged 40 years or older, increasing with age, such that 5% of people above 65 years of age and 12% of people above 80 years of age have AMD. It was previously thought that AMD was less frequent in Asians, but this is no longer true as recent studies have reported that the prevalence of AMD in Asians is comparable to that in Caucasians.

There are two forms of AMD: early and late AMD. Late AMD may be further divided into two sub-types: atrophic AMD (geographic atrophy) and neovascular ("wet") AMD. Only 10% of people with early AMD will develop late AMD. However, If patients with neovascular AMD are left untreated, progressive visual loss will occur, with 75% becoming blind by three years. While AMD by itself does not lead to complete blindness, it causes loss of central vision and thus has a significant impact on the activities of daily living and the quality of life.

Although AMD is not curable, severe vision loss can be prevented because the "wet" form of AMD responds favourably to treatment with intravitreal injections, making early detection crucial.

The exact cause of AMD is unknown. AMD risk factors include older age, cigarette smoking, a family history of AMD and previous cataract surgery. One strategy for prevention of AMD is based on modification of nutrient intake. An increased intake of foods rich in lutein and zeaxanthin (i.e. spinach, kale and other greens) is associated with a decreased risk of AMD. Dietary supplements containing antioxidant vitamins such as vitamins C and E, β-carotene and zinc may delay the progression of AMD from the early to advanced stages.

Physicians should refer at-risk patients (persons over 60 years old, cigarette smokers, persons with a first-degree family history of AMD, and persons with previous cataract surgery) to be screened for

AMD with regular dilated fundus examination. Additionally, patients identified as high-risk should be given an Amsler grid to detect any macular pathology at home.

GLAUCOMA

Glaucoma is another major cause of irreversible blindness in older people, affecting 60–80 million people worldwide.

Primary open-angle glaucoma (POAG) has been shown to be seen in 3% of the global population but people of African ancestry are three times more likely to have it than Caucasian people. In patients of African descent, it is the most common cause of blindness, with a higher prevalence, earlier age of onset, and greater severity of optic nerve damage than other racial groups.

Since glaucoma progression can be effectively reduced when treated, identifying individuals at a higher risk of developing the disease could potentially prevent vision loss. Physicians should refer high-risk patients (persons over 50 years old, with a family history of glaucoma or African ancestry) for a dilated funduscopic examination of the optic nerve head.

The other major form of glaucoma, primary angle closure glaucoma (PACG), constitutes about 30% of glaucoma cases worldwide. However, PACG is responsible for a larger number of patients with severe vision loss than POAG. It is the major form of glaucoma in Asia, accounting for nearly 50% of all glaucoma patients. About 20% of PACG patients suffer from the acute version, which is almost always unilateral; at-risk persons are the elderly, women, those of Asian ethnicity (i.e. Chinese) and long-sighted individuals.

DIABETIC RETINOPATHY

Diabetes mellitus can affect the eye in many ways (retinopathy, cataract and cranial nerve palsies). Diabetic retinopathy (DR) is the most common and significant vision-threatening complication of diabetes, and because diabetes affects middle-aged people, DR is the leading cause of blindness in working age people between 20–74 years of age worldwide. About a third of the people with diabetes have DR at any one point in time, so about 100 million people have DR, and 10% have more severe forms of vision-threatening DR.

The risk factors for DR are well-established and are longer duration of diabetes and increased levels of hyperglycaemia. It has been recommended that the glycosylated haemoglobin (HbA1c) should be kept ≤ 7% for optimal glycaemic control in most patients. Other risk factors include hypertension and dyslipidemia.

DR can progress from mild to more severe stages when there is no intervention. Patients with diabetes should be regularly screened for DR with a dilated eye examination soon after the diagnosis of diabetes and subsequently on an annual basis. Physicians should help patients understand the importance of annual dilated eye examination even though the patient may be asymptomatic. These patients must be informed that timely detection and appropriate intervention of DR can result in the saving of sight.

UNCORRECTED AND UNDER-CORRECTED REFRACTIVE ERROR

Uncorrected or under-corrected refractive error is the leading cause of visual impairment even in developed countries. Myopia, the inability to see far clearly, has been estimated to affect 20–30% of the global population. Along with presbyopia, the inability to see clearly at near, these are the common refractive errors that can be corrected with spectacles. Myopia generally starts in children and is associated with a lack of outdoor activities and an increasing number of near-work activities, such as reading. Genetics is also an important risk factor for myopia.

Age is the common risk factor for presbyopia. However, the exact age where near-vision glasses are required may be earlier for individuals who have underlying hypermetropia or certain conditions, such as diabetes or neurological disease. Medications can also accentuate presbyopia.

INDEX

5-fluorouracil, 54, 87

Acetazolamide, 87, 90, 92
Acne rosacea, 156
Acute glaucoma, 2, 3, 47, 64, 95f, 237
Acycloguanosine, 232
Aciclovir, 33, 54, 232
Adenine, 232
Adie's tonic pupil, 174
AIDS, 99, 100, 153
Alkaline burns, 209
Amblyopia (lazy eye), 35, 189, 192–195, 197, 235
    prevention and treatment of, 194, 197, 235
AMD, 115, 116, 120, 131–136, 236, 239, 240, 242, 243
Anhidrosis, 174
Anisometropia, 195
Ankylosing spondylitis, 99
Anophthalmos, 199
Antenatal infection, 199
Anterior chamber, blood in (hyphaema), 219f
Anterior segment, examination of, 18f, 25f

Anti-vascular endothelial growth factor (anti-VEGF), 108–111, 114, 116, 124, 134, 137, 138, 144, 145, 148, 149, 160, 162–165, 191, 192
Antiviral drugs, 33
Aphakia, 228
    intraocular implants, 228
Applanation tonometry, 12, 25f
Arabinoside, 232
Arachnodactyly, 207f
Arcus juvenilis, 57
Arcus senilis, 57, 71f
Argyll Robertson pupil, 174, 175
Arteriosclerosis, 109, 110, 150, 172, 175
Arthritis
    dry eyes and, 155
    juvenile rheumatoid, 99
    rheumatoid, 50, 155
        scleromalacia, 155, 169f
Astigmatism, 2, 53, 59, 75, 195, 224, 226, 228
    corrected, 224f
Atropine, 11, 56, 99, 194, 223, 235, 237
Azathioprine, 99f

Figures & tables denoted by letters — "f" – figures & "t" – tables

Basal cell carcinoma, 37, 45*f*
   treatment of, 37
Beta adrenergic blocker, 86, 232
Bevacizumab, 116, 121*f*, 122*f*,
   149, 159*f*, 236
Bilateral red eye, 47–49, 62*f*
Binocular microscope, 12
Binocular single vision, 12, 193
Binocular slit-lamp microscopy, 12
Bitemporal hemianopic field
   defect, 170, 173, 184*f*, 185*f*
Bjerrum screen, 13
Blepharitis, 3, 31, 32, 34, 42, 49,
   50, 156
     squamous, 42*f*
     ulcerative, 42*f*, 55
Blepharospasm, 213, 226, 235, 238*t*
Blindness
     causes of, 47, 72*f*, 144, 145,
       154, 196, 223, 239
     glaucoma and, 83, 243
     legal, 4, 114
     macular degeneration, 114
     opaque cornea, 52
     preventing, 64, 77, 144, 148,
       149, 152, 154, 197, 239
     sudden, 64
     total, 5–6
Blind spot, 13, 171, 180*f*
Blood erythrocyte sedimentation
   rate (ESR), 109, 172
Blowout fracture, 213, 221*f*
Blue field entoptoscope, 16
Blunt injuries, 174, 213, 219*f*,
   220*f*, 221*f*
     blowout fracture, 213, 221*f*
     commotio retinae, 211, 220*f*
     hyphaema, 211, 219*f*

     iridodialysis, 211, 220*f*
     subconjunctival haemorrhage,
       220*f*
     traumatic mydriasis, 174
Blurred vision, 1, 6, 48, 51, 55,
   89–91, 98, 99, 110, 111, 118,
   138*f*, 172, 222
Bourneville's disease, 198
Buphthalmos (ox eyes), 197, 203*f*
Burns
   alkaline, 209, 215*f*
   chemical, 209, 215*f*

Canaliculus, 38, 218*f*
Canalisation, 196
Cancer, nasopharyngeal, 40, 156
Candida albicans, 100
Capillary haemangioma, 40, 198,
   205*f*
Carbonic anhydrase inhibitors, 86,
   87, 232, 233
Carcinoma, eyelid, 37, 45*f*
Cataract, 2, 73–75, 78*f*, 79*f*, 80*f*,
   81*f*, 82*f*, 145, 154
   congenital, 73, 80*f*, 189, 191,
     194, 196, 200, 203*f*
   dense, 7, 14, 73, 197
   diabetes and, 145
   extraction, 59, 74, 76, 228
   glaucoma, 74
   retinal detachment in, 76
   secondary, 98, 192
   senile, 73
   surgery, 14, 50, 74–77, 88,
     112, 197, 223, 228, 236,
     240, 242
   treatment of
       anterior capsulectomy, 74

extracapsular technique, 75
phacoemulsification, 75
post-operative complications, 76
Cataract blindness, worldwide, 77
Catarrh, spring, 49, 66f
Cavernous sinus thrombosis, 39
Cellulitis, orbital, 38, 39, 46f, 156
Cellulitis, preseptal, 39
Central retinal artery occlusion, 108–109, 120f, 173, 182f
Central retinal vein occlusion, 96f, 109, 120f, 121f, 152, 167f
Central scotoma, 171t, 172, 178
Cephazolin, 55, 231
Cerebrovascular occlusion, 173
Chalazion cyst, 32, 42f
Chemical burns, 215f
Chemosis, 38, 46f
Chiasmal lesions, 170, 173, 184f
Children, eye diseases in, 189–207
    amblyopia (lazy eye), 189, 193, 195
    anisometropia, 195
    anophthalmos, 199
    astigmatism, 195
    Bourneville's disease, 198
    buphthalmos (ox eyes), 197, 203f
    capillary haemangioma, 198, 205f
    choroidal angioma, 198
    Coats' disease, 190, 192
    congenital cataract, 189, 191, 196, 200, 203f
    congenital cyst, 199
    conjunctivitis, 189, 195, 196
    craniofacial dysostosis, 199
    Descemet's membrane, 197
    developmental abnormalities, 199, 206f, 207f
    double vision, 193, 195
    endophthalmitis, 190
    examinations, difficulties in, 6, 190
    eyes, watering, 196, 197, 204f
    glasses for children, 193, 194, 202f
    glaucoma, congenital, 197, 198, 203f
    hypermetropia (long sightedness), 193, 195
    hyperplastic vitreous, primary, 192
    intraocular malignancy, 190
    lacrimal drainage system, 196
    leukocoria, 189, 201f
    management of, 191
    mandibulofacial dysostosis, 199
    meningoencephalocele, 199
    microphthalmos (small eye), 199
    myopia and, 193
    neurofibromas, 198
    neurofibromatosis, 198
    ocular pathology, 75, 194, 195
    ophthalmia neonatorum, 195, 204f
    squints, 192–194
    vitamin A deficiency (Keratomalacia), 154
Chlamydia, 51, 52, 196
"Chlamydia trachomatis", 51
Chloroquine, 155

Figures & tables denoted by letters — "f" – figures & "t" – tables

Chorioretinal atrophy, 117, 118, 138*f*
Chorioretinal scar, 99, 105*f*, 152, 155, 200
Chorioretinitis, 99, 100, 103*f*, 104*f*, 105*f*
Choroidal melanoma, 101
  benign, 100, 106*f*
  malignant, 101, 107*f*
  retinal detachment, 101
Choroidal metastasis, 101, 107*f*
Choroidal tumours, 100–101
  naevus, 100
Choroidal vessel, 22
Cicatricial ectropion, 36
Ciprofloxacin, 48, 55, 232
Closed-angle glaucoma, 50, 64*f*, 83, 89, 91, 95*f*
CMV retinitis, 100
Coloboma, 199, 206*f*
Colour vision, test for, 13
  Farnsworth–Munsell 100-hue, 13
  Ishihara, 13
  Lantern colour matches, 13
Commotio retinae, 211, 220*f*
Confrontation test, 6, 12, 23*f*
Conical cornea *see* Keratoconus
Conjunctiva, 7, 47–72
Conjunctival follicles, 7, 66*f*
Conjunctival lesions, raised, 53, 67*f*
  astigmatism, 53
  melanoma
    benign, 53, 67*f*
    malignant, 53
  pingueculum, 53
  pingueculum, nasal, 67*f*
  pterygium, 53

pterygium, nasal, 67*f*
subconjunctival haemorrhage, 51
  treatment of, 53
Conjunctivitis, 4, 204*f*
  acute, 51
  allergic, 48, 62*f*
  bacterial, 47–48, 62*f*
  chronic, 36, 49, 156, 238
  exposure, 36
  follicular, 34, 66*f*
  infectious, 195–196
  non-specific, 49, 234
  papillary, 227, 229*f*
  trachoma inclusion, 51
  unilateral, 51
  vernal (spring catarrh), 49, 66*f*
  viral, 48, 62*f*
Contact dermatitis *see* Dermatitis, contact
Contact lenses, 10, 11, 12, 55, 56, 59, 68, 118, 156, 197, 222–229
Convergent squints *see* Squints
Cornea, 47–72
  conical, 59, 70*f*, 224
  diagnostic equipment,
    Orbscan, 30
  opacity, 57, 71*f*, 72*f*
  upper, 52
Corneal abrasion, 36, 211, 238
Corneal dystrophies, 58, 69*f*, 70*f*
  astigmatism and, 59
  Fuchs' endothelial, 59
  Grafts, corneal, 60, 72*f*
  keratoconus in, 59
  light reflex, 8
  opacities, 47, 57, 60, 61, 71*f*, 72*f*

Figures & tables denoted by letters — "*f*" – figures & "*t*" – tables

trauma, 60
treatment of, 59
ulcers, 54–56, 65f, 68f
  bacterial, 55
  dendritic, 54
  examination of, 55
  fluorescein dye, 68f
  fungal, 56
  herpes simplex infection and, 54
  severe, 55
  treatment of, 55
Cryoapplication, 113
Cryotherapy, 36, 54, 113, 125, 152, 191, 192, 198
CT scan, 15, 29f, 153, 156, 174, 212
Cup–disc ratio, 22, 84, 85, 94f
Cyclophosphamide, 99
Cycloplegics, 99, 194, 209, 235
Cyclosporine, 50, 61, 99, 234
Cyst, 32, 130f, 173, 199
Cytomegalovirus (CMV) retinitis, 100

Dacryocystitis, 38
Dacryocystorhinostomy, 38, 196
Dandruff, 31, 32
Degenerative myopia see Myopia, high
Demyelinating lesions, detection of, 15
Dendritic ulcer, 33, 54, 65f
Dermatitis, allergic, 34
Dermatitis, contact, 34
Descemet's membrane, 59, 61, 72f, 197
Developing countries
  blindness in, 154
  malnutritional, 154
Developmental abnormalities, 199, 206f, 207f
  anophthalmos, 199
  coloboma, iris of, 199
  craniofacial dysostosis, 199
  cyst, congenital, 199
  homocystinuria, 199
  hyperplastic primary vitreous, 199
  mandibulofacial dysostosis, 199
  Marfan's syndrome, 199
  meningoencephalocele, 199
  microphthalmos (small eye), 199
  persistent hyaloid (embryonic vitreous), 199
Diabetes see also Diabetic retinopathy
  and eye disease, 144
  mellitus, 144, 243
  refractive changes in, 144
  retinal changes and, 148
Diabetic maculopathy, 146, 147, 158f
Diabetic retinopathy, 96, 114, 120, 145–149, 157f, 158f, 159f, 160f, 161f, 162f, 163f, 164f, 165f
  background, 146, 157f, 158f
  classification of, 146–147
  diagnosis of, 147
  in developing countries, 145
  maculopathy, 146, 147, 158f
  management of, 148
  photocoagulation and, 149
  proliferative, 96, 113, 146, 147, 160f, 161f
  treatment of, 148–149

Figures & tables denoted by letters — "f" – figures & "t" – tables

Diathermy, 198
Diplopia, 2, 11, 39, 40, 153, 170, 176
   binocular, 2
   monocular, 2
   tests for, 11
      red–green goggles, 11
      synoptophore, 11
Discharge, mucopurulent, 1, 47, 55, 62*f*
Divergent squints *see* Squints
Double vision, 1, 2, 40, 175, 176, 193, 195, 213
Drugs *see* Ocular drugs
Drusen, 2, 115, 131*f*, 132*f*, 133*f*, 172, 181, 186*f*
Dry eyes, 49–50
   idiopathic, 50
   Sjoegren's syndrome, 50
   Stevens–Johnson syndrome, 50
   tear substitutes, 50
   treatment of, 50
Dystrophic conditions, 59
   hyphaema, 219*f*

Eales disease, 111, 123, 152
Ectropion, 7, 36, 37, 44*f*, 154
   cicatricial, 36
Electrooculography (EOG), 16
Electrophysiological
   clinical, 16
   electrooculography (EOG), 16
   electroretinography (ERG), 16
   visual evoked response (VER) study, 16
Electrophysiology, 16
Electroretinography (ERG), 16, 119

Endophthalmitis, 3, 52, 56, 76, 190, 236
Entoptoscope, blue field, 16
Entropion, 7, 36, 52
   keratitis, exposure, 44
EOG *see* Electrooculography
Epicanthal folds (eyelids), 9, 195
Epiphora (tearing), 31, 36, 37
Episcleritis, 155
ERG *see* Electroretinography
Esotropia, 193 *see also* Squints
ESR *see* Blood erythrocyte sedimentation rate
Examinations *see* Eye examinations
Excimer laser, 15, 227, 228, 230*f*
Exophthalmos, 46*f*, 153
   bilateral, 168*f*
   keratitis, exposure, 168*f*
   thyroid complications of, 153
      keratitis, exposure, 153
Exotropia, 193 *see also* Squints
Extracapsular cataract technique, 75
Extraocular muscles, 8, 175–176
   examination of, 8–9, 19*f*
   paralysis, 2, 9, 145, 175–176, 187*f*
   tests for, 11
      binocular slit-lamp microscopy, 12
      cover–uncover, 11
Eyeballs
   diseases of, 2
   protrusion of, 39
Eye diseases, 52
   developing countries, in, 52
   thyroid, 168*f*
Eye drops
   antibacterial, 231

Figures & tables denoted by letters — "*f*" – figures & "*t*" – tables

antibiotic, 47, 55, 196, 210, 212, 231, 238
antihistamine, 49, 234
anti-infection, antibacterial, 231
anti-infection, antiviral, 232
atropine, 223, 237
broad spectrum antibiotics, 231
contaminated, 237
cycloplegic, 99, 235
decongestive, 49
diagnostic, 238*t*
glaucoma, 232
homatropine, 235
misuse of, 237–238
mydriatic, 11, 145, 174, 175, 235
steroid, 54, 99, 156, 237
Eye examinations, 1, 4–30, 7
 applanation tonometry, 25*f*
 colour vision, test for, 13
 CT scan, 15
 difficulties in, 6
 E chart, 6
 external, 7
 eyeballs, 8
 fundal fluorescein angiography, 26*f*
 gaze, position of, 9, 19*f*
 indocyanine green angiography (ICGA), 27*f*
 industrial vision, 6
 Jaegar test, 6
 ocular movements, 9
 ophthalmoscopy, 9–11, 20*f*
 optical coherence tomography (OCT), 28*f*
 pinhole, 6
 pupil responses, 8
 Schiotz tonometry, 12
 slit-lamp microscopy, 12, 25*f*
 visual acuity, 4–6
Eye injuries *see* Ocular injuries
Eyelashes
 crusting, 7, 31, 42*f*, 43*f*
 inturned, 3, 36, 51, 52
Eyelid deposits, 37
Eyelid inflammation, 31–32, 42*f*
 blepharitis, 31–32
  squamous, 42*f*
  ulcerative, 42*f*
 chalazion cyst, 32, 42*f*, 43*f*
 dandruff and, 31–32
 dermatitis, contact, 34
 granulomatous lesion, 32, 43*f*
 herpes zoster ophthalmicus, 33, 42*f*
  treatment of, 33
 oedematous lids, 34
 seborrhoeic conditions and, 31
 stye, 33, 42*f*
Eyelid malposition, 35–36, 44*f*
 ectropion, 36
 entropion, 36
 lid retraction, 35
 surgical eversion, 36
 tarsorrhaphy, 36
 trichiasis, 36
Eyelids
 epicanthal, 9, 195
 eversion of, 7, 18*f*
 sticky, 47
Eyelid tumours, 37–38
Eye movement, restriction of, 39, 153

Eye operations, 97*f*
    trabeculectomy, 97
Eye pain, 3
Eyes, itching of, 1, 3, 48, 227
    allergy and, 3, 34
    blepharitis, 3
Eye strain, 225
Eyes, watering of, 1, 3, 4, 7, 31, 38, 48, 54, 55, 59, 62*f*, 98, 212, 213, 225, 226
    in adults, 4
    in infants, 3
    surface irritation, 4

Farnsworth–Munsell 100-hue, 13
Filarial worm infestation, 144
Fixation point, 13
Flashes, 1, 3, 119
Floaters, 1, 2
Fluorescein angiography, fundal, 13, 26*f*, 116, 117, 161*f*, 170, 179*f*
Fluorescein dye, 7, 14, 236, 238
    staining with, 7
Fluoroquinolones, 55, 211, 231, 232
Fluorouracil, 54, 87
Foreign bodies, 3, 210–211, 216*f*
    detection of, 15
    intraocular, 217*f*
Fuchs' endothelial dystrophy, 58, 59, 69*f*
Fundal background, 9, 22
Fundal examination, 1
Fundal photography, 13, 101, 148
Fundus
    description of, 22
        macular area, 22
        optic disc, 22

    retinal vessels, 22
    examination of, 10, 13
        difficulties in, 10–11

Gaze, position of, 9*f*, 176, 177, 192
Gentamicin, 55
Gentamycin, 231
Geographical atrophy, 116
Glasses, 223
Glaucoma, 83–97
    acute, 2, 3, 64
    acute closed-angle, 50
    blindness and, 83
    chronic, 2
    closed-angle, 95*f*
    congenital, 3, 203*f*
    diagnosis of, 83–85
    hereditary and, 85
    intraocular pressure and, 83, 84
    neovascular, 92, 96*f*, 110
    ocular hypertension and, 84
    open-angle, 83, 84–89, 94*f*
    prevention, 85
    primary closed-angle glaucoma, 89–91
    retinal vein occlusion and, 96*f*
    secondary, 33, 91, 96*f*
    secondary neovascular, 110
    treatment of, 86–90
        acetazolamide, 87
        beta adrenergic blocker, 86
        latanoprost, 86
        prostaglandin agonists, 232
        timolol, 86

Figures & tables denoted by letters — "*f*" – figures & "*t*" – tables

travoprost, 86
visual field loss and, 84, 85
Glaucomatous cupping, 197
Gliomas, 198
Glycerol, 90
Goldmann Applanation Tonometer, 12
Goldmann bowl perimetry, 12
Gonioscopy, 12, 84, 91
Gram stain, examination of corneal ulcers, 48, 55
Granulomatous lesion, 43
Graves' disease, 153

Haemangioma, 205*f*, 207*f*
    elevated, 205*f*
Haemophilus, 55, 196
Haemorrhage, subconjunctival, 51
Halos, seeing, 91
Headaches
    causes of, 177
    eye pain and, 3
    migraine, 3
Herbert's pits, 52, 66*f*
Hereditary defective genes, 199
Herpes simplex infection, 47, 196
    corneal ulcers and, 54
Herpes zoster ophthalmicus, 33, 42*f*
    ocular complications, 33
    treatment of, 33
Histoplasmosis, 99, 105*f*
HLA-B27 gene, 99
Homatropine, 11, 99, 235
Homocystinuria, 199
Homonymous hemianopia, 174
Homonymous quadrantic, 174
Hordeolum *see* Stye

Horner's syndrome, 35, 174
Hypermetropia (long sightedness), 22, 172, 181*f*, 193, 195, 224
Hyperplastic primary vitreous, 189, 192, 199
Hypertension, 150–152
    hypertensive retinopathy, 150–151, 166*f*
    pre-eclamptic, 151
Hypertensive retinopathy, 150–151, 166*f*
Hyperthyroidism, 35, 153
    treatment of, 153
Hypertrophy, papillary, 52, 66*f*
Hyphaema, 211, 219*f*

ICGA *see* Indocyanine green angiography
Idoxuridine, 232
Imaging techniques, non-invasive, 14, 15
Immunosuppressive drugs, 99, 155
    azathioprine, 99
    cyclophosphamide, 99
    cyclosporine, 99
    methotrexate, 99, 155
Implants
    lens, 74, 77
    posterior chamber, 77, 81*f*
Indocyanine green angiography (ICGA), 27*f*
Industrial vision, 4, 6
Infections, 154–155
    antenatal, 199
    bacterial, 32, 50, 52, 54, 55
    "chlamydia trachomatis", 51
    opportunistic, 100

Figures & tables denoted by letters — "*f*" – figures & "*t*" – tables

prevention of, 48, 210
spread of, 39, 48
staphylococcal, 68f, 229f
viral, 99
Inflammatory conditions, 2, 105
Injuries, ocular see Ocular injuries
Interstitial keratitis see Keratitis,
  non-ulcerative
Intracranial aneurysms, 175, 177
Intracranial tumours, 171, 173
Intraocular haemorrhage, 212
Intraocular lens
  implant, 74, 82f, 228
Intraocular pressure (IOP), 12, 25f,
  83, 84, 90, 92
  control of, 86
  in children, 197
Intraocular surgery, 228
Intravitreal injections, 99, 116,
  149, 231, 236
IOP, 12, 25f, 83, 84, 90, 92, 197
Iridocyclitis, 98–99, 102f
  see also Iritis
  recurrent, 99
Iridodialysis, 220
Iris, 7
  abnormalities, 145
  defects, congenital, 175
  prolapsed, 212
Iritis, 3, 33, 47, 50, 64f, 102f
Ischaemia, 172
Ischaemic optic neuropathy, 145,
  172, 179f
Ishihara, 13
Itching (eyes), 1, 3, 34, 227

Jaegar test, 6
Jinja fly, 154

Kaposi sarcoma, 100
Keratitis, 4, 33, 36, 48, 57, 155
  interstitial, 57, 71f
  non-ulcerative, 57
Keratoconjunctivitis, 49, 63f
Keratoconus (conical cornea), 59,
  60, 70f, 224
Keratomalacia, 57, 144, 154
Keratopathy, banded, 58, 71
Keratotomy
  photorefractive, 227
  radial, 227

Lacerations, corneal, 218f
Lacrimal disease, 31
Lacrimal drainage system, 31, 36,
  38
  blockage, 38
Lagophthalmos, 7, 153, 154, 168f
Lantern colour matches, 13
Laser-assisted intrastromal
  keratomileusis see LASIK
Laser interferometer, 16
Laser iridotomy, 95f
  peripheral, 90
Laser trabeculoplasty, 87
LASIK, 50, 227, 228, 230
Latanoprost, 86, 232, 233
Lazy eye, 189, 193
Lens, 73–82
  dislocation, 207f, 211, 220f
Leprosy, 57, 99, 154
Lesions
  chiasmal, 170, 173–174
  choroidal, 100–101
  granulomatous, 43f
  post-chiasmal, 170, 173, 184f
  space-occupying, 40, 41, 153

Figures & tables denoted by letters — "f" – figures & "t" – tables

254

third nerve, 175
Leukocoria (white pupils), 189, 201f
Lid see also Eyelids
Lid conditions, 31–46
    entropion of, 36
    oedema, 38, 47
    retraction, 7, 35
Lid margin, 7
Light, perception, 5, 175
Limbus, 7, 8
    follicles at, 52
Lower lid, entropion, 36, 44f
Lupus, systematic, dry eyes and, 50
Lymphangioma, 40
Lymphoma, 37, 40, 103

Macula, 9, 10
    examination of, 10, 15
Macular conditions, 114
Macular degeneration (AMD), 2, 114–115
    age-related, 14, 115–116, 131f, 132f, 231, 236, 239, 242
Macular diseases, 1, 114–119, 225
Macular dystrophy, 114, 127f, 128f, 129f, 130f
Macular hole, 14, 114, 117, 118, 139f, 140f, 211
Macular potential acuity, 15
Maculopathy, 155 see also Macular degeneration
Magnetic resonance imaging (MRI), 15
mandibulofacial dysostosis, 199
Mannitol, intravenous, 90
Marcus–Gunn pupil, 175

Marfan syndrome, 76, 80f, 199, 207f
Medial epicanthal lid folds, 9, 195
Meibomian cyst see Chalazion cyst
Melanoma, 45f
Meningioma, 40, 173
meningoencephalocele, 199
Merck, 154
Metastasis, choroidal, 101
Methotrexate, 99, 155
Methyl cellulose, 234
Microphthalmos (small eye), 199, 206f
Microscope
    operating, 77, 80f
    slit-lamp, 12, 57
Middle age see Presbyopic age
Migraine, 3, 177
Mitomycin C, 54, 87
Molteno, 89
Monocular, 2
Monocular diplopia, 2
Morphine, 174
MRI, 15
Mucocutaneous diseases, 156
    acne rosacea, 156
    Stevens–Johnson syndrome, 156
Multiple sclerosis, 15, 171, 172, 178f
Myasthenia gravis, 2, 35, 176, 187f
Mydriatic eye drops, 145, 174, 235
Myopia (short sightedness), 2, 84, 193, 195, 222–223
    corrected, 223f
    high, 10, 11, 112, 117, 229f
Myopic maculopathy, 223

Figures & tables denoted by letters — "f" – figures & "t" – tables

Naevus, 45f, 53, 100, 106f
Nasociliary nerve, 33
Nasolacrimal duct, 3, 38, 51, 189, 196, 204f
Nasopharyngeal cancer, 40, 156
"N" chart, 6
Neomycin, 231
Neovascular glaucoma, 92, 96f, 145
Neuritis, optic, 2, 173, 174
Neurofibromas, 198
Neurofibromatosis, 198
Neuro-ophthalmic disorders, 15
Neuro-ophthalmic investigations, 174
Neuro-ophthalmic lesions, 100
Neuro-ophthalmology, 170–188
Neuroprotective agents, 87
Nodular scleritis, 169f
Normal vision, 4
Nuclear magnetic resonance (NMR) scan, 174
Nystagmus, 11, 177

Occlusion
    cerebrovascular, 173
    double vision, 2
    retinal artery, 2, 108–109
    retinal vein, 2, 109
OCT, 14, 28f
Ocular conditions
    examination of, 11–16, 47
Ocular diseases, cataract, 73
    symptoms of, 2
Ocular drugs
    diagnostic
        fundal fluorescein angiography, 236, 238t

        phenylephrine, 235, 238t
        tropicamide, 235, 238t
    eye drops, 231–238
    therapeutic, 231–235
Ocular emergency, hyphaema as, 211–212
Ocular hypertension, 84
Ocular injuries, 208
    alkaline burns, 209
    blunt injuries, 211–212, 219f
    burns, 209
    chemical burns, 209, 215f
    flying objects, 210
    foreign bodies, 210–212, 216f
        intraocular, 217f
    head injuries and, 213, 221f
    penetrating wound, 212
        intraocular haemorrhage, 212
    prevention of, 208–209
    sharp instruments, 212, 218f
Ocular media, 9, 13, 14, 27f
Ocular movements, 9
Ocular pain, 1, 237
Ocular symptoms, 1–4
    decreased visual acuity, 2
    double vision, 2
    flashes, 3
    floaters, 2
    headaches, 3
    itching, 3
    ocular pain, 1
    watering, 3
Oedema, 7, 178f, 179f, 180f
    corneal, 197, 226
    disc, 39
    epithelial, 90
    lid, 34, 38

Figures & tables denoted by letters — "f" – figures & "t" – tables

macular, 14, 110
retinal, 108, 150
vitreous, 99
Onchocerciasis (river blindness), 144, 154, 240
Open-angle glaucoma, 83, 94f
visual field loss, 93f
Ophthalmia neonatorum, 195, 204f
Ophthalmic drugs, 231–238
diagnostic, 235, 238t
eye drops, 231–238
therapeutic, 231–235
Ophthalmoscope, 10, 109
Ophthalmoscopy, 9–11, 21f
fundus, examination of, 10
indirect, 13, 25f
red reflex, 9
Opportunistic infections, 100
Optical coherence tomography (OCT), 14, 28f
Optical correction, 75–77
aphakic, 228
cataract extraction, 76
posterior chamber implants, 75
Optic atrophy, 85, 94f, 170, 173, 182f, 183f
ischaemia and, 172
optic cup, 85
papilloedema and, 171
syphilis, 155
Optic disc, 9, 172
Optic disc cup, 85, 94f
Optic disc, swelling of, 170–172
Optic neuritis, 2, 174
Orbit, 31, 38–41, 46f
Orbital cellulitis, 38–39, 46f, 156

Orbital tumours, detection of, 15
Orbscan, 30f
Ox eyes see Buphthalmos

Pachymetry, 14, 84
PAM, 16
Pannus, 52
Panretinal dystrophy, 118
Papillae, 66f, 227
Papillary conjunctivitis, 227, 229f
Papillitis, 170–172, 178f
diagnosis, 171t
Papilloedema, 150, 151, 166f, 170–172, 178f
diagnosis, 171t
Papillomas, 37
Paranasal sinuses, 39, 156
PCAG, 89–91
Perimetry, 12–13, 23f, 24f, 141f
computerised, 13
Goldmann, 12
Peripheral retinal vasculitis, 152
Persistent hyaloid (embryonic vitreous), 199
Phacoemulsification, 75, 81f, 228
Phakomatoses, 198, 205f
Phenylephrine, 234, 235, 237, 238t
Phoropter, 14
Photocoagulation, 101, 149, 152, 161f, 162, 192, 198
laser, 110, 111, 117, 144, 148, 157f, 160f
Photodynamic therapy, 116, 117
Photophobia, 1, 4, 48, 59, 98, 197, 210, 212, 213, 214, 226
Photorefractive keratectomy, 227
Pilocarpine, 90, 174, 232, 233, 237

Figures & tables denoted by letters — "f" – figures & "t" – tables

Pingueculum, 53
    nasal, 67f
Pinhole, 6, 15, 17f, 222
Pneumococcus, 196
Pneumocystis carinii, 100
Polymyxin, 231
Polyvinyl alcohol, 234
Post-chiasmal lesion, 170, 173, 184
Posterior synechiae, 56, 98, 99, 102f, 175, 235
Post-herpetic neuralgia, 34
Potential visual acuity meter (PAM), 16
Presbyopia (old-age sightedness), 2, 225
Presbyopic age, 6 see also Middle age
Preseptal cellulitis, 39
Primary closed-angle glaucoma (PCAG), 89–91 see also Glaucoma, closed angle
Proptosis, 38, 39, 40, 41, 153, 156
Prostaglandin agonists, 232
Pseudomonas aeruginosa, 55
Pseudopapilloedema, 172, 181f
Pseudosquint, 8, 9, 195
Pterygium, 53
    nasal, 67f
Ptosis, 7, 44f, 187f, 188f
    types of, 35, 199
Punctum, 38, 50
Pupillary sphincter (traumatic mydriasis), 174, 175
Pupil responses, extraocular muscles, 8–9
Pupils, 9, 174–175
    abnormalities, 145
    Adie's tonic, 174
    Argyll Robertson, 174, 175
    light, reaction to, 175
    Marcus–Gunn, 175
    small, 11

Radial keratotomy, 227
Radiotherapy, 37–41, 101–102, 191–192
Ranibizumab, 116, 149, 236
Red eyes, bilateral, 47, 48, 62f
    conjunctiva, bacterial, 47
    watering, 48
Red eyes, unilateral, 47, 50–51, 64f, 65f
    acute closed-angle, 50
    corneal ulcer, 50
    eyelashes, inturned, 51
    foreign bodies, 50
    iritis, 50
    keratitis, 50
    nasolacrimal duct, blocked, 51
    trichiasis, 51
Reflex
    corneal light, 8, 195
    light, 22, 150, 171
    red, 9, 20f, 112, 189
    ring, 117
    white, 7, 190
Refraction, 14
Refractive errors, 2, 6, 10, 222–230
    corrected, 227
        excimer laser, 227
        myopia (short sightedness), 222–223
        photorefractive keratectomy, 227
        radial keratotomy, 227
        surgery, 227

Figures & tables denoted by letters — "f" – figures & "t" – tables

uncorrected, 3, 225
Refractive surgery, 230f
Retina, 12, 108–143 see also
    Retinal detachment
Retinal arterioles, 108
Retinal artery occlusion, 108
    arteriosclerosis, 109, 150
Retinal detachment, 2, 3, 10, 13,
    112, 113, 117, 124f, 211
    cataract and, 76
    exudative, 113
    rhegmatogenous, 112–113
    traction, 113
Retinal diseases, 28f, 108
Retinal dystrophy, diagnosis of, 16
Retinal periphery, examination,
    13, 25f
Retinal tears, 3, 112
Retinal vein occlusion, 2, 231, 236
Retinal vessel occlusion, 120f
    branch, 122f
Retinal vessels, 9, 22, 119
Retinitis pigmentosa, 16, 118–119,
    119, 141f, 173
Retinoblastoma, 189, 190–191,
    201f, 202f
    management of, 191
Retinopathies, other, 152–153, 167f
Retinopathy
    central serous, 114, 117, 140f
    diabetic, 108, 114, 144,
        145–149
    hypertensive, 150–151, 166f
    hyperviscosity, 152, 167f
    maculopathy, 158f
Retinopathy of prematurity, 113,
    189, 191, 201f
Retinopathy, other, 167f

Retinoscopy, 235
Retrobulbar neuritis, 172
Retrolental fibroplasia, 189, 201f
Rhegmatogenous retinal
    detachment, 112, 113
Rheumatoid disease, 169f
    nodular scleritis, 169f
River blindness, 154
Rodent ulcer see Basal cell
    carcinoma
Rubeosis iridis, 96f, 109, 110, 145,
    192

Sarcoidosis, 50, 99
Scar
    chorioretinal, 99, 105f, 200
    corneal, 195, 210
    tissue, 36, 164
Schiotz indentation tonometer, 12
Sclera, 7, 47–72, 218
Scleritis, 3, 50, 105, 155, 169
Scleromalacia, 155, 169
Sebaceous cysts, 37
Sickle cell anaemia, 152
Single vision, binocular, 12, 193
Sinuses, X-ray of, 39
Sjoegren's syndrome, 50
Slit-lamp microscopy, 25
    keratitis, non-ulcerative and, 57
Snellen chart, 4
Spring catarrh, 49, 66f
Squamous cell carcinoma, 37, 38,
    67f
Squints, 8–9, 11, 189, 192
    convergent (esotropia), 8, 175,
        187f, 193, 194, 202f
    divergent (exotropia), 8, 187f,
        193, 194

Figures & tables denoted by letters — "f" – figures & "t" – tables

259

non-paralytic, 193
paralytic, 175–176, 193
pseudo, 9, 195
vertical, 8, 193, 194
Staphylococcus, 55, 196
Steroids
   complications of, 237
   cream, 34
   eye drops, 49, 54, 56, 99, 156, 235, 237
Stevens–Johnson syndrome, 50, 63, 87, 156
   conjunctivitis and, 156
Still's disease, 99
Strabismus, 40, 176, 189, 192
Streptococcus, 55, 196
Sturge–Weber syndrome, 92, 198, 205f
Stye, 33, 42f
Subconjunctival haemorrhage, 51, 220f
Subretinal fluid, 113, 140f
Suprasellar cyst (craniopharyngioma), 173
Synechiae
   prevention of, 56, 99, 102f, 235
Synoptophore, 11
Syphilis, 57, 60, 99, 104f, 155, 173, 174, 199, 200
Systemic diseases, 73, 98, 111, 144, 225

Tangent screen, 13
Tarsal plate, inflamation of, 32
Tarsorrhaphy, 36, 168f
Tear replacement, 234
Tetracycline, 231

Third nerve paralysis, 44f, 187f, 188f
Thyroid disease, 31, 39, 144, 153, 168f
   Graves' disease, 153
   lid retraction, 35, 46f, 168f
Thyroid exophthalmos, 46f, 153
Timolol, 86, 90, 232, 233, 237
Tobramycin, 48
Tomography
   computerised, 15, 174
   optical coherence tomography (OCT), 14, 28f, 148
Tonometers
   Goldmann applanation, 12–13
   non-contact, 12
   Schiotz indentation, 12
Tonometry, 12, 25f
Toxaemia, pre-eclamptic, 113, 151
Toxocariasis, 190
Toxoplasma gondii, 100
Toxoplasmosis, 73, 99, 192, 199
Trabeculectomy, 87–89, 91
Trachoma, 7, 36, 51–52, 66f, 231, 240
   endophthalmitis and, 52
   entropion and, 52
   treatment of, 52
      corneal graft surgery, 52
      trichiasis, 52
Trachoma inclusion conjunctivitis (TRIC), 51, 196
Traumatic mydriasis, 174
Travoprost, treatment of, bimatoprost, 86
Triamcinolone, 99, 236
TRIC see Trachoma inclusion conjunctivitis

Figures & tables denoted by letters — "f" – figures & "t" – tables

Trichiasis, 4, 32, 36, 44, 51, 52
Trifluorothymidine, 232
Tropicamide, 11, 235, 238
Tuberculosis, 57, 99, 105, 111, 152, 155
Tuberous sclerosis, 198, 205*f*
Tumours
    basal cell carcinoma, 37, 45*f*
    choroidal, 100–101
    congenital, 207*f*
    eyelid, 37–38, 45*f*
    intracranial, 171, 173
    lymphoma, 37
    melanoma, 45*f*
    optic nerve, 40
    orbital, 15
    pituitary, 13
    squamous cell carcinoma, 37
    subcutaneous, 198
    xanthelasma, 37, 45*f*

Ulceration, 36, 52, 153, 236
Ulcerative blepharitis, 42*f*
Ulcers
    corneal, 54–57, 68*f*, 227, 229*f*
    dendritic, 54, 65*f*
Ultrasonic disintegration, 75
Ultrasonography, 14, 27*f*
Unilateral red eye, 36, 47, 50–51, 64*f*, 65*f*, 89
Uveal tract, 98–101
Uveitis, 98–101, 102*f*
    acute, 2

Vascular occlusion, 108–110
    central retinal artery, 108–109
    central retinal vein, 109–110
Vascular retinopathies, 152

Vasculitis, 100, 103, 111, 152
VER *see* Visual evoked response
Vernal conjunctivitis *see* Spring catarrh
Vision loss
    gradual, 2, 74, 114
    sudden, 2, 64, 83, 108, 110, 112, 116, 120, 172
Visual acuity, 4–6, 17*f*, 173
    assessment of, 4–6
    confrontation, 6
    decreased, 2
    distant, 4–5
        Snellen chart, 4
    near, 6
Visual acuity table, 5*t*
Visual evoked response (VER) study, 16
Visual field
    charts, 24*f*
    defects, 184*f*, 185*f*
    glaucoma and, 85
    loss, 93*f*
    testing of, 13, 24*f*
Visual function, testing, 1
Visual pathway, 16, 170, 174
Vitamin A deficiency, 57, 144, 154
Vitrectomy, 113, 119, 164*f*
    in progress, 126*f*
Vitreoretinal surgery, 126*f*
Vitreous conditions, 119
Vitreous degeneration, 112, 119
Vitreous detachment, 3, 119
    posterior, 112, 118
Vitreous haemorrhage, 112, 120, 149, 152, 160*f*
    sudden vision loss and, 2, 110, 112, 120

Figures & tables denoted by letters — "*f*" – figures & "*t*" – tables

Vitreous opacities, 99, 119, 143*f*
Von Hippel–Lindau disease, 198, 205*f*
Von Recklinghausen's disease, 198

Watering (eyes), 3–4, 7, 31, 38, 48, 54, 55, 59, 62*f*, 98, 196, 197, 204*f*
    in adults, 4
    in infants, 3
    surface irritation, 4
Welding flash injury, 213
White pupils, 189–191, 199, 201*f*
Worm infestation *see* Toxocariosis

Xanthelasma, 37, 45*f*
X-ray of sinuses, 39

Figures & tables denoted by letters — "*f*" – figures & "*t*" – tables